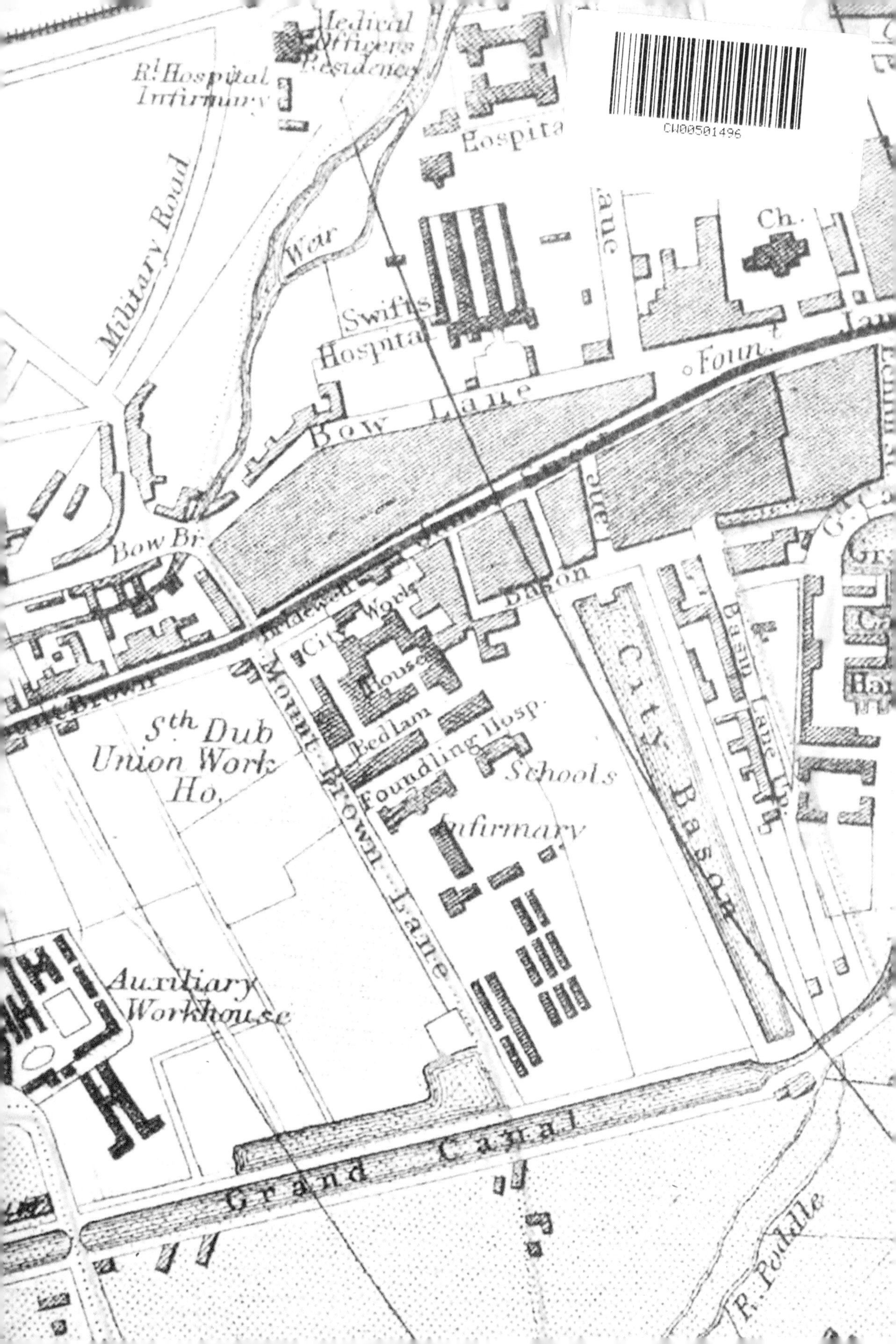

Medical Officers Residence

Rl. Hospital Infirmary

Military Road

War

Hospital

Lane

Ch.

Swifts Hospital

o Foun.

Bow Lane

Lane

Bow Br.

Basin

City Works House

Bedlam

Foundling Hosp.

Schools

Sth Dub Union Work Ho.

Mount Brown Lane

Infirmary

City Basin

Basin Lane

Auxiliary Workhouse

Grand Canal

R. Poddle

THE HISTORY AND HERITAGE OF ST JAMES'S HOSPITAL, DUBLIN

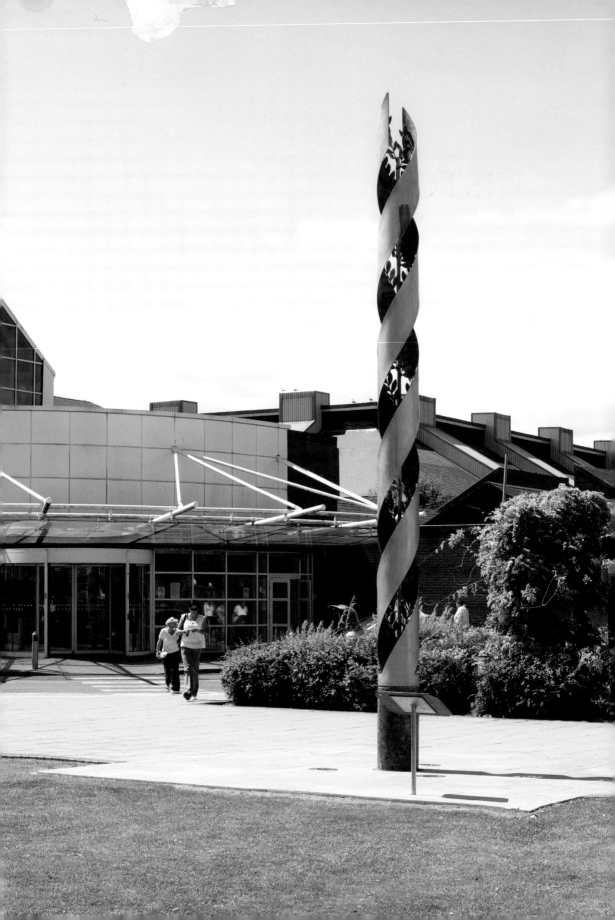

The

HISTORY AND HERITAGE

of

ST JAMES'S HOSPITAL, DUBLIN

DAVIS COAKLEY & MARY COAKLEY

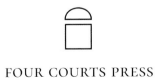

FOUR COURTS PRESS

Set in 11 pt on 14 pt Cormorant Garamond by
Catherine Gaffney for
FOUR COURTS PRESS LTD
7 Malpas Street, Dublin 8, Ireland
www.fourcourtspress.ie
and in North America for
FOUR COURTS PRESS
c/o IPG, 814 N Franklin St, Chicago, IL 60622

A catalogue record for this title is available
from the British Library.

ISBN 978-1-84682-607-8

Endpapers: Detail from map of Dublin City. Published by Letts, Son & Co., London 1883.

Printed in Spain by Castuera, Navarra.

For the staff, past and present, of St James's Hospital

Contents

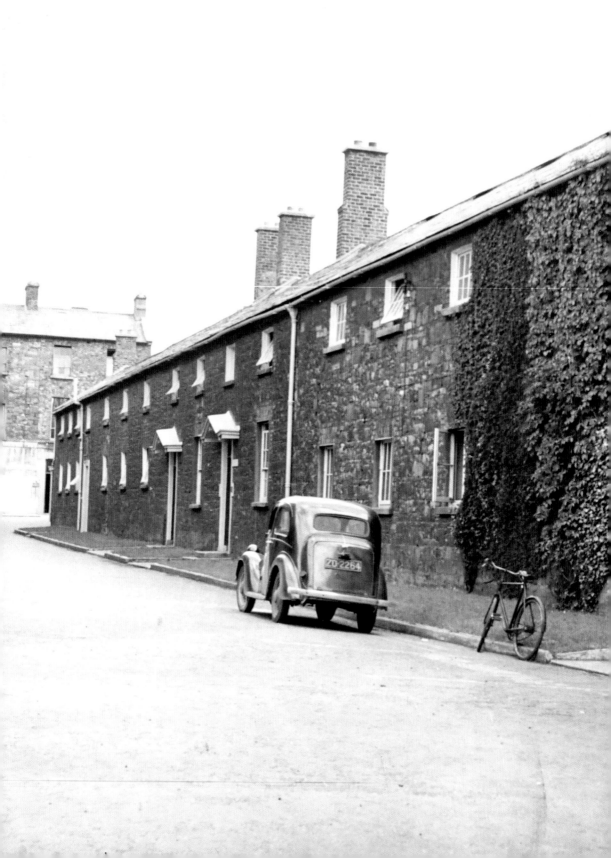

Acknowledgments

We would like to thank all those who helped with our research for this book and with its preparation for publication. Over several years we have drawn on the expertise, support and patience of old friends and have also made many new friends. We were heartened by the number of people who shared our interest in St James's Hospital and its history.

We are very grateful to Ian Howie, former chairman of the board of St James's Hospital and John O'Brien, former CEO, for inviting us to write this history. The former CEOs Ian Carter and Brian Fitzgerald, and the current CEO Lorcan Birthistle, have been very encouraging and supportive. Paul Gallagher, director of nursing, could not have been more helpful.

We owe a great debt of gratitude to Tom Mitchell, former chairman of the board of St James's Hospital and former provost of Trinity College Dublin, for the considerable amount of time he gave to reading the manuscript and for his many constructive suggestions. Particular thanks are due to John Moynihan, Maria Mulrooney and Stephen Coakley for their help in editing the text. We are also grateful to Peter Daly and John Reynolds, who helped with sections of the manuscript and made very relevant observations.

Anthony Edwards, clinical photographer at St James's Hospital, has made a major contribution to this book. He gave generously of his time and expertise, and he is responsible for the quality of most of the images that appear in the book. David Coleman searched the archives of Bobby Studio Photographers for photographs of early events and staff that were taken by his father Bobby Coleman during the years following the establishment of St James's Hospital.

We have been collecting material and working on this book for many years. During this time several people gave us information which has subsequently proved to be very valuable. We would like to acknowledge the late James Nolan, deputy CEO of the Eastern Health Board, who entrusted to us a collection of photographs and documents relating to the formation of St Kevin's Hospital, and the late Victoria Coffey, paediatrician, who gave us papers and notebooks relating to her time on the staff of

St Kevin's Hospital. Caoimhghín S. Breathnach, medical historian and physiologist, shared his memories of working in St Kevin's Hospital and in the Rialto Chest Hospital. His interesting and thoughtful contributions are much appreciated.

The late John Prichard, associate professor of medicine, developed a chronology of St James's Hospital, covering the years between 1971 and 1989, which was circulated with the annual report of St James's Hospital for 1988/9. We have developed and updated this chronology.

We would like to acknowledge the support of the following people, who made the writing of this book easier for us: Sr Aine Barrins, Gerard Boyle, Yvonne Brophy, Paul Browne, Cathal McSwiney Brugha, Helen Burke, Luke Clancy, Pádraigín Clancy, Ian Fraser Clark, David Clarke, Peter Coakley, John Davis Coakley, James Coakley, Robert Coen, Bryn Coldrick, the late Frank Corrigan, Adele Crowder, Hugh Daly, the late Desmond Dempsey, Cuimin Doyle, Alan Duncan, Sean Duffy, James Enyangu, William Fennell, David FitzPatrick, Seamus Fitzpatrick, Bob Fitzsimons, Patrick Freyne, Eoin Gaffney, Mary Gallagher, Barbara Galligan, the late Peter Gatenby, the late Eamon L. Gavin, Jane Grimson, Joe Harbison, John Hanlon, Gerry Heffernan, Miriam Hogan, Susan Hood, Frances Houlihan, Dermot Hourihane, Conor Keane, Joseph Keane, Margaret Kelleher, John Kelly, Liam Kenny, Rose Anne Kenny, Ron Kirkham, William Laffan, Emer Lawlor, Tim Lyne, Shaun McCann, Niall McElwee, Alva MacGowan, Maccon Macnamara, Edward McParland, Joseph McPartlin, Eamonn MacSearraigh, James Mahon, Dermot Malone, Jim Malone, Niamh Marnham, Berni Metcalfe, Irene Moran, Fiona Mulcahy, Susan Mullaney, Carol Murphy, Caoimhe Nic Allabroin, Chris Pigott, the late Aideen Pittion, Patrick Plunkett, James O'Beirne, the late Sr Catherine of Siena O'Brien, Therese O'Connor, the late James O'Dea, Colum O'Riordan, John O'Rourke, Niamh O'Sullivan, Judy Oxley, John Reynolds, Neasa Rowan, Stephen Ryan, Catherine Scuffil, the late Keith Shaw, Carol Sommerville, David Sweeney, the late Ian Temperley, Robert Towers, Donald Weir, Stephen Weir, J. Bernard Walsh, the late Michael Walsh, and Barry White.

Mary O'Doherty, archivist, Mercer's Library, RCSI, and Harriet Wheelock, keeper of collections, RCPI, have given us unfailing support from the beginning. We would also like to express our gratitude to the following archivists: Mary Clark and Enda Leaney, Dublin City Library and Archives; Sr Marianne Cosgrave, Mercy Congregational Archives; Brian Crowley, curator of the Pearse Museum; Aisling Dunne, archivist, Irish Architectural Archive; Siobhan Fitzpatrick, librarian RIA; Brian Donnelly, senior archivist, National Archives of Ireland; Jane Maxwell, principal curator, manuscripts and archives, TCD; Lydia Ferguson and Helen McGinley, Department of Early Printed Books and Special Collections, TCD; Catherine Giltrap, curator of the college art collections, TCD; Mary Higgins, Research Library TCD; Jason McElligott, keeper of Marsh's Library; David Power, Decade of Centenaries project consultant, South Dublin County Libraries.

We wish to thank the director of the National Archives of Ireland for permission to quote from the minutes of the meetings of the board of guardians of the South Dublin Union and of the Dublin Union. Thomas Kinsella kindly gave us permission to quote stanzas from his poem 'Dick King'. We wish to acknowledge the trustees of the estate of the late Katherine B. Kavanagh, through the Jonathan Williams Literary Agency, for permission to quote the poem 'The Hospital'. Excerpts from 'Hospital Notebook', a recording made by Kavanagh and broadcast on 4 September 1955 on Radio Éireann, are reproduced courtesy of RTÉ Archives.

We are hugely indebted to Sheila McCarthy for her secretarial skills and for her patience in working through numerous drafts of the manuscript. She knew the text so well that she was able to point out errors and repetitions to us. Finally, we would like to thank the great team at Four Courts Press for their help and advice.

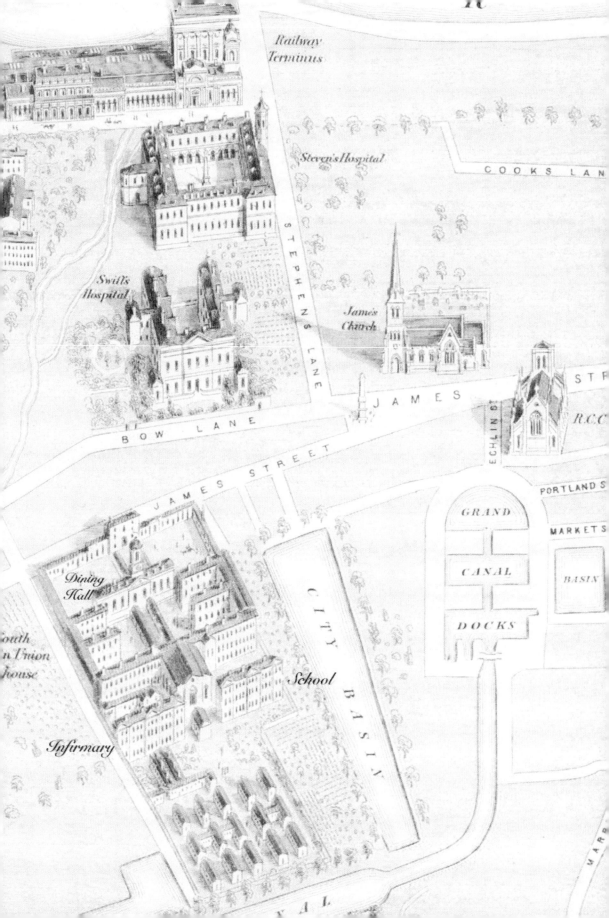

Introduction

One of the first things a contemporary visitor to St James's Hospital will notice is the variety in age and architecture of the buildings on its grounds. These were built in the eighteenth, nineteenth, twentieth and twenty-first centuries and connect St James's Hospital in a tangible way with all the institutions that have occupied the site since the establishment of the City Workhouse in 1703. The history of these institutions forms one strand of the history and heritage of St James's Hospital. Another strand is formed by the heritage of the four old and distinguished voluntary hospitals – Mercer's, Sir Patrick Dun's, the Royal City of Dublin (also known as Baggot Street Hospital) and Dr Steevens' – that amalgamated with St James's Hospital in the 1980s. A third strand is formed by the historic medical school of Trinity College Dublin, which needed a large, modern teaching hospital for its students. These three interwoven strands form the fabric of this book.

Like a mirror, the history of the various institutions that stood on the St James's site reflects the challenges faced by successive generations of Dubliners as they struggled to cope with the social, health and political challenges of their times. War and recurrent famine impoverished many Irish people living in rural areas during the seventeenth century. Often they had no option other than begging in order to survive. A significant number made their way to Dublin, where they joined other starving people begging on the streets. After numerous complaints from harassed citizens, the city assembly decided, in 1697, to build a workhouse on James's Street, outside the western gate of Dublin, in an attempt to stem the flow of destitute beggars entering the city from the west of Ireland. The workhouse admitted its first inmates in January 1706, when 124 vagrants were apprehended on the streets of Dublin.

The abandonment of infants left at the doors of wealthy citizens, in churches and on the banks of the canal, was another issue that gave rise to public scandal at the beginning of the eighteenth century. After a number of parish-based solutions failed, legislation was enacted in 1730 obliging the governors to admit all abandoned children to the City Workhouse. The name of the institution was changed to the Foundling Hospital and Workhouse of the City of Dublin. A revolving basket was placed at the entrance so that infants could be left anonymously at the hospital. Infants were transported to the institution from all over Ireland, and many of them died en route or were moribund on arrival. Unfortunately, the infants did not receive the necessary standard of care and many died in appalling conditions giving rise to inquiry after inquiry throughout the eighteenth century. In 1772, the Irish parliament decided to remove the beggars and vagrants to the House of Industry, which had just been opened on the north side of the city. As a result, the care of abandoned infants became the sole responsibility of the Foundling Hospital and Workhouse and the name was changed to the Foundling Hospital. The hospital continued to admit children until parliament decided to stop all further admissions in 1829.

The activity of the Foundling Hospital was wound down and in 1839 the buildings were acquired by the poor law commissioners to form the workhouse of the South Dublin Union. The workhouse, which itself became known as the South Dublin Union or 'the Union', was one of over a hundred workhouses which were placed around Ireland after the British government decided, against strong advice to the contrary, to introduce the workhouse system in Ireland. The philosophy behind the workhouse system was to make the conditions within the workhouses so harsh that only those who were unable to get work would seek admission. However, destitution existed in Ireland not because able-bodied men and women did not want to work but because there was no work to be had.

Just a few years after the system was introduced, famine spread across the country and workhouses provided shelter and food for the starving population. The South Dublin Union, which had a maximum capacity of around 2,000 inmates, struggled to cope with over 3,000 at the height of the Great Famine. This overcrowding led to the transmission of infectious diseases throughout the institution and to the death of many inmates. Towards the end of the Famine, when the people had little resistance to infection, a cholera epidemic spread throughout the city. Fever sheds were placed at the Rialto end of the South Dublin Union in an attempt to deal with the crisis. The victims were treated and nursed by individuals who placed their own lives at risk. Within a short time, the facilities were overwhelmed and very ill patients lay on the ground outside the sheds waiting for admission.

The number of inmates in the South Dublin Union continued to rise significantly during the 1850s because of the social distress and poverty in the country following the Famine. According to the medical officers, the institution was functioning as a 'vast hospital'. The board of guardians established a committee to make recommendations on how to deal with the overcrowding. The committee reported in 1854 and recommended a significant increase in the accommodation for inmates and also proposed the development of a general hospital in the grounds, capable of accommodating 800 patients, which would be distinct from the other buildings. Although the latter recommendation was not implemented at the time, it was the first proposal to build a general hospital in the grounds of the South Dublin Union Workhouse.

The original function of the infirmary of the South Dublin Union was to treat sick inmates, but in the latter half of the nineteenth century it also began to admit sick poor patients specifically for treatment. During the same period there were complaints about the general standard of care within the Union. Aware of these complaints, the board of guardians responded by inviting the Mercy order of nuns to take over both the care and management of some of the wards. The order accepted the challenge, and ten nuns began working in the Union in 1881. At around the same time, two Protestant deaconesses, who were trained nurses, were appointed to work in the Protestant wards. The South Dublin Union was run along strict sectarian lines, and was divided into Catholic and Protestant sections. It was also divided into hospital and welfare areas, and men and women were housed in separate accommodation.

In the opening years of the twentieth century, there were around 1,200 medical patients in the wards and two medical residents delivered the day-to-day care. Tuberculosis was a major cause of death in young people at this time. The voluntary hospitals were reluctant to admit patients with advanced tuberculosis as there was no treatment and they 'blocked' beds. As a consequence, many of these patients had no option but to seek refuge in the Union. The care of patients with tuberculosis became a major undertaking for the South Dublin Union, and there were several male and female wards for patients with the condition.

At this time the South Dublin Union had the appearance of a medieval town surrounded by high walls. The original buildings of the City Workhouse and of the Foundling Hospital were still standing, together with a number of tall grey buildings that were erected during the nineteenth century. Intersecting lanes and alleys connected these buildings and the atmosphere was unhurried. Many of the more senior staff lived in houses on the grounds with their families. This scene was shattered by the Easter Rising, which began on Easter Monday 1916. The South Dublin Union was occupied by the 4th Battalion of the Irish Volunteers, under the command of Éamonn Ceannt. Within hours of the beginning of the rebellion, the Union was surrounded by troops from the Royal Irish Regiment. Intense fighting ensued throughout the week as the soldiers attempted to gain access to the grounds. They eventually succeeded and began to move through the institution attacking buildings occupied by Volunteers. A nurse named Margaret Kehoe was mortally wounded in one of the hospitals. Eventually, the Volunteers were surrounded in the night nurses' home, which they were using as their headquarters. They managed to hold out until the general surrender at the end of Easter Week. Staff remained in the Union throughout the conflict to care for the inmates. The bakery continued to function, and food was distributed to the different hospitals by staff carrying a white flag. Arrangements were also made to feed the residents of the local community, who were cut off by the fighting.

Two years after the Easter Rising, the South Dublin Union faced another crisis, one of far more deadly proportions, as the great influenza pandemic of 1918–19 swept through Dublin. The influenza was very virulent, and young adults were particularly vulnerable. People living in large institutions were greatly at risk of infection and this was borne out in the Union. In this period, under normal circumstances, the number of deaths in the South Dublin Union ranged from fifteen to twenty each week, but at the peak of the epidemic this rose to around fifty, and many of these were young adults. The inmates were terrified, yet a number of them volunteered to help care for the sick. Their contribution was very valuable as, at any one time, more than half the staff of the workhouse had influenza and was absent on sick leave.

In 1918, the military authorities acquired the North Dublin Union as winter quarters for troops. The staff and inmates of the North Dublin Union were moved to the South Dublin Union, and the unions were amalgamated to form the Dublin Union. Some years after Irish independence, the name of the Dublin Union was changed to St Kevin's Institution. However, the role of the institution did not change, and it continued to fulfil most of the functions of a workhouse. This was largely due to the financial difficulties of the new state in the years following independence. There was an aspiration to develop St Kevin's Institution into a large municipal hospital that would serve the sick poor of the city. The Department of Local Government, which held the health portfolio at the time, was fully supportive, but the onset of the Second World War delayed progress. In 1952, work began with the purpose of changing St Kevin's Institution into an acute general hospital. This involved the demolition of some of the old Workhouse and Foundling Hospital buildings and the extensive refurbishment of others. The hospital became known as St Kevin's Hospital. The clinical services were delivered by a small but dedicated group of consultants who provided a high standard of medical care.

Throughout the twentieth century a number of attempts were made to amalgamate the small voluntary hospitals, which were traditionally linked to the medical school of Trinity College Dublin, to form one large hospital. As medicine and surgery began to subspecialize, it became obvious that none of these hospitals would be able to employ the full range of specialists necessary to provide an appropriate level of clinical care and student teaching. The growing cost of an expanding range of equipment was another factor. Following negotiations in 1961, seven of the hospitals formed a federation with a view to ultimate amalgamation. The hospitals that made up the federation were the Adelaide, Mercer's, the Meath, Dr Steevens', Sir Patrick Dun's, Baggot Street and the National Children's Hospital. The hospital group became known as the Federated Dublin Voluntary Hospitals.

In the 1950s, the Irish Medical Association invited the American Medical Association to send a team to assess standards in Irish medical schools. The resulting report was highly critical of the schools, and for a while Irish medical qualifications were not recognized in some states in America. The adverse findings relating to the school of medicine in Trinity College centred on the small size of the teaching hospitals and the lack of coordination between the medical school and these hospitals. The poor pathology services and the absence of any significant research were other criticisms. Trinity realized that if its medical school was to survive, it would need to be associated with a large teaching hospital. As a result, the board of Trinity College placed the development of the medical school and its integration with a teaching hospital high on its list of priorities and became a powerful player in the development St James's Hospital.

A number of sites for the new hospital were proposed by the Federated Hospitals, but the Department of Health insisted that it should be built on the grounds of St Kevin's Hospital. Three of the seven Federated Hospitals – Sir Patrick Dun's, Baggot Street and Mercer's – agreed to move to the site following the completion of the new hospital, and they became known as the 'designated hospitals'. St James's Hospital was established on the site of St Kevin's Hospital in 1971. There were no new facilities, and the hospital began to develop busy clinical services in the old wards of St Kevin's. A teaching agreement was signed between St James's Hospital and Trinity College Dublin that recognized the hospital as the primary teaching hospital of the university. This led to the development of strong academic departments in medicine, surgery, psychiatry and pathology. The transfer of the adult haematology service and the National Haemophilia Centre from the Meath Hospital to St James's Hospital in 1976 also strengthened the clinical and research profile of St James's. Research in the hospital received a major boost with the opening of the Sir Patrick Dun's Research Laboratory in 1983. This made St James's the first hospital in Ireland to have a dedicated clinical research laboratory on its campus. It was funded by the sale of the nurses' home of Sir Patrick Dun's Hospital. Mercer's Hospital closed in 1983, and most of the patients and staff moved to St James's Hospital. Mercer's was sold, and a major part of the income from the capital that accrued from its sale was used to establish the Mercer's Institute for Research on Ageing at St James's in 1988. St James's Hospital continued to develop new specialties, and its willingness to confront health crises such as HIV/AIDS and hepatitis C head-on, strengthened its working relationship with the Department of Health and the Eastern Health Board.

It was envisaged that Baggot Street and Sir Patrick Dun's, the two remaining hospitals designated to move into St James's Hospital, would do so when the building of the new hospital was completed. However, as a consequence of the financial crisis in the country in the 1980s, Sir Patrick Dun's was closed precipitously in 1986. This was followed in 1987 by the rapid closure of Baggot Street and Dr Steevens' Hospitals. Some of the funding from the sale of Sir Patrick Dun's, Dr Steevens' and Baggot Street Hospitals was used to build the Trinity Centre for Health Sciences in St James's Hospital, which provided accommodation for the clinical professorial units, a library, a teaching laboratory and a 250-seat lecture theatre.

The final chapter of this book describes the remarkable developments in St James's Hospital over the last twenty years. These include the construction of clinical and research institutes and centres of excellence that have placed St James's among the leading European hospitals of the twenty-first century. The range and expertise of the specialties within the hospital were major factors in the choice of St James's Hospital as the site for the new national children's hospital, which is currently under construction, and for the planned relocation of the Coombe Women and Infants University Hospital. The chapter also describes how the hospital and staff battled successfully to maintain both general and specialist clinical services to patients during the catastrophic financial crisis that began in 2008.

The history of St James's Hospital has been presented in a narrative form in this book. This precluded the authors from including detailed histories of the development of the many departments in the hospital. In order to compensate for this, we have added a chronology of the major events and senior appointments since the establishment of St James's Hospital in 1971.

1

A workhouse in the city of Dublin

[A] house should be built to put idlers to worke in.[1]

At the end of the seventeenth century Dublin was the fifth biggest city in Europe with a population of fifty thousand, exceeded only by London, Paris, Amsterdam and Venice. Following the restoration of Charles II, the city began to expand outside its walls. New bridges were constructed over the Liffey, quays were built and residential areas began to develop on the north side of the river. The Royal Hospital at Kilmainham, the first great public building of the city, was completed in 1685, the Phoenix Park and St Stephen's Green were laid out as pleasure grounds and Dame Street was built connecting Trinity College to Dublin Castle. However, Dublin was still in many ways a medieval city, with gable-fronted timber houses and narrow streets and laneways. The city already had its slums where people lived in dire poverty. There was no support for the destitute and they had little option but to resort to begging, stealing and prostitution.

Policy under successive kings had made it exceedingly difficult for the Irish, whether Catholic or Protestant, to compete against English merchants and manufacturers. During the reign of Charles II the importation of Irish meats and dairy products into England was prohibited. As a consequence, the Anglo-Irish landowners turned from cattle farming to sheep farming, and they began to export wool instead of meat and dairy products. They produced very good quality wool and became serious competitors to the English wool producers. Restrictions were then enforced against the Irish woollen industry and in 1699 the English parliament prohibited the export of Irish wool to any country other than England and imposed a high tariff on Irish woollens entering England. This caused great hardship for the weavers in the Liberties of Dublin, who numbered nearly 1,700.[2] Further economic difficulties, with depressed export prices, unhelpful currency adjustments and poor harvests, exacerbated the situation.³ It was this state of affairs that in 1720 prompted Jonathan Swift, dean of St Patrick's cathedral, to write his pamphlet, *A proposal for the universal use of Irish manufacture in clothes and furniture of houses, etc., utterly rejecting and renouncing everything wearable that comes from England.*

The medieval Hospital of St John the Baptist

Hospital care for the sick poor of Dublin was inadequate in the extreme; it had been better in medieval times when the city was smaller. The Hospital of St John the Baptist was founded in the twelfth century by Ailred the Palmer on a site in Thomas Street now occupied by the Augustinian priory and church, and the National College of Art and Design. Ailred was inspired to establish the hospital during a pilgrimage to the Holy Land, where he visited a monastery of Italian Hospitallers caring for sick pilgrims in Acre. Ailred became the first master of the Hospital of St John the Baptist and for many years it was richly endowed by the Anglo-Norman lords.

In the fourteenth century the hospital had 155 beds in constant use for the sick poor. The hospital was suppressed by Henry VIII in 1539.⁴ The building continued to have a medical use for a time under a lease granted in 1539 to Edmund Redman, a surgeon. It is thought that the institution probably functioned as a private charity without endowments.⁵ In 1629, the tower of the Hospital of St John the Baptist was rented by the city authorities and used as a house of correction for 'rogues, vagabonds and sturdy beggars'.⁶ There was a hospital for mendicants in Back Lane.⁷

In England, Elizabethan poor law made the English poor the responsibility of the parish in which they resided.⁸ This law formed the basis of the English poor law system but a similar law had not been introduced in Ireland. There was no obligation on local communities to maintain and support their poor, with the result that many of the poor in Ireland migrated from their own localities to the cities. The suppression of the monasteries in the sixteenth century, together with the failure to develop poor law relief, meant that there was scant support for the sick and poor in Ireland.⁹

Migration of the rural poor

Many landowners showed little interest in their tenants and some landlords, attracted by a better life in London, decided to leave the country; others left because of disillusionment with legislation that prohibited them from improving their lands and the welfare of their tenants; the absentee landlord came into being, and estates were often managed in Ireland by ruthless agents. These landlords and their agents squeezed as much income as they could out of leasing and subletting. There was also a significant rise in the population of Ireland in the latter half of the seventeenth century. It increased from 1.1 million to 2 million between 1672 and 1712. This rise

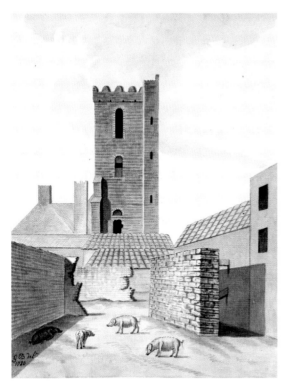

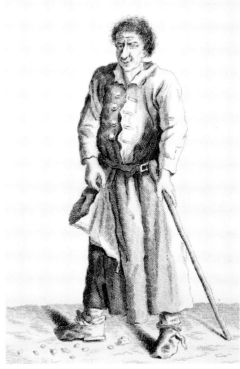

1.1 The tower of the medieval Friary and Hospital of St John the Baptist in Thomas Street by Gabriel Beranger. The tower was demolished in 1800. By permission of the Royal Irish Academy © RIA.

1.2 Jack Haugh (alias 'Mill-Cushin'), an eighteenth-century Dublin beggar. Reproduced from J. Caulfield, *Portraits, memoirs and characters of remarkable persons* (London, 1819).

placed great pressure on the agricultural system, which began to collapse, forcing an increasing number of hungry and impoverished people to gravitate towards urban centres.[10] For most of the impoverished, according to Jonathan Swift, the search for food and a better life led to Dublin.[11] The migration of rural poor into the city increased during periods of crop failure in the early eighteenth century.[12] For the majority, the journey was made in the vain hope of improvement, and many joined the throng of wretched beggars who roamed the streets of Dublin seeking subsistence.

Several efforts were made to rid the city of 'strange beggars'. In 1682 the lord mayor of Dublin, Humphrey Jervis, attempted to solve the problem by introducing the English practice of compulsory badges for local beggars. Anyone found begging without a badge was to be sent to the house of correction.[13] However this strategy did not result in any significant change.

First foundations

In 1680, certain hackney coachmen approached the city assembly and petitioned that the number of hackneys in the city should be limited to forty and that these should be licensed.[14] The city assembly agreed and also decreed that the funding obtained from the licences should be set aside for the erection and maintenance of a workhouse for the relief of the poor of the city. The proposal also had the support of the duke of Ormond, who was lord lieutenant of Ireland at the time.[15] The first attempt to build a workhouse took place in 1687, when the city spent £800 on foundations for a building in James's Street, in the grounds of what is now St James's Hospital. The land had been bestowed on the city by King James II and William Dungan, earl of Limerick.[16] James's Street formed part of an early medieval route known as An Slighe Mhór (the Great Way), which linked Galway and Dublin. The western suburb of the city had begun to develop shortly after the Norman conquest in 1190. Allotments of land, known as burgage plots, were sold along Thomas Street and James's Street to attract settlers from England, and as a result there was a ribbon of development along James's Street as early as the middle of the thirteenth century. An archaeological assessment of the St James's Hospital site fronting James's Street, carried out in 2000, revealed the remains of medieval garden soil containing pottery from that period. The location of the site for the workhouse, just outside St James's Gate, was chosen so that the poor could be stopped at the gate and all those without visible means of supporting themselves could be taken there. However, the building of the workhouse had to be abandoned with the outbreak of the war between William and James in 1688.

Dishonour and disturbance

Bristol faced similar problems with beggars and had responded with the establishment of the Bristol corporation of the poor under an act of parliament in 1696. This corporation established a workhouse to accommodate the destitute. Other cities began to follow Bristol's lead, establishing similar corporations and workhouses.[17] After William's victory over James, the Dublin city assembly again came under increasing pressure to do something about the large number of vagrants in the city. The vagrants posed a threat to the safety of Dublin's affluent citizens and it was this consideration, rather than any altruistic motive, which stimulated the debate. Many of those begging were children who had sought support without success from relatives and friends who had already moved to Dublin.[18] Begging children were regarded as a nuisance by the wealthy inhabitants of the city, 'crying at their doors at unreasonable hours in the night to excite them to give them reliefe'.[19] In 1695, the city assembly was informed that 'beggars are seen in great numbers in all parts of the city to the great dishonour of the government thereof, and the disturbance of all the inhabitants'.[20] The city assembly was alerted to the problem again in August 1697 and this time a decision was taken to proceed with the building of a workhouse outside St James's Gate.[21] The purpose was to take the beggars off the streets and to make them work:

> This citty swarms with beggars, who, for want of learning to get their livelyhood, are become a great nuisance, and will more and more encrease if some course be not taken to put them to worke; that it has been the care of the government to make good lawes to prevent idlenesse, which brings poverty; that it was designed that a house should be built to put idlers to worke in.[22]

A proposal to accommodate 'lunatics' near the same location as the workhouse was discussed at the assembly in 1699:

> Whereas certaine of the commons preferred their petition to the said assembly, setting forth that there is a proposall made to the government of this honorable citty for the erecting an hospitall therein for the reception of aged lunaticks and other diseased persons, there being noe citty in the world soe considerable as this citty of Dublin where there is not some such; that doctor Thomas Mullineux (Molyneux), on the behalf of a gentleman, who desires to be nameless, offers two thousand pounds, sterling, towards the maintenance of such an hospitall when it shall be built ...[23]

Thomas Molyneux was a graduate of Trinity College Dublin and had studied medicine in Leiden. He was later appointed professor of physic (medicine) in Trinity. The city assembly agreed to grant £200 and land near St James's Gate for an asylum but the proposal was not developed further at that time.

After the defeat of King James at the battle of the Boyne in 1690, the original land designated for the workhouse had been given to Lady Orkney and part of it was farmed by a man named Periam Poole. Lady Orkney was quite happy to hand over her land to the city for the building of a workhouse but Poole resisted attempts to acquire the land. Poole was obviously a strong-minded individual as he 'commanded his under-tenants to keep the same by force'.[24] However, his objections were to no avail as the city assembly ordered that the land should be taken from him by force if necessary. Lady Orkney sold the land to Sir Mark Rainsford, who was lord mayor of Dublin between 1700 and 1701, and the city acquired the property from him in 1703.[25]

For the use of the poor

An act of parliament in 1703 entitled 'An Act for erecting a Workhouse in the City of Dublin, for employing and maintaining the poor thereof', identified the walled-in fourteen-acre site on the south-west end of James's Street as the location for the new building and the site was settled forever for the use of the poor.[26] The City Workhouse was to be run by a body of nearly 200 people, to be known as the Governors and Guardians of the Poor of the City of Dublin, which consisted of the

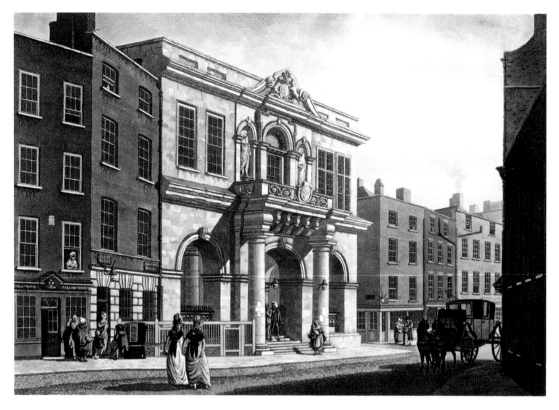

1.3   The Tholsel by James Malton, 1793. Courtesy of the National Library of Ireland.

lord lieutenant, the lord mayor, the lord chancellor, the archbishop of Dublin, the sheriffs, the justices of the peace, members of the corporation and a great many others. A donor of £50 and upwards was eligible to become a governor. The governors were charged with 'relieving, regulating, and setting at work, all vagabonds and beggars which shall come within the city or liberties'.[27] They were also 'to detain and keep in the service of the said corporation until the age of 16, any poor child or children found or taken up within the said city or liberties above 5 years of age, and to apprentice out such children to any honest persons, being Protestants'.[28] The governors held their meetings at the Tholsel (merchants' hall), which stood opposite Christ Church cathedral and was some distance from the workhouse in James's Street. As a consequence, the governors were remote from the institution and this contributed to the very poor management that led to several scandals during the eighteenth century. Moreover, with the passage of time the governors met infrequently.

There was a bridewell associated with the workhouse, in which beggars could be incarcerated if necessary. The act of 1703 provided various taxes to maintain

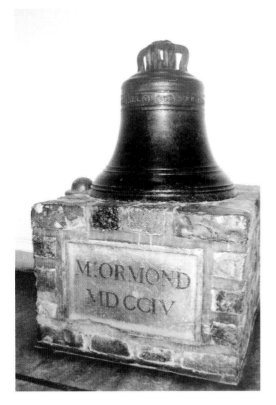

1.4   The foundation stone of the City Workhouse and the bell of the Foundling Hospital. Reproduced with permission of the Dublin County Council/Civic Museum collection.

the City Workhouse, which included a licence fee for all sedan chairs, carts, cars and brewers' drays. In addition, a house tax was levied at three pence in the pound of the total yearly value of each house in the city. This income was supplemented by the interest on land granted with the original site for the workhouse, which included about fourteen acres adjacent to the site, known as 'the pipes', 'on which are built several houses called George's Folly'.[29] The act establishing 'a Workhouse in the City of Dublin' was very significant as it was the first act in Ireland to recognize the principle of taxing the public for the relief of the destitute.

Voluntary contributions and subscriptions were made by several individuals and groups towards funding the construction of the workhouse. Mary, wife of the 2nd duke of Ormond, encouraged her aristocratic friends to contribute to a subscription. She supported the project 'not only by her own liberality, but by a singular and unwearied application in exacting several of the nobility and others of quality in that kingdom to the like charity'.[30] She raised £910, which would be the equivalent of over £100,000 today. Others who made donations included Trinity College Dublin and Lady Dun, wife of Sir Patrick Dun.[31] These contributions have a particular resonance today as the Trinity Centre for Health Sciences and the Sir Patrick Dun's Research Laboratory both stand on the site of the City Workhouse in St James's Hospital.

The foundation stone of the City Workhouse was laid on 12 October 1704 by the duchess of Ormond.[32] Walter Harris concluded his *History and antiquities of the city of Dublin*, published in 1766, with a description of the event:

> Oct. 12th (1704). This year the foundation stone of the city work-house, at the west end of St James's-street, was laid by Mary, duchess of Ormond attended by the lord mayor, recorder, aldermen and sheriffs; the lord mayor, Sir Francis Stoyte, invited her grace to a splendid entertainment prepared by him upon that occasion ...[33]

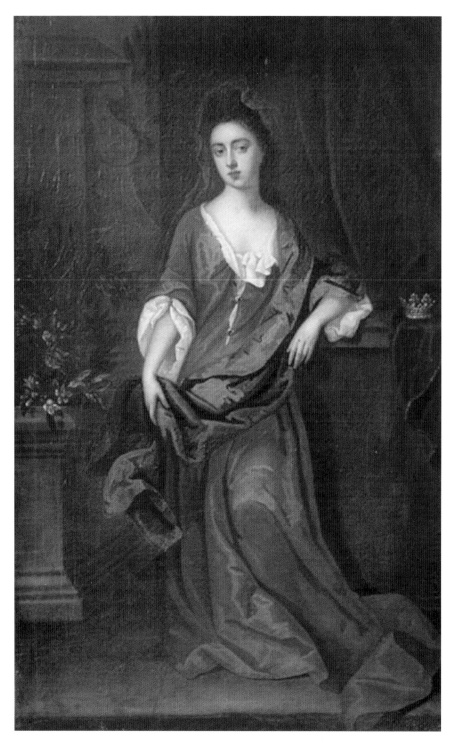

1.5 Mary Somerset, duchess of Ormond, artist unknown. Reproduced with permission of the Butler Collection, Kilkenny Castle.

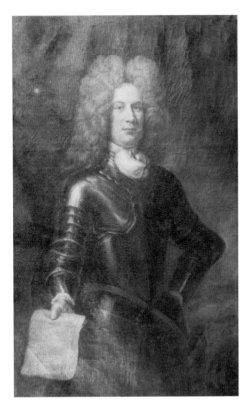

1.6   Thomas Burgh, surveyor general and architect of the City Workhouse. Courtesy of Hubert de Burgh.

1.7   Façade of City Workhouse. Reproduced from Charles Brooking, *A map of the city and suburbs of Dublin* (London, 1728).

Building of the workhouse

Thomas Burgh, the surveyor general, is credited with being the architect of the workhouse.[34] He contributed 'a pile of stone-work at his own cost at the entrance into the work-house' at the time of its construction.[35] It is likely that this refers to the wall in front of the workhouse on James's Street. Burgh served as a governor of the workhouse, which in 1710 still had an outstanding debt to him for timber.[36] He was the architect of the Royal Barracks (later Collins Barracks, and subsequently the National Museum of Ireland), Dr Steevens' Hospital and the Old Library in Trinity College Dublin. The plan for the workhouse was based on a U-shaped structure open to the rear. A large east-west-orientated dining hall with high, round leaded windows flanking an impressive entrance modelled on Michelangelo's Porta Pia in Rome faced James's Street. The façade was framed by the blind gables of the side ranges.[37]

Burgh's plans for the workhouse were influenced by the Royal Hospital in Kilmainham, which was designed by

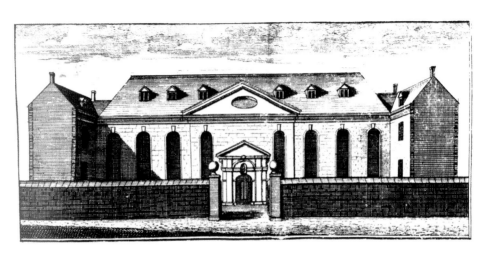

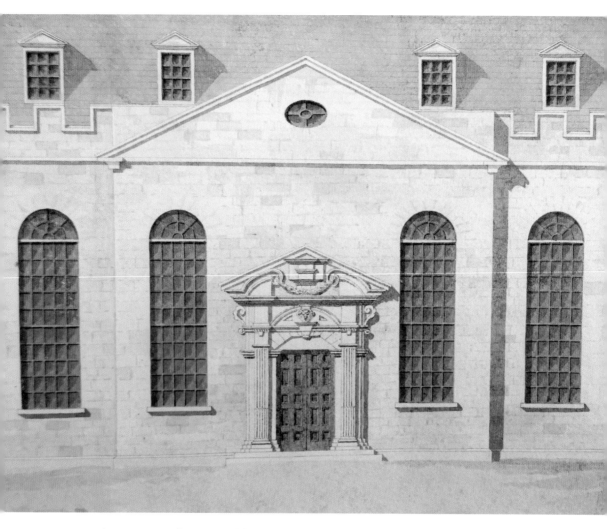

1.8   The entrance to the City Workhouse, which was modelled closely on the Porta Pia in Rome. Reproduced from the RIAI Murray Collection with permission of the Irish Architectural Archive.

William Robinson, whom Burgh succeeded as surveyor-general of Ireland in 1700. The façade of the dining hall was similar to the courtyard façade of the hall in the Royal Hospital. The deeply coved ceiling of the dining hall also resembled that of the hall in Kilmainham. According to a progress report made by the lord mayor in June 1705, two large buildings 300 feet long and 20 feet broad were finished except for glazing. These buildings were two storeys high with garrets and large vaults 'proper for stores and setting the poor to work in'. Another building to house about six hundred poor was in progress and there were two kitchens 'ready for roofing'. Vaults underneath the

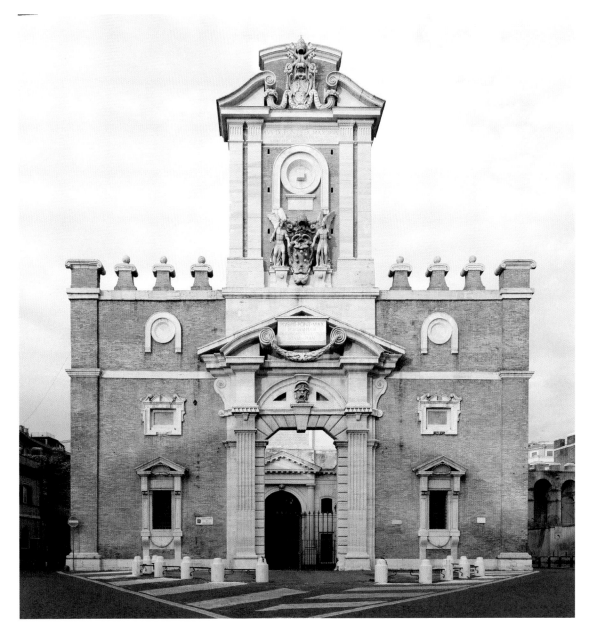

1.9   Façade of the Porta Pia, a gateway in the walls of Rome, which was designed by Michelangelo in 1561.

dining hall were almost completed and work on the rest of the hall was proceeding. It was estimated that the building should be finished by Christmas 1705 'provided there be a sufficient sum of money to answer the weekly charge'.[38] At this stage the cost of construction was estimated at £6,000, with a further £2,000 required for a bedlam and

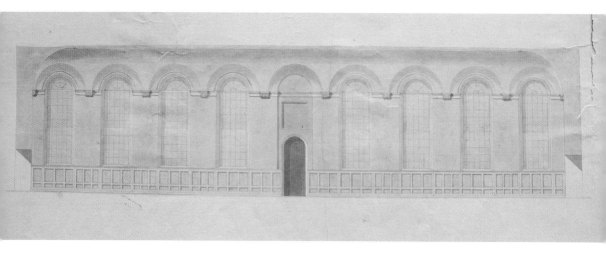

1.10   The interior of the front wall of the dining hall of the City Workhouse. Reproduced from the RIAI Murray Collection with permission of the Irish Architectural Archive.

infirmary and £2,500 for furnishings. This brought the total cost to £10,500. Voluntary contributions of around £4,000 were received.[39] The buildings included a linen manufactory, which was equipped with ten looms. Stone from a quarry in Dolphin's Barn was used to build the workhouse.

First inmates

The City Workhouse opened in January 1706 when 124 vagrants were apprehended in the streets of Dublin and brought to the new institution.[40] The beggars could be kept in the workhouse for any length of time not exceeding three years and only able-bodied vagrants were to be admitted. The admission of 'disabled poor people' and those suffering from the 'falling sickness' was prohibited. Beggars were 'to be employed and to work', but if they refused they were to be flogged and imprisoned and to receive 'severe usage'. Finally, if this approach failed to change their ways, they were to be transported overseas to the colonies.[41] In the first two years after it opened the average occupancy of the workhouse was 324. The accommodation for vagrants was in the vaults underneath the dining hall. These vaults, or cellars, were 240 feet long and 17 feet wide, with what was described as an 'airy' sunk along the outside of the building to provide light and to drain rainwater. Light entered through a series of arched windows at basement level in the north and south walls. In these dark and damp vaults there was a double row of two-tiered bunks to accommodate 100 men and 60 women.[42] Others were accommodated in buildings above ground level. Many of the beggars on the streets of Dublin were children and these, when apprehended,

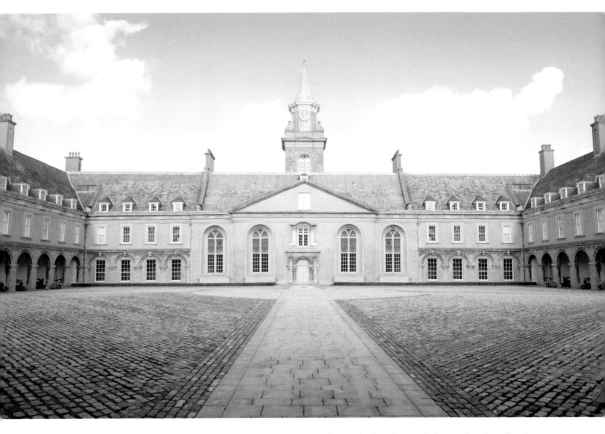

1.11   The courtyard façade of the Royal Hospital Kilmainham, which influenced de Burgh's plans for the City Workhouse. Photograph: Anthony Edwards.

were admitted to the workhouse where special accommodation had been set aside for them. The boys and girls were lodged in the workhouse until they could be boarded out to farmers and tradesmen as apprentices. The number of children grew and by 1725 approximately half the inmates in the workhouse were children from the age of five years upwards.[43]

William Fownes, lord mayor of the city in 1708, a wealthy landowner and *ex officio* governor, had six cells for the insane built in the City Workhouse. However, because of the lack of alternative accommodation, the number of mentally ill people within the workhouse increased significantly, as described by William Fownes in a letter to Jonathan Swift in 1732:

> When I was lord mayor I saw some miserable lunatics exposed to the hazard of others, as well as to themselves. I had six strong cells made at the workhouse for the most outrageous, which were soon filled, and by degrees, in a short time, those few

drew upon us the solicitations of many, till by the time the old corporation ceased (1727) we had in that house forty and upward.[44]

The diet for the adult inmates of the workhouse was gruel, bread, milk, porridge and 'burgoo'. The latter consisted of some oatmeal stirred up in cold water and 'seasoned with salt and enlivened with pepper'.[45]

Work

It was a fundamental principle of the workhouse that all adults and children should work. Rooms for weaving were installed and ten boys worked at each loom, supervised by a master. These children could earn enough to support themselves and also generate a profit for the workhouse. This was an ideal situation, according to the governors, who believed that 'the poor must eat whither they work or no, but being employed, their work feeds themselves and many others too'.[46] On the same principle, facilities were also made available for spinning so that the child spinners could become self-supporting. Spinning and weaving were skills that could also provide employment for children when they were old enough to leave the workhouse. Adult inmates, whose work included sawing logs and picking fibres out of old hemp ropes, were entitled to some extra food and to 8 pence as wages for a hard day's work.[47] Every year about sixty boys and girls were sent out as apprentices to various trades. From the outset the City Workhouse assumed a national character even though it was financed by a tax levied on Dublin properties alone. Children were sent from all over the country to the new institution and they often arrived in a very weakened condition. This state of affairs was deeply resented by Swift, who charged:

> As the whole fund for supporting this hospital is raised only from the inhabitants of the city, so there can hardly be anything more absurd, than to see it mis-employed in maintaining foreign beggars and bastards or orphans.[48]

Early financial difficulties

The income of the City Workhouse was not sufficient to run the institution and by 1726, according to a document now preserved in Marsh's Library, it was in very significant financial trouble. Drastic action was necessary and the governors decided:

> to maintain all the poor now in the house (in number two hundred and eleven) until the first day of May next ensuing and no longer, unless each parish makes a provision to be paid down monthly for supporting such of their poor in said house as must otherwise be returned to the parishes, and it is computed that an

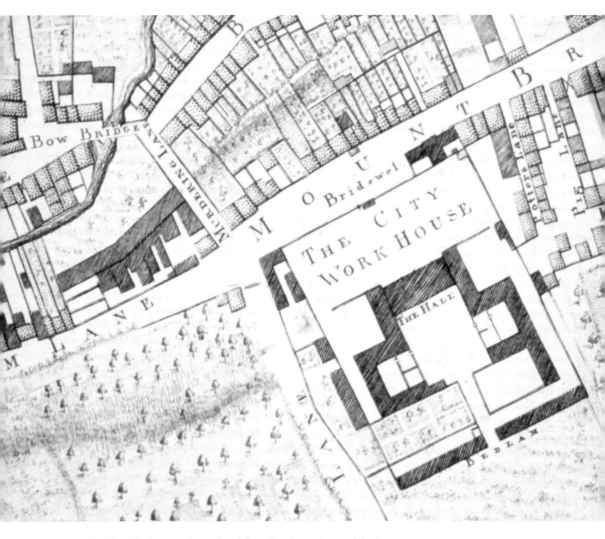

1.12 The City Workhouse. Reproduced from Brooking, *A map of the city.*

allowance of one shilling and ninepence per week will be necessary for feeding each poor person, and fourpence per week more for their clothing, if the house be desired to furnish it.[49]

The governors took this approach because they thought 'it especially incumbent upon them to subsist as many of the lunaticks and such sort of poor as are most miserable and helpless and if turned out would be most inconvenient to the publick until the next session of parliament, or as near as they can'.[50]

A list was drawn up of the inmates of the workhouse who would be returned to their respective parishes should it have to close. This list gives an interesting insight into the type of person housed within the institution at that time. Despite the strict admission rules, significant numbers of those admitted were elderly and disabled.[51]

Inmates in 1725[52]

	Number	Per cent
Superannuate	30	13.5
Infirm	26	11.7
Bed-rid	7	3.2
Mad	16	7.2
Fools	14	6.3
Has fits	3	1.4
King's evil (scrofula)	6	2.7
Blind	9	4.1
Dumb	4	1.8
Lame	7	3.2
Healthy adults	7	3.2
Healthy children	93	41.9

From the beginning the City Workhouse had a significant role in caring for older infirm adults.[53] The average age of adults housed in the workhouse in 1725 was 51 years. However, the average age of the three groups listed as 'superannuate', 'bed-rid' and 'infirm', was 63 years and they formed nearly 30 per cent of the inmates.

A solution was found to contain the financial crisis, and it did not become necessary to evict the inmates of the workhouse. A new act was introduced in 1727 as the authorities concluded that the foundation act of 1703 had not met 'the good end and design proposed thereby'.[54] The legislation dissolved the old governance and established a new one, the Governors of the Workhouse of the City of Dublin.[55] The new powers provided by the act were draconian, giving the governors full power and authority to seize any sturdy beggar or vagabond 'begging or strolling, or frequenting any of the streets ... of Dublin' and to commit them to the workhouse for any term not longer than four years with hard labour. Any children found on the streets over the age of 6 and without means of support were also to be sent to the workhouse, where they were to be instructed 'in the principles of the Protestant religion'.[56] Abandoned infants were to be the responsibility of the parish, but they could be admitted to the workhouse after the age of 6 years if they were still dependent on parish support.[57]

1.13 'Observations on the present state and condition of the Workhouse', 6 Apr. 1726. Reproduced with permission of Marsh's Library, Dublin.

The lack of more suitable accommodation for the mentally ill, or as they were termed at the time 'lunatics', put great strain on the resources of the workhouse. The governors decided to run the number down either through death or discharge and not to admit any more. The governors took a firm stand and 'the first denial was to a request of the earl of Kildare, which put a full stop to further applications'.[58] The resultant lack of any accommodation for the mentally ill was one of the factors that prompted Jonathan Swift to announce in November 1731 that he was going to provide

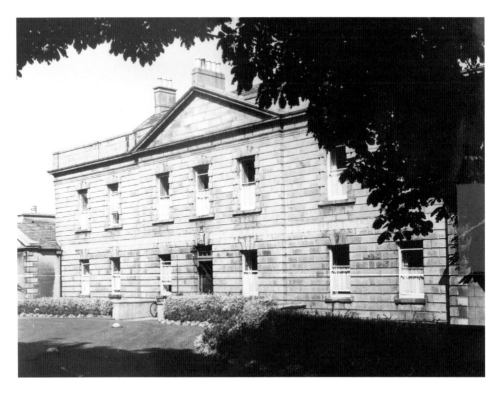

1.14   St Patrick's Hospital. Private collection.

in his will for the provision of a 'lunatic asylum'. The announcement was contained in the famous quatrain of his poem *Verses on the death of Doctor Swift*:

> He gave the little wealth he had,
> To build a house for fools and mad:
> And shew'd by one satiric touch,
> No nation wanted it so much:[59]

The asylum was established in 1746, a year after Swift's death, on a site very close to the workhouse.[60] The hospital, which became St Patrick's Hospital, still stands on its original grounds and is a teaching hospital for the medical school of Trinity College Dublin.

Workhouse of little benefit

According to Swift, many people considered that the workhouse was of little benefit in controlling the number of beggars on the streets of the city. As dean of St Patrick's cathedral, Swift was one of the governors of the institution but he had no hesitation in pointing out its failures. He wrote in 1729 that although the principal

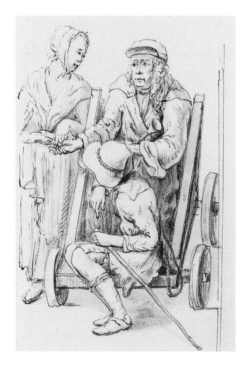
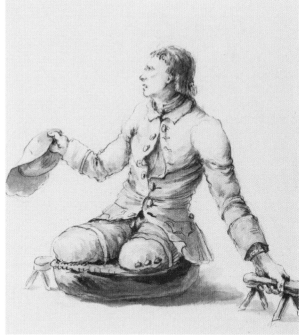

Left 1.15 'Hackball, king of the beggars', from W. Laffan (ed.), *The cries of Dublin, drawn from the life by Hugh Douglas Hamilton, 1760* (Dublin, 2003). Reproduced with permission.

Right 1.16 'A cripple beggar', from Laffan (ed.), *The cries of Dublin*. Reproduced with permission.

purpose of the poor house was to reduce the number of beggars and orphans, in reality 'Dublin is more infested since the establishment of the poor house, than it was ever known to be before.'[61] This was not entirely due to a failure of the work-house to fulfil its function. Poor harvests during the 1720s had reduced the rural community to penury and near starvation. At the end of the decade the situation was further exacerbated by an extremely cold winter.[62] In 1732 the mayor responded to the crisis by ordering that all the beggars should be apprehended and sent to the workhouse.[63]

Unwanted children

In the seventeenth century illegitimate children were seen as a burden on society and subjected to appalling neglect.[64] Unwanted children were often murdered and frequently infants were left exposed on the banks of the canals.[65] There was little tolerance in society for any woman who became pregnant outside of marriage. She

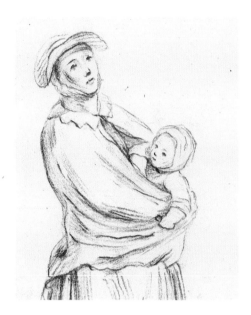

1.17 'A beggar woman and her baby', from Laffan (ed.), *The cries of Dublin*. Reproduced with permission.

was despised and shunned by the community and often by her family, and she might be forced to leave her neighbourhood. A girl in this situation might have no options to support herself and her child apart from begging or prostitution. Under these circumstances it is not surprising that some young women decided to abandon their babies.[66] Parishes in Dublin showed little enthusiasm for supporting abandoned infants. A parish tax to support illegitimate children was levied by Protestant church wardens on Catholic and Protestant householders. Many of the Catholic householders refused to contribute as they were not members of the vestries levying the tax. Parish officials also tried to transfer the responsibility for supporting abandoned infants to neighbouring parishes. The practice of covertly moving babies from one parish to another in the dark,

known as 'dropping', became so common that in 1722 the Protestant archbishop of Dublin, William King, found it necessary to write to his ministers and their church wardens asking them to suppress such a 'wicked practice'.[67] The archbishop's plea had no effect, and in 1727 the government enacted the legislation that made each Dublin parish responsible for the care of children abandoned in their parish until they reached the age of 6, when they were to be admitted to the City Workhouse. Women were to be employed to care for the children under the supervision of an overseer.[68] These new rules were ignored and the practice of 'dropping' continued as before. It was in this context that Jonathan Swift wrote his satirical essay that bore the title *A modest proposal for preventing the children of poor people from being a burthen to their parents or country, and for making them beneficial to the publick.*

Swift's *Modest proposal*

For many years Jonathan Swift had been writing about the need for action to alleviate the appalling living conditions of the poor, which forced them and their children to become beggars. Swift was very critical of those landlords who were ruthless in their dealings with their tenants. He was particularly angered by the predicament of foundlings and the children of beggars, and he abhorred 'that horrid practice of

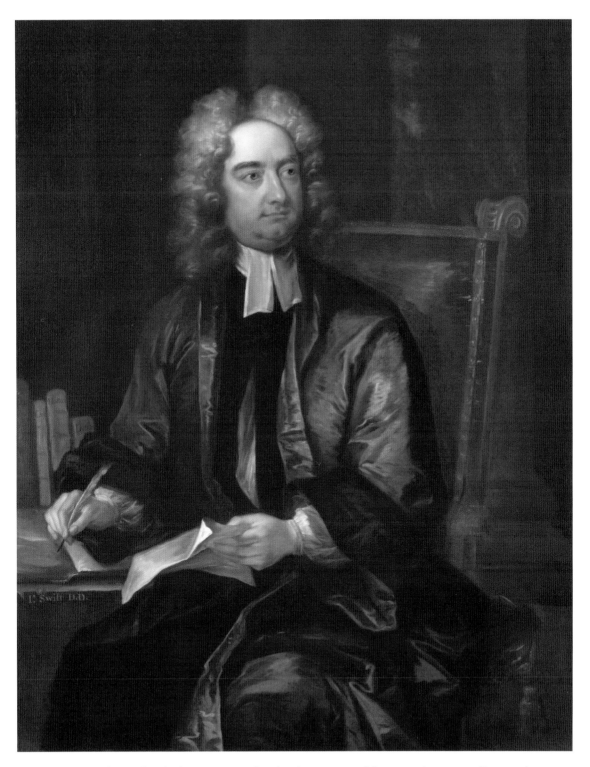

1.18　Jonathan Swift c.1718 by Charles Jervas. Reproduced with permission of the National Portrait Gallery, London.

women murdering their bastard children, alas! too frequently among us, sacrificing the poor innocent babes'.[69] He suspected that mothers did this more because of a lack of means to support their children rather than from shame. Swift vented his anger in what has been described as one of the most famous and savage satires in the English language.[70] The essay was published anonymously in 1729. Readers are still shocked by the 'modest proposal', which suggested that the infants should be fattened over the course of a year and then sold as food. However, as there would be a certain expense in feeding the infants, the food would have to be sold as a delicacy:

> I grant this food will be somewhat dear, and therefore very proper for landlords, who, as they have already devoured most of the parents, seem to have the best title to the children.[71]

Swift lists several advantages that would result from his proposal, which included a reduction in the number of 'papists', whom he described as being 'the principal breeders of the nation as well as our most dangerous enemies'. The scheme would also provide a source of funds for the poorer tenants and enable them 'to pay their landlord's rent, their corn and cattle being already seized, and money a thing unknown'.[72] Towards the end of the essay Swift pretends to reject out of hand his genuine proposals to alleviate the problem:

A MODEST PROPOSAL

by

Jonathan Swift

FOR PREVENTING THE CHILDREN OF POOR PEOPLE IN IRELAND FROM BEING A BURDEN TO THEIR PARENTS OR COUNTRY, AND FOR MAKING THEM BENEFICIAL TO THE PUBLICK

DUBLIN, IRELAND

PRINTED AND FOR SALE AT THE YORK & STEVENSON

PRINTING-OFFICE

Directly opposite the Bank of Dublin.

1729

1.19   Title page of J. Swift, *A modest proposal* (Dublin, 1729).

> Therefore let no man talk to me of other expedients: of taxing our absentees at five shillings a pound: of using neither cloaths, nor houshold furniture, except what is of our own growth and manufacture: of utterly rejecting the materials and instruments that promote foreign luxury ... of teaching landlords to have at least one degree of mercy towards their tenants.[73]

One cannot be sure how much Swift's *Modest proposal* influenced the thinking of the ruling class, but in December 1729, following a complaint by the earl of Cavan about the practice of moving abandoned infants from one parish to another, the Irish house of lords established a committee to investigate the problem. Elizabeth Hyland, a nurse from St John's parish, was one of the parish officers who appeared before the committee. She described how she had managed twenty-seven foundlings. Seven had died and two had been taken back by their mothers. She 'dropped' the remaining eighteen in other parishes. The infants were given a substance called diacodium, a syrup of poppies, when they were being 'dropped', to ensure that they did not make any noise. The parish warden in St Mary's parish admitted that the parish employed a 'lifter' whose role was 'to move foundlings to other parishes under the cover of darkness'.[74] When the findings of the committee were published, no one could deny the extent of the problem or the need for an urgent solution.

The establishment of the Foundling Hospital and Workhouse

The Irish parliament responded to the ensuing public outcry by passing legislation that obliged the governors of the workhouse to admit all children, irrespective of age, abandoned in Dublin from March 1730.[75] The institution now adopted the name Foundling Hospital and Workhouse of the City of Dublin, and it was to be governed by a new corporation known as the Governors of the Poor of the City of Dublin. Due to the increased demands and responsibilities placed on the institution, two additional wings were added on either side of the original buildings. Swift was critical of the new governance structure, which almost trebled the number of governors. He pointed out that several of the new governors 'live at a great distance, and cannot possibly have the least concern for the advantage of the city'. He thought that very little was achieved at the general meetings of the governors 'except one or two acts of extreme justice, which I then thought might as well have been spared'. He was similarly unimpressed by the work of the court of assistants, a subcommittee of the board of governors, charged with the responsibility of overseeing the day-to-day running of the Foundling Hospital and Workhouse. He found the members 'usually taken up in little brangles about coachmen, or adjusting accounts of meal and small beer; which however necessary, might sometimes have given place to matters of much greater moment'.[76]

Apart from Swift, several other celebrated individuals served for a time as governors of the institution, such as Lord Mornington (father of the duke of Wellington), Arthur Guinness, who founded his famous brewery in 1759, and the politician and patriot Henry Grattan. In his history of the Foundling Hospital and Workhouse, William Wodsworth reproduced from the minute books a facsimile of some of the signatures of the governors, including the earl of Kildare (1732), Lord Mornington (1746), Lord Shelburne (1758) and Arthur Guinness (1807).[77]

Welsh Prunty and *Wuthering Heights*

The decision not to send one particular child to the Dublin workhouse in the early years of the eighteenth century has left its mark on literary history. If the boy had been sent, *Wuthering Heights* would probably not have been written by Emily Brontë. The boy was discovered in the hold of a ship on a journey between Liverpool and Warrenpoint, Co. Down. Someone suggested that the child may have been abandoned because he was sick and there was immediate agitation to throw him overboard. Among the passengers was a cattle dealer named Prunty, who was accompanied by his wife. Mrs Prunty protected the boy and bought food and clothing for him

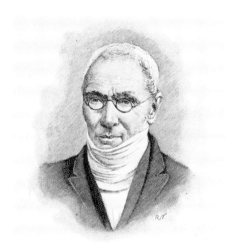

1.20 Patrick Brontë. Reproduced from W. Wright, *The Brontës in Ireland* (London, 1894).

when the boat docked, with the intention of sending him back to Liverpool. However, the captain refused to take the child on board again. This created a dilemma for Mrs Prunty because, even though there was a vestry tax at the time to cover the cost of carrying a child to the workhouse in Dublin, no funding was made available. The other option was to take the child to the workhouse herself, but this was a long and arduous journey, so she decided to take the child home. It was thought the child might be from Wales because of his dark colouring so he was named Welsh.[78]

As he grew up, Welsh developed a close relationship with Prunty and gradually displaced the other children in the old man's affection. A sinister figure, Welsh eventually gained control over the family home and farm, bringing tragedy and jealousy to his adoptive family. Patrick Brontë, who was born in 1777 in Co. Down, was the grandson of one of the displaced brothers. Patrick became a clergyman in the Church of England, and he changed his name from Prunty to Brontë. He settled in Haworth near Bradford and there, during the long winter nights, he told his four children the story of Welsh Prunty. Later, Emily Brontë would use the story when she described the circumstances of Heathcliff's adoption by the Earnshaw family in *Wuthering heights*.[79] One evening when Earnshaw returned to his home after a business trip to Liverpool, the family was amazed to find him carrying a child, bundled up inside his greatcoat, whom he had found starving and homeless in the streets of Liverpool.

In this way Welsh, the little boy whom the Prunty family decided not to send to the workhouse in James's Street, was transformed by Emily Brontë into Heathcliff, one of the most enigmatic characters in English literature.[80]

2

The Foundling Hospital and Workhouse of the City of Dublin

[A] charity peculiarly suited to this kingdom, situated in a metropolis abounding with Papists of the lowest rank.[1]

Pope Innocent III is credited with establishing the first foundling hospital in Rome in 1198. The pope was horrified by the number of drowned infants being recovered from the Tiber in fishermen's nets. In the thirteenth century a growing number of Italian cities opened institutions for abandoned infants, and over subsequent centuries foundling hospitals were established throughout Europe. The Ospedale degli Innocenti (Hospital of the Innocents) in Florence was one of the best known of these early institutions. Infants were left in a special basin, similar to a baptismal font, which was placed near the entrance to the hospital. This was replaced in 1660 by a turning wheel mechanism in the wall near the entrance.[2] The number of foundling hospitals mushroomed in the eighteenth century. They were established to reduce infanticide and the abandonment of infants, however, 'paradoxically, tragically, and, from a modern point of view, predictably, gathering so many infants in one place in societies with very little awareness of hygiene and almost no real medicine resulted in an appalling death rate'.[3]

Infants in Dublin's Foundling Hospital and Workhouse

Infants up to the age of 12 months could be admitted to Dublin's Foundling Hospital and Workhouse. During the first year following its opening in 1730, 265 infants were admitted. Fifty-eight of these children came from St Michan's parish, which was one of the poorest in the city. Archbishop Hugh Boulter, Protestant archbishop of Dublin, ordered that a 'turning-wheel should be placed near the gate of the workhouse'.[4] An

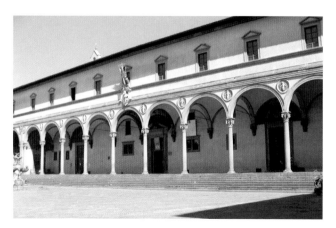
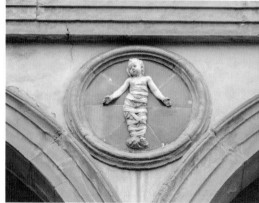

Left 2.1   One of Europe's oldest and best-known foundling hospitals, Ospedale degli Innocenti in Florence, which was designed by Filippo Brunelleschi.

Right 2.2   A baby wrapped in swaddling clothes, in a terracotta relief by Andrea della Robbia on the façade of Ospedale degli Innocenti in Florence.

infant could be placed in a basket attached to the wheel at any time, day or night, and there was a bell to attract the attention of the porter. The porter rotated the wheel, bringing the infant inside. He was instructed to take in all infants delivered at the gate or left in the cradle and not to have any conversation with the individuals who brought the children.[5] The anonymity of the system was designed to encourage mothers to bring unwanted children to the hospital rather than to abandon them. Some babies carried a token on their person as an enigmatic indicator of their identity. These items were carefully registered by the official who recorded the admission of the babies. Such talismans were the only means by which parents could identify an abandoned child should they wish to claim him or her in the future. A register was kept in the hospital that recorded the date of admission of an infant, the state of health, the distance carried to Dublin, the date sent out to a nurse and the date of return to parents or the date of death.

All infants admitted were assessed, and those who appeared to be ill were sent to the infirmary. The chances of infants surviving the first few days after being abandoned depended on the ability of the hospital to secure an adequate number of wet nurses to feed the infants within the institution while awaiting placement with a wet nurse in the country. Safe and effective artificial feeds for infants had not yet been developed. There were difficulties in recruiting a sufficient number of wet nurses to care for the children within the hospital and, as a result, individual nurses frequently had to breast feed several infants. It was not easy to attract women of 'decent character', and often the institution ended up recruiting unscrupulous women as wet nurses.

Many women were afraid they would contract syphilis from an infected baby, as a significant number of foundlings were the children of prostitutes. Some of these infants had congenital syphilis and could, while suckling at the breast, pass the disease to their wet nurses. Officials reacted to this situation by trying to identify infants with syphilis on admission so that they would be admitted directly to the infirmary.

As soon as it could be arranged, the healthy infants were given to wet nurses in the country, who were paid an annual fee to care for them. Country air was regarded as healthy, so women from rural areas were preferred as wet nurses. Women arrived at the hospital each day seeking children they could nurse. These nurses came mainly from counties Dublin, Wicklow and Meath. The children remained with their wet nurses until their eighth year. They were then readmitted to the Foundling Hospital and Workhouse to be educated and given a skill that would later help them to find employment. Some nurses became attached to the children under their care and refused to part with them when they reached the age of 8.

Wet nurses outside the institution received an advance of 3s. 4d. for each infant under their care and a further £1 16s. 6d. when an infant was presented for inspection after twelve months. However, this system was open to abuse, and some nurses killed the infants soon after they received the advance payment. In order to prevent another child being presented at the annual inspection in place of the foundling it was necessary to place some form of identity on each foundling that could not be removed easily. In Continental foundling hospitals, infants were fitted with necklaces or earrings. This had the effect of stigmatizing the children, and in many foundling hospital archives there are impassioned letters from foster parents asking for permission to have the necklace taken off the child for some special holiday or occasion. The branding or tattooing of children on the inside of one arm was another method of identification and this was used in the Dublin Foundling Hospital.

Staffing of the Foundling Hospital and Workhouse

A small number of senior staff positions were created in the Foundling Hospital and Workhouse. The occupants of these positions were described as officers and all others working in the institution were servants. The officers included a treasurer, who also functioned as the chief administrator of the institution, a matron (resident), a clerk of foundlings, a nurses' superintendent, a butler, a surgeon, a physician and a resident apothecary.

The matron had overall responsibility for the children in the Foundling Hospital, and she was instructed to ensure:

> that the children rise every morning at the hour appointed by the board, to be washed and combed, taught their prayers before breakfast and to take care the provisions are properly distributed and that the nurses be kept clean and sweet.[6]

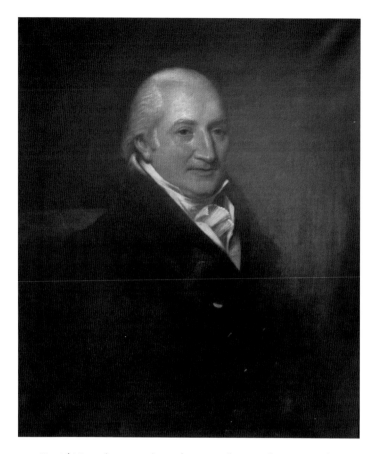

2.3   Daniel Moore (1750–1847), apothecary to the Foundling Hospital c.1770.
Reproduced with permission of the Royal College of Physicians of Ireland
and of the Apothecaries' Hall of Ireland.

Apothecaries formulated medicines for physicians and surgeons but they could
also prescribe independently. The duties of the apothecary included admission of the
sick and responsibility for their care between the visits of the surgeon and physician.
The apothecary was also responsible for the preparation of medicines. One of the
apothecaries, Daniel Moore, who worked in the Foundling Hospital and Workhouse
around the year 1770 became a leading figure in the development of the profession.
Moore was born in 1750 and was trained by his uncle, John Clarke, a distinguished
apothecary with a business on Capel Street. Before his appointment to the Foundling
Hospital and Workhouse, Moore spent some years as an apprentice to John Whiteway,
surgeon to Dr Steevens' Hospital. Whiteway, who was a cousin of Jonathan Swift,
served as president of the Royal College of Surgeons in Ireland (RCSI) in 1786. Daniel
Moore played a central role in the foundation of the Apothecaries' Hall of Dublin and
several of his descendants would play leading roles in Irish medicine over the follow-

ing two centuries. One of his descendants, his great, great, great grandson, Richard Stephens, was appointed as surgeon to St James's Hospital in 1982.[7]

From the early years of the Foundling Hospital and Workhouse, unscrupulous staff defrauded it. 'Yet I confess I have known an hospital', Swift wrote in 1727, 'where all the household officers grew rich, while the poor, for whose sake it was built, were almost starving for want of food and raiment.'[8] In 1737, the treasurer, Nicholas Grueber, and his son George, whom he had appointed as his assistant, were caught embezzling the hospital's funds. The butler, who was in charge of the stores, was also stealing from the hospital. When some of the workhouse boys became aware of these activities, the treasurer had the boys convicted on a false charge and transported to the West Indies. However, the malpractices were eventually discovered and the guilty staff were dismissed.[9]

Religion

At the beginning of the eighteenth century Dublin was a Protestant city. Over 70 per cent of the population was Protestant and the majority of these were members of the Church of Ireland.[10] In their regular submissions to the Irish parliament for support, the governors of the Foundling Hospital and Workhouse emphasized the importance of the institution as a 'Charity peculiarly suited to this kingdom, situated in a metropolis abounding with papists of the lowest rank'.[11] The institution had as one of its principal objectives the education of children 'in the reformed or Protestant faith … to strengthen and promote the Protestant interest in Ireland'.[12] According to Wodsworth, the hospital's first historian, 'the tenets of the Christian religion were flogged into the boys and they were caned into the girls'.[13] The use of foundling hospitals to increase the numbers adhering to a particular faith was a common practice. At around the same time as the Dublin Foundling Hospital and Workhouse was established, Jesuit missionaries in Peking ran a similar institution for the reception of infants found abandoned on the streets. These children were cared for by the Jesuits and received a Catholic education in order to increase the numbers of Chinese Christians.[14] From the beginning, the religious objective was frustrated in Dublin. Not enough Protestant nurses could be found to nurse the infants, so many had to be given to Catholic nurses. Under the influence of these nurses a significant number of the children adopted the Catholic faith. Within the Foundling Hospital and Workhouse, on Fridays and fast days, the children were made to eat broth with meat. According to Catholic teaching at the time it was considered a serious sin to eat meat on Fridays and fast days. The edict that the children should all be brought up as Protestants attracted considerable public animosity. Concern was expressed in the minutes of the governors' meeting in 1774 about a secret society known as the 'Whitefeet', which threatened the lives of employers if they continued to hire Protestant apprentices from the Foundling Hospital.[15]

Once admitted to the institution, further contact between the children and their parents was forbidden. Some Catholic parents found ways of subverting this rule in order to frustrate the governors' policy of rearing all children as Protestants. Mothers were known to collude with those employed to find wet nurses in the parishes, so that the mothers would be employed as nurses to their own children.[16] The governors were so determined to enforce their policy on religion that special legislation was introduced to allow the transfer of children between the foundling hospitals in Dublin and Cork so that, when considered necessary, mothers could be separated from their children by a prohibitive distance.[17] Some children between the ages of 6 and 8 years were exchanged between Cork and Dublin but there was no enthusiasm for the scheme and the legislation soon fell into disuse.

Education

Schools were established in the institution for children over the age of 8. The purpose of these was:

> to rear the children to habits of industry … and with that design the females are taught plain work, knitting, spinning and to make their own clothes; and the boys employed every second day at different trades, as weavers, scribblers, taylors, carpenters, shoemakers, and gardeners; and those employments, with the instruction in reading, writing, arithmetic, a perfect knowledge of the scriptures, and the principles of the Protestant religion, complete the general system of education.[18]

Emphasis was placed on physical activity for the boys whereas the girls were given more sedentary tasks. With the passage of time, the Foundling Hospital and Workhouse developed an extensive nursery garden and workshops. Net making and lace making were other skills fostered in the institution.

Diet

The diet of the infants consisted of a mixture of bread and water with some milk. There were frequent problems with the milk suppliers and a number of contractors were prosecuted for supplying milk diluted with water. The supply of adulterated milk and contaminated food continued throughout the existence of the Foundling Hospital and Workhouse and of its successors, the Foundling Hospital and the South Dublin Union. In 1775, the College of Physicians drew up a special diet for the older children in the Foundling Hospital, which included beer. This diet remained the regular fare for twenty years. The ordering of the beer was given great attention by the governors and there were lively debates on the merits of different brews. In July 1772, tenders for beer were received from Lady Taylor, Ambrose Cox and Arthur Guinness. Lady Taylor was awarded the contract because her beer was the cheapest. However, it was soon noted that the beer 'made the wet nurses' stomachs ache'.[19] The arrangement with Lady Taylor was cancelled and Ambrose Cox was awarded the contract.

Punishment

The punishment of children was extremely harsh in the institution, particularly in its early years. Boys were flogged and girls were caned when they wet their beds and when they were caught stealing food. Corporal punishment was used frequently in the classrooms. From time to time children ran away, and if they were caught they were punished severely. In August 1732, two boys ran away and one of them, William Mills, was apprehended. His punishment was to be 'confined in the house of correction, and whipt three several days; that he be then brought to the work-house, put in the dungeon, and tyed with a chain to a piece of logg'.[20] Sometimes boys were 'publickly whipt through the workhouse yard'.[21] In 1754, the governors of the workhouse had a whipping post erected at the Tholsel,[22] so that the public 'may see their sentences properly executed upon delinquents in High Street after which punishment, the offender is to be taken through the city at a cart's tail with his back bare, to show that justice has been executed on him'.[23] Children were also punished by placing them in the vaults underneath the Foundling Hospital and Workhouse, or by locking them for long periods in a dark room. In later years punishments were ameliorated and were brought under the surveillance of the chaplain.

Indecent behaviour

In February 1744, Margaret Hayden, seamstress to the hospital, complained to the board that the treasurer, Joseph Pursell, 'had used her in an indecent manner'.[24] She made her case before a meeting of twenty-seven governors chaired by Lord Lanesborough and as a result Pursell was summarily dismissed.[25] Pursell lobbied intensively after the meeting and at the next assembly of governors on 12 March there was an attendance of sixty-six. The whole issue was debated again and the majority voted to reinstate Pursell but to issue him with a reprimand. It is likely that many of the female staff and foundling girls were subjected to harassment by the male staff and Margaret Hayden's experience did little to encourage complaint. There were occasional dismissals, such as that of John Johnston, who was dismissed for abusing a foundling named Charlotte Grey. In the later years of the Foundling Hospital and Workhouse, when a group of lady governesses took control, abuse of this nature was dealt with much more effectively.

Inadequate resources to support two objectives

Due to a significant increase in the number seeking admission to the Foundling Hospital and Workhouse, successful petitions for additional assistance were made to parliament by the governors in 1743 and 1746. A further petition was made in 1752, which pointed out that children were being brought to Dublin from around the country and abandoned so that they had to be admitted to the Foundling Hospital.[26]

The governors received a sympathetic response but no material assistance. The following year the governors again informed parliament of the growing number of children being admitted and of the urgency of erecting new buildings. On this occasion their appeal was successful and they were granted £2,000.[27] A further grant was made when the governors claimed that children had to stay with their wet nurses for longer periods because there was insufficient space in the Foundling Hospital. This was considered undesirable as most of the wet nurses were Catholics.

The governors were struggling to meet the two major objectives with which they had been charged. The first was to provide admission to all abandoned infants and destitute children, and the second was to accept all the beggars and vagrants apprehended on the streets of the city. It was apparent to Swift, as early as 1737, that the institution was unable to deliver on these objectives. Swift's own answer to the problem was to revert to the previously unsuccessful solution of badging the indigenous poor in every parish. He published his views in 1737 in a pamphlet entitled *A proposal for giving badges to the beggars in all the parishes of Dublin*. All 'foreign' beggars without exception were to be driven out. It would then be reasonable for charitable people to support the small number of poor in their own neighbourhood. Swift had little sympathy for the hungry and starving people that thronged to the city to seek relief:

> To say the truth, there is not a more undeserving vicious race of human kind than the bulk of those who are reduced to beggary, even in this beggarly country. For as a great part of our publick miseries is originally owing to our own faults (but, what those faults are I am grown by experience too wary to mention) so I am confident, that among the meaner people, nineteen in twenty of those who are reduced to a starving condition, did not become so by what lawyers call the work of God, either

A

PROPOSAL

FOR GIVING

BADGES

TO THE

BEGGARS

IN ALL THE

PARISHES of DUBLIN.

BY THE

DEAN of St. *PATRICK's*

LONDON,
Printed for T. COOPER at the *Globe* in *Pater Noster Row*.
MDCCXXXVII.

Price Six Pence,

2.4   The title page of the first edition of *A proposal for giving badges to the beggars in all the parishes of Dublin* (London, 1737), by 'the dean of St Patrick's'. Image courtesy of Whyte's, Dublin and Bernard Quaritch, London.

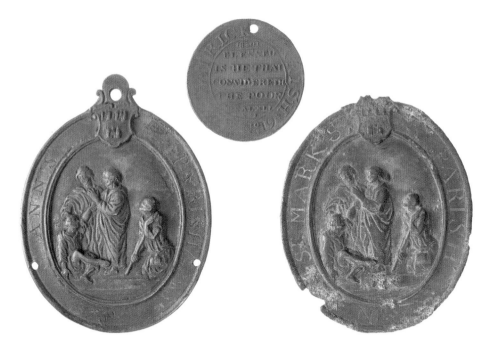

2.5   Badges worn by Dublin beggars in St Patrick's, St Anne's and St Mark's parishes. Reproduced with permission of the National Museum of Ireland.

upon their bodies or goods; but merely from their own idleness, attended with all manner of vices, particularly drunkenness, thievery, and cheating.[28]

The badges were to be made from brass, copper or pewter and were to be securely attached to the beggar's coat. Swift had no empathy for those who objected to wearing them:

As I am personally acquainted with a great number of street beggars, I had some weak attempts to have been made in one or two parishes to promote the wearing of badges; and my first question to those who ask an alms, is, Where is your badge? I have in several years met with about a dozen who were ready to produce them, some out of their pockets, others from under their coat, and two or three on their shoulders, only covered with a sort of cape which they could lift up or let down upon occasion. They are too lazy to work, they are not afraid to steal, nor ashamed to beg; and yet are too proud to be seen with a badge, as many of them have confessed to me, and not a few in very injurious terms, particularly the females.[29]

Swift believed that previous attempts to deal with beggars by a policy of badging had failed because the citizens had not enforced it:

Wherefore, I do assert, that the shopkeepers who are the greatest complainers of the grievance, lamenting that for every customer, they are worried by fifty beggars, do very well deserve what they suffer, when an apprentice with a horse-whip is able to lash every beggar from the shop, who is not of the parish, and does not wear the badge of that parish on his shoulder, well fastened and fairly visible; and if this practice were universal in every house to all the sturdy vagrants, we should in a few weeks clear the town of all mendicants, except those who have a proper title to our charity: as for the aged and infirm, it would be sufficient to give them nothing, and then they must starve or follow their brethren.[30]

Swift was scathing about the practice of English justices of the peace and parish officers who were 'exporting hither their supernumerary beggars' under the specious reasoning that they would contribute to 'the English Protestant interest' in Ireland. Sometimes, when he was travelling by ship from Chester to Dublin, he found 'large cargoes' of English beggars on board.[31] Swift made no effort to conceal his authorship of *A proposal for giving badges to beggars in all the parishes of Dublin*, as 'Dean of St Patrick's' was printed on the title page. This indicated that the views expressed were his own and, unlike in *A modest proposal*, on this occasion there was no irony or satire.[32]

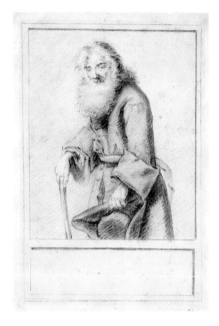

2.6   William Thompson, a Dublin beggar, reputedly aged 114 in 1744, by Rupert Barber. Reproduced with permission of the National Gallery of Ireland.

Cold and famine

Between December 1739 and September 1741, European countries experienced arctic weather conditions.[33] It was the longest period of extreme cold in modern European history. In December 1739 the river Liffey froze within days of the drop in temperature. The cold placed a great demand on fuel, and coal became so expensive that many could not afford it. Mill wheels stopped functioning because the water froze and there was a resultant shortage of wheat for the bakers. Water power also drove machinery for weaving, which meant that many of the weavers in Dublin were unable to work. For nearly seven weeks Ireland was in the grip of frost. Potatoes in storage were destroyed by the freezing weather and this caused great hardship as even at that time the potato was very important in the diet of the poor. The situation was exacerbated by low temperatures and little rainfall throughout 1740. Crops were destroyed and there was a shortage of fodder for cattle and sheep, so the animals began to die in the fields. Food became very scarce in Dublin and the poor could not afford it.

The frost returned in December 1740 and the Liffey froze again, this time for ten days. As Christmas approached, food prices soared and it was feared that many people would starve. The archbishop of Dublin, Hugh Boulter, launched an appeal for money to buy food for the poor of the city. Only residents of Dublin were to be fed as the authorities did not want to increase the influx of starving paupers from the countryside. Boulter decided to centre his relief effort in the Foundling Hospital and Workhouse as the institution was convenient to the Liberties, where most of those in distress lived. The governors were instructed to sign meal tickets which would enable each ticket holder to procure one meal per family member per day. Soon nearly 3,000 Dubliners were being fed every day at the hospital, and in May the number rose to 4,400.[34] By early summer the pressure for food was so great that ticket holders were restricted to three meals per week. Boulter continued to appeal for funds to support the scheme and appeals were also made by Dean Swift, Dean Delany and Viscount Mountjoy.

The weather began to improve in the second half of 1741, and even though there was a drought in the early summer there was not a resultant food crisis.[35] In order to show their appreciation of Boulter's efforts on behalf of the poor, the lord mayor of Dublin and a group of citizens commissioned the painting of a portrait of the archbishop, which was to be hung in the dining hall of the Foundling Hospital and Workhouse. The large painting, which was the work of the artist Francis Bindon, depicted Boulter surrounded by poor supplicants. It was placed over a large fireplace at the eastern end of the dining hall where the children, sometimes as many as a thousand of them, would eat and pray under the watchful eye of Archbishop Boulter.[36] It now hangs in the provost's house in Trinity College Dublin.[37]

The Hospital for Incurables

In 1743 members of the Dublin Charitable Musical Society decided to donate their funds to establish the Hospital for Incurables in rented rooms in Fleet Street. It was hoped that the initiative would lessen the pressure on the Foundling Hospital and Workhouse by providing 'several such miserable objects' with accommodation, food and the attention of physicians and surgeons. In 1749, an act of parliament gave the governors of the Foundling Hospital and Workhouse power 'to commit beggars and vagrants labouring under disease, and exposing their infirmities, to the workhouse, and upon the certificate of the physicians or surgeons that the disorder was dangerous or incurable, to confine them in some house in the city, or send them to the Hospital for Incurables'.[38] The governors continued to hold these powers until 1772,

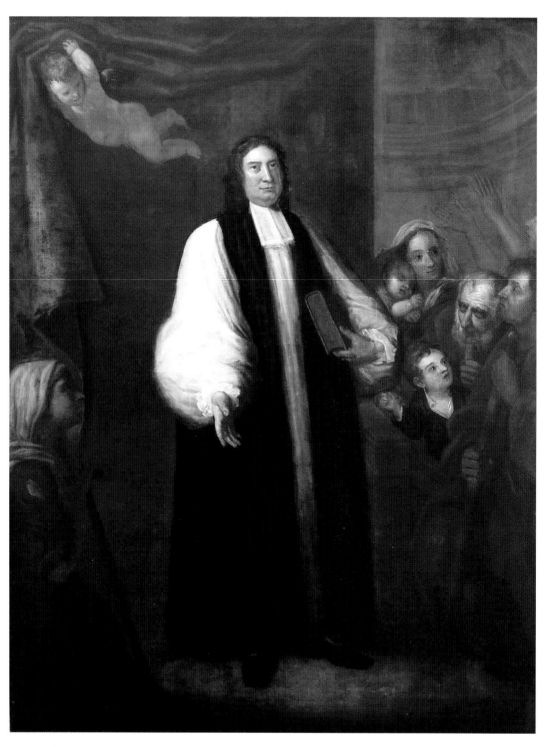

2.7 Hugh Boulter, archbishop of Dublin, by Francis Bindon. Reproduced with permission of the Board of Trinity College, the University of Dublin.

when the whole system was reorganized. The governors cut back on the admission of adult beggars to the Foundling Hospital and Workhouse in 1755 in an attempt to create more space for the children. This action brought a strong response from the merchants of Dublin, who claimed that there were, as a result, so many beggars on the street that it was a scandal 'in the eyes of all foreigners and strangers'.[39] However, the standards within the institution seemed to have been even more scandalous, and in 1758 a parliamentary committee of inquiry was established to investigate them.

Evidence of neglect

At a time when infant mortality was extremely high among the poor right across Europe, infants admitted to foundling hospitals had a mortality rate about twice as high as those cared for at home. In the foundling hospital in Florence, between 1755 and 1773, over 15,000 babies were admitted and two-thirds died before reaching their second year. It is estimated that 80 per cent of children sent to the Hôpital des Enfants Trouvés in Paris died en route or within three months of admission.[40] The infant mortality rate was also very high within the Foundling Hospital in Dublin. Between the years 1750 and 1760, 3,797 infants died, out of a total of 7,781 admitted. The governors claimed that the death rate was so high because many of the infants were moribund on admission, and that others died from diseases such as measles, smallpox and scrofula. The infants were buried inside the north wall of the Foundling Hospital fronting James's Street.[41] Sometimes six to eight children were buried at a time by placing them in a hole and then covering them with lime.[42] The chaplain, Revd Hill, read the funeral service from the safe distance of the main gate so that he would not be at risk of any infection.

Two physicians, Knox and Blackhall, and a surgeon named Stone, together with two surgeon apprentices, Morris and Fitzgerald, were on the staff of the Foundling Hospital and Workhouse in 1758, when the parliamentary committee of inquiry into the state and management of the institution took place.[43] The committee was informed by Blackhall that wet nurses had to care for as many as four or five infants at a time. Blackhall claimed that many of the infants were suffering from venereal disease and were dying because they were too ill to be breastfed or because there were not enough nurses to feed them. The matron of the hospital was under instructions to examine all children on admission, and if they were 'sound', to give them 'to the nurse that had least in number, to be washed in warm water if needful'. The children who were considered 'unsound' were to be kept apart and fed with a spoon until examined by the surgeon, who then decided which infants were to be sent to the infirmary.[44] Blackhall told the inquiry that the infirmary was overcrowded and that he had 'attended four children in the same bed all ill at the time with fevers'.[45] Sixty children were found lying in miserable conditions in the infirmary and were being looked after by two elderly women.[46] At the time of the inquiry the institution was under the control of the treasurer, Joseph Pursell, assisted by the butler, John Faucey.

Under Pursell's management, the children congregated in the cold hall in the winter and fires were only lit at Christmas or on an occasional Sunday. Most were barefoot and wore flimsy clothes. The hands of the children were swollen because of the cold, and many had sores. The building was also in bad repair – there was no glass in the windows of the children's dormitories and there were some holes in the roof. Children were malnourished and those who complained were treated harshly. A number of older boys who attempted to complain to the governors were given twenty lashes each and placed in the stocks. Children were also confined to the bedlam for running away. A contemporary described the bedlam as being so nauseous, dirty and wet that the physicians refused to enter it.[47] The inquiry found that Pursell was equally cruel to the adult inmates. On one occasion he kicked a mentally disturbed woman in the abdomen because she was throwing stones in the garden. She subsequently died from her injuries. Servants who objected to Pursell's regime or displeased him in any way were also liable to receive very harsh treatment and to be locked up with the inmates of the bedlam. The housekeeper, Mary Whistler, was Pursell's sister and this strengthened his control over the institution. The governors also bore a large responsibility for the ill-treatment of the children. Their meetings were infrequent and it was often difficult to get a quorum of five governors.

As a result of the findings of the committee of inquiry, Pursell, Faucey and Whistler were dismissed in 1758. After Pursell's dismissal it was discovered that he had embezzled well over £2,000 of the hospital's funds.[48] The committee of inquiry made several recommendations to improve the running of the Foundling Hospital, including the appointment of more suitable wet nurses. It also recommended that the hospital buildings should be improved and that the management of the Foundling Hospital should be separated from that of the Workhouse.

Scenes of wretchedness

Conditions in the eighteenth century were extremely harsh for the many people living in poverty. The statistician and philanthropist, Revd James Whitelaw, described the conditions of the poor in the Liberties of Dublin in the eighteenth century:

> The streets [in this part of the city] are generally narrow; the houses crowded together; the rears or back-yards of very small extent, and some without accommodation of any kind. Of these streets, a few are the residence of the upper class of shopkeepers or others engaged in trade; but a far greater proportion of them, with their numerous lanes and alleys, are occupied by working manufacturers, by petty shopkeepers, the labouring poor, and beggars, crowded together to a degree distressing to humanity. A single apartment in one of these truly wretched habitations, rates from one to two shillings per week, and to lighten this rent two, three, or even four families become joint tenants. As I was usually out at very early hours

on the survey I have frequently surprised from ten to sixteen persons, of all ages and sexes, in a room not 15 feet square, stretched on a wad of filthy straw, swarming with vermin, and without any covering, save the wretched rags that constituted their wearing apparel ...[49]

At this time the poor were regarded as inferior and it was a common belief that they were poor either through the will of God or because of their own lack of effort.[50]

The importation of children

The number of children admitted annually to the hospital rose dramatically in the mid eighteenth century, increasing from 274 in 1752 to over 1,000 in 1757, and it remained at an annual average of 870 for the following decade.[51] The governors appealed for extra support from the house of commons and they received £4,252. In their submission they claimed that military campaigns were in part responsible for the increased numbers, as children of soldiers fighting in North America, India and in the West Indies were being admitted in large numbers to the institution.[52]

Admission numbers were inflated by the number of illegitimate children being sent across the Irish sea to Dublin, mainly from Wales and the west of England.[53] It was reported that some women were making a living by bringing children across in the boats at two guineas per child. A writer in the *Freeman's Journal* commented, 'Our masters on the other side of the water are not satisfied at the vast sums drawn from this poor kingdom but are resolved that we should maintain their illegitimate offspring as well as their whores.'[54] This practice became so common that it was given statutory recognition by an act of 1772.[55] The resultant growth in admissions led to financial difficulties and the governors had to appeal for donations. In response George III sent £1,000 from his 'private purse'.

New buildings

The rise in numbers led to a period of expansion at the Foundling Hospital and Work-house in the latter half of the eighteenth century, and four new buildings were erected. A two-storey linen factory was built along the western perimeter on a north-south axis backing onto Cut Throat Lane. A long, narrow dormitory range was erected on an east-west axis, replacing the bedlam and enclosing the courtyard behind the dining hall of the Foundling Hospital and Workhouse. A chapel was built in 1764 behind this range on the same axis, with a hemispherical vault above the sanctuary at its eastern end. A fine three-storey Georgian building was erected north of the linen factory to serve as an infirmary. This Georgian building and the linen factory have survived and are now listed as protected structures.

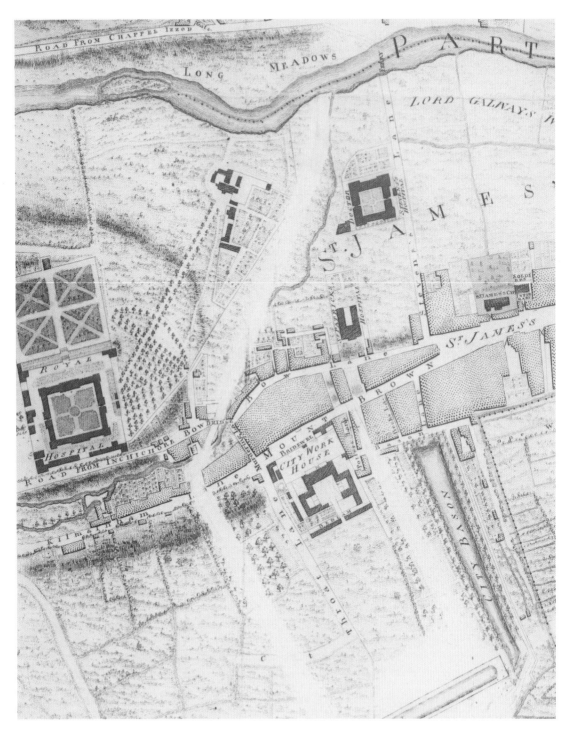

2.8   Section of a map of Dublin in 1756, showing the Foundling Hospital and City Workhouse, with adjacent Cut Throat Lane and Murdering Lane. The Royal Hospital Kilmainham, St Patrick's Hospital and Dr Steevens' Hospital are also shown. Reproduced from John Rocque, *An exact survey of the city and the suburbs of Dublin* (London, 1756).

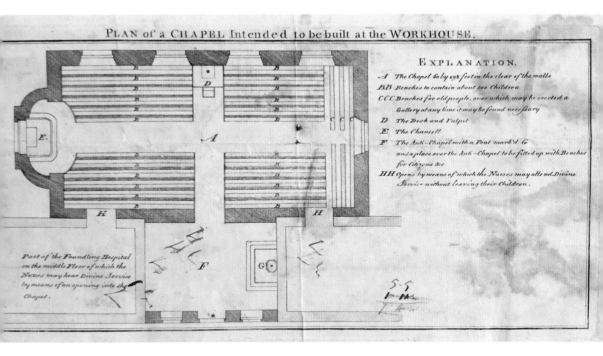

2.9   Plan for the chapel built in 1764. Reproduced from the RIAI Murray Collection with permission of the Irish Architectural Archive.

The voluntary hospital movement

During the eighteenth century, Dublin began to develop as a city and there was increased political stability. Prominent individuals began to show concern for the sick poor and as a consequence a strong voluntary hospital tradition developed. It led to the foundation of hospitals such as the Charitable Infirmary, Jervis Street (1718), Dr Steevens' Hospital (1733), Mercer's Hospital (1734), the Royal Hospital for Incurables (1744), the Rotunda Lying-in Hospital (1745), St Patrick's Mental Hospital (1746) and the Meath Hospital (1753). After its foundation, the Foundling Hospital and Workhouse did not attract the attention of philanthropic individuals until well into the eighteenth century. Robins, in his book, *The lost children*, cites a number of reasons for this, including the attitude of society at that time towards illegitimate children and the belief that the Foundling Hospital and Workhouse, being a public institution, was staffed by individuals who were lacking in compassion.[56] Robins also mentions the religious proselytism of the Foundling Hospital and Workhouse, which was notably absent in the voluntary hospital system of the period. However, the shocking reports in the late 1750s, detailing appalling standards of care, prompted one of the most influential women of the time, Lady Arbella Denny, to take a direct interest in the affairs of the Foundling Hospital.

A N

INTRODUCTION

To the READING of the

HOLY BIBLE,

Compoſed for the USE of the

Foundling-Hoſpital in Dublin,

AND THE

Charter Schools of Ireland,

And offered as

A PRESENT to Them.

D U B L I N:

Printed by and for S. POWELL and SON,
in *Dame-Street,* oppoſite *Fownes's-Street,*

MDCCLXV.

2.10   Title page of *An introduction to the reading of the Holy Bible, composed for the use of the Foundling Hospital in Dublin and the charter schools of Ireland* (Dublin, 1765), which was published anonymously 'to guard our young people against the pains that may be taken by the popish clergy to convert them to their faith'.

Lady Arbella Denny

Lady Arbella Denny was the second daughter of Thomas Fitzmaurice, 21st lord of Kerry. The Fitzmaurice family was one of the oldest of the Norman families that came to Ireland with Strongbow, and owned 100,000 acres in Kerry. Her mother, Ann, was the daughter of the famous physician, Sir William Petty, who had come to Ireland as physician in Cromwell's army. Petty was responsible for the Down Survey of confiscated land in 1654, and he acquired an estate of 50,000 acres in Kerry. Arbella was

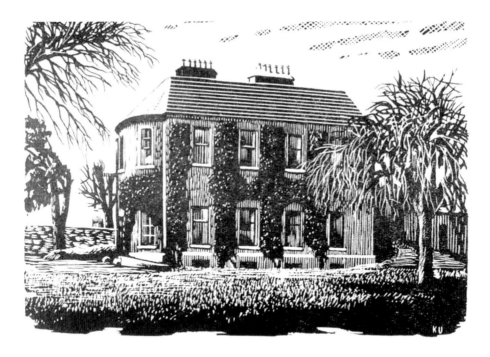

2.11 Peafield Cliff (now Lios-an-Uisce), the residence of Lady Arbella Denny on Rock Road, Blackrock. Frontispiece of *Lios-an-Uisce* by Mary Pat O'Malley (Dublin, 1981).

born in 1707 and grew up at Lixnaw, the family estate near Listowel. In 1725, Arbella married Arthur Denny of Tralee Castle. Arthur represented Kerry in the Irish parliament and the couple spent much of the year in Dublin.

When her father became Viscount Clanmaurice and the 1st earl of Kerry in 1722, he acquired Kerry House, an imposing property on St Stephen's Green in Dublin that stood on the site now occupied by the Shelbourne Hotel. After her husband's death in 1742 Arbella lived in Kerry House with her brother's family for three years. She acquired a fine house on the corner of St Stephen's Green and Dawson Street in 1745 and nine years later she purchased Peafield Cliff (now Lios-an-Uisce), a house on the seafront at Blackrock. She devoted much of her time to the education of her nephew William Fitzmaurice. According to Wodsworth, Arbella was:

> singularly free (and especially in those times), from sectarian religious bigotry, her ladyship was bigoted only where abuses were to be reformed and improvements introduced; when she brooked no delays, shortcomings, or interference.
>
> She was one of those personages capable of influencing for good all with whom she came in contact; having a remarkable capacity for comprehending great principles and attending at the same time to matters of minute detail and management.[57]

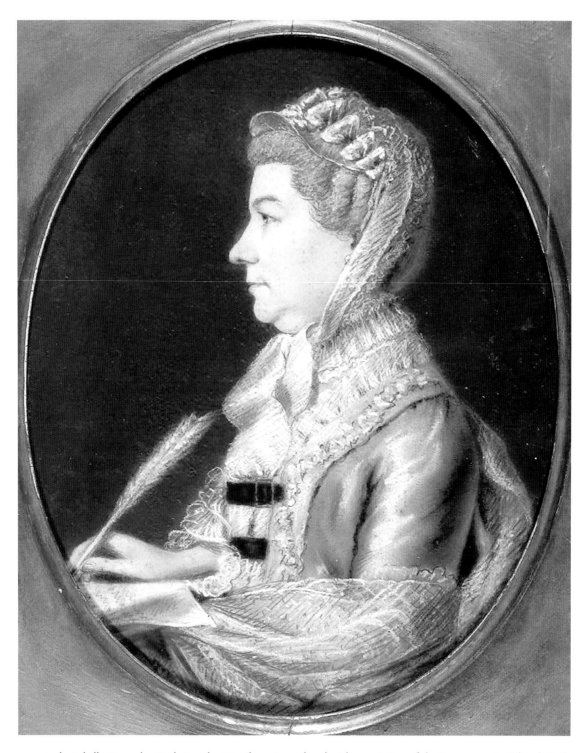

2.12 Lady Arbella Denny by Hugh Douglas Hamilton. Reproduced with permission of the Representative Church Body Library.

Her work for the Foundling Hospital

Lady Arbella began to visit the Foundling Hospital and Workhouse in 1759 and she encouraged ladies of similar rank to become involved. The enthusiasm of many of these ladies soon waned but Arbella became deeply committed to the reform of the institution. Her work was complemented by the work of two physicians attached to the hospital at that time. In a petition to the house of commons in 1763 for arrears of remuneration, the physicians Edmund Blackhall and Clement Archer pointed out that the death rate had fallen considerably between 1757 and 1761 and that this was in no small measure due to their efforts.[58]

Throughout the eighteenth century, sermons were organized in Dublin churches to raise support for a specific charity or charities and they were attended by members of the nobility, the professions and wealthy Dubliners.[59] It was important to have a good and well-known preacher to fill the church, and the congregation was expected to contribute generously. The Foundling Hospital was a beneficiary of these sermons, which were held on a chosen day every year. In 1760, Sunday 27 April was the day chosen to support the 'orphans in the Foundling Hospital'. William Henry, who was both a doctor of divinity and a fellow of the Royal Society, delivered the sermon in the parish church of St Michael. The sermon was subsequently published under the title *The cries of the orphans*, and it was dedicated to Lady Arbella, the protectress of the orphans, whom the preacher praised fulsomely:

> Your ladyship has the great honour and comfort to maintain the cause of pure Christianity, even in the midst of a thoughtless generation; and both by your conversation, and uniform example, to render it amiable: and almost restore religion to be fashionable, among persons of high rank.[60]

Lady Arbella gave generously from her own resources and because of the level of her commitment to the hospital she also received support from wealthy friends and admirers. The *Freeman's Journal* announced in 1766 that the countess of Hertford had given Lady Arbella £50 for the Foundling Hospital.[61] In May 1769, a notice appeared in the same journal stating that Lady Arbella had received 'from a lady who desires to be concealed, twenty pounds ... for the use of the Foundling Hospital'.[62] Such donations

THE

Cries of the Orphans.

A

SERMON

PREACHED

In the Parish CHURCH

OF

St. MICHAEL,

On SUNDAY *April* 27th.

Being the Day appointed for a General Collection throughout all the Churches in *Dublin*, for the Support of the ORPHANS in the FOUNDLING HOSPITAL.

BY

WILLIAM HENRY, D. D. F. R. S.

DUBLIN:

Printed by S. POWELL, in *Crane-lane*,

MDCCLX.

2.13 Title page of *The cries of the orphans* by William Henry (Dublin, 1760).

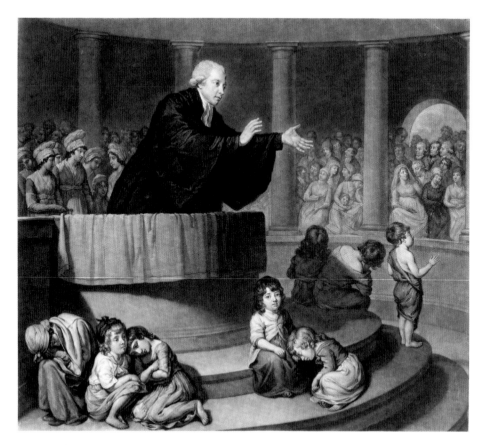

2.14 *Revd Dean Kirwan Pleading the Cause of the Destitute Orphans* by Hugh Douglas Hamilton.
Reproduced with permission of the National Gallery of Ireland.

were worth a considerable amount of money at that time and no doubt the announce-
ments in the press were calculated to encourage others to do the same. Lady Arbella's
work in the Foundling Hospital was not confined to patronage, as she became directly
involved in the day-to-day affairs of the institution. She personally engaged the wet
nurses who cared for babies at home and who were paid at the end of the year when
they brought the infants to the hospital for inspection. Her niece and companion,
Catherine Fitzmaurice, invented 'a most useful bottle, resembling a human breast'
for infants where a wet nurse was not available.[63] Arbella had an organ erected in
the chapel of the Foundling Hospital and she had a special clock made by Alexander
Gordon of Temple Bar, which was placed in the nursery of the hospital.[64] An inscription on the clock explained her reason for donating it:

> For the benefit of infants protected by this hospital Lady Arbella presents this
> clock, to mark, that as children reared by the spoon must have but a small quan-

tity of food at a time, it must be offered frequently; for which purpose this clock strikes every twenty minutes, at which notice all the infants that are not asleep must be discretely fed.

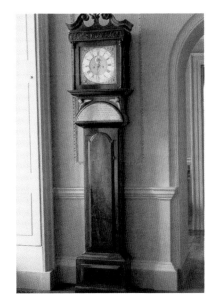

2.15   The clock presented by Lady Arbella Denny to the Foundling Hospital in 1760. Private collection.

The clock was purchased by Lord Iveagh in 1829 and is still in the possession of the Guinness family. The 'suck nurses' were instructed that one of them should 'sit up every night to waken any nurse whose child cries in the night and to take their turns daily to wash the clouts for the whole nursery'.[65]

The ordinary people of Dublin were also becoming aware of the compassion shown by Lady Arbella for foundling children. In October 1765, a baby boy was found abandoned in the hall of a house in Back Lane. He was taken by the parish beadle of St Nicholas Within to the Foundling Hospital, where the following note was found on his clothing:

> Frederick Gustavus Johnston is this child's name and the cruelty of fortune causes this desolation upon his infancy.
> Let innocent maids take care
> And not let perjured men their hearts ensnare,
> To Lady Arbella Denny
> Whom God preserve.[66]

The children in the Foundling Hospital were taught reading, writing and arithmetic, and there was a special emphasis on religious teaching. In 1765, a book was written to provide an introduction to the Bible for the children of the Foundling Hospital and the charity schools of Ireland. The master or mistress would read a story to the children 'by way of amusement' when they were involved in any practical work. The last two chapters were dedicated to teaching the children about the 'absurd' beliefs and errors of the Roman Catholics.[67]

Lady Arbella encouraged the female children to acquire skills such as knitting, lace making and spinning cotton and flax, so that they would be able to support themselves when they left the hospital. The boys became proficient at spinning worsted.[68] She presented gloves knitted by the children to her friend Queen Charlotte, wife of King George III, and encouraged her aristocratic relatives and friends to purchase lace and gloves.[69] Lady Arbella also took relations and friends to visit the Foundling

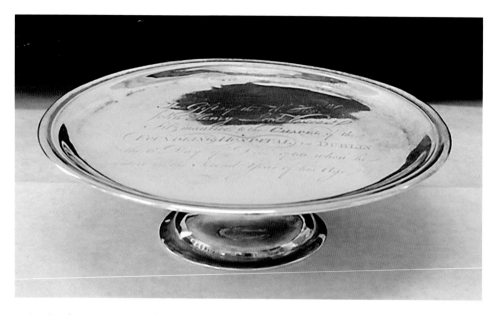

2.16   The silver paten presented to the chapel of the Foundling Hospital by William. Fitzmaurice, earl of Shelburne, in 1766. Reproduced with permission of the Dublin County Council/Civic Museum collection.

Hospital so that they would see the reforms that she had implemented. In this way she hoped to gain their empathy and support for the children. Arbella was particularly close to her nephew, William Fitzmaurice, the earl of Shelburne, later marquess of Lansdowne and prime minister of England. He visited Dublin and donated an Irish Georgian silver paten to the chapel of the Foundling Hospital in 1766 to mark the birth of his son, John Henry, whose name is inscribed on the paten. Four years later Fitzmaurice visited Dublin again to inspect his Irish estates. He was accompanied by his wife Sofia, and John Henry. Lady Arbella took Sofia and her son to visit the Foundling Hospital. At the time, there were 886 children in the hospital, most of whom were waiting to be fostered out. Sophia recorded her impressions in her diary, noting that the children 'were all healthy, well clad and served with great regularity', and that they 'were learning crafts such as spinning, knitting and lace making, as well as being taught to read'. Arbella presented Sophia's son with 'a child's library, a catechism, a map of Ireland and a writing set, devised by her in conjunction with Dr Thompson, one of the guardians, for use by the foundling children'.[70]

On parade

The children were provided with Windsor uniforms that were blue with red collars and cuffs. The boys wore cloth jackets and knickerbockers and the girls wore a woollen outer garment with a plaited bodice and full skirt. The children wore these uniforms when they marched from time to time to Dublin Castle for inspection by the lord lieutenant and his wife. In 1764 the earl of Northumberland and his wife viewed 200 children from the front window of the castle and they ordered that each child should receive 'a new schilling of his present majesty's coin'.[71] The earl and countess of Hertford responded in a similar fashion when they reviewed the children two years later. These parades raised badly needed funds for the maintenance of the children. The children were also marched to the Mansion House twice a year. On these occasions the streets were lined by soldiers to protect the Protestant boys and girls from insult or molestation.

In 1767, the Dublin Society, later known as the Royal Dublin Society (RDS), voted that £34 2s. 6d. should be donated to Lady Arbella to be given as awards to the most deserving children in the Foundling Hospital who make bone (bobbin) lace 'in such a manner as will in her Ladyship's opinion be conducive to the improvement of the manufacture'.[72] This gift was repeated in 1768 and 1769. Lady Arbella recognized that many of the children in the Foundling Hospital were abandoned because their parents did not have the means to support them. She realized the importance of providing jobs and she worked with the Dublin Society to encourage Irish industry. Her name is recorded frequently in the minutes, and in 1766 she was unanimously elected the first honorary member of the society. It would be over 150 years before another woman was elected a member. Lady Arbella Denny continued her involvement in the administration of the Foundling Hospital until 1778 when she was over 70 years old. During that time the mortality within the institution fell to less than 25 per cent of the admissions: over a ten-year period 8,726 infants were admitted and 1,990 died. Lady Arbella enlarged and improved the buildings of the Foundling Hospital and spent over £4,000 on the institution, derived mainly from her own and her friends' resources. She also took an active part in helping Protestant 'fallen women' and prostitutes, and she established the Magdalen Asylum in Leeson Street, where they were given accommodation, food, clothes and religious instruction. The asylum also provided training in a skill so that the women would become economically independent when they left.[73]

The freedom of the guild of merchants of the city of Dublin was conferred on Lady Arbella in 1765 'as a mark of their esteem for her ladyship, for her many great charities and constant care of the poor foundling children in the City Workhouse'.[74] The presentation was enclosed in a silver casket, an honour reserved for people of the highest rank.[75] Lady Arbella Denny was the first woman to have her achievements acknowledged in this way. In 1770 she left the country for a short period and when she returned the governors asked her to resume her involvement with the Foundling Hospital. Although she continued to take an interest until her death in 1792, Lady Arbella did not play an active part in the administration of the institution and, despite the lessons learned, as soon as she withdrew, the infant mortality rate began to rise and management deteriorated. As a result of mismanagement, by 1788, a decade after Lady Arbella Denny's retirement, the Foundling Hospital had a debt of almost £10,000.[76]

3

The Foundling Hospital

A void in the heart ... aching to be filled.[1]

In 1768, Richard Woodward, dean of Clogher, published *An argument of the right of the poor in this kingdom to a national pension.* Woodward put forward three propositions:

1. That the poor are so inadequately provided for by voluntary contributions in Ireland that they should be given a legal title to maintenance;
2. That it is the duty of the rich to provide a competent maintenance for the poor;
3. That it is in the interests of the Commonwealth that this duty be discharged.[2]

This document was the first proposal to advocate national provision for the Irish poor, although it had been the right of the English poor for 167 years.[3] An act of the Irish parliament in 1772 decreed that the governors of the Foundling Hospital and Workhouse were no longer to keep children and beggars in the same institution and that they were to source accommodation for the beggars elsewhere.[4] In the same year, legislation was passed providing for the establishment of houses of industry in every county in Ireland, but this was not followed through and institutions were only established in Dublin, Cork, Waterford and Limerick. Their purpose was to provide accommodation for beggars and paupers. The house of industry in Dublin was opened in 1773 in Channel Row, North Brunswick Street. From then on, beggars and paupers were admitted to it rather than to the Foundling Hospital and Workhouse, and the name of the latter institution was shortened to the Foundling Hospital.

New governance

The 1772 act relating to the Foundling Hospital set up a new corporation to govern the institution, with a board consisting of nearly 300 of the leading church and lay men in Ireland, including the lord lieutenant, the lord primate, the lord chancellor, the lord archbishop of Dublin, the speaker of the house of commons, the chancellor of the exchequer, the secretary of state, the lord chief justice and the attorney general. The state physician and the state surgeon were also on the board, as well as several other leading ecclesiastical and civil dignitaries from around the country. Fifteen governors were to be elected every year to act as a court of assistants to ensure that all the laws and rules passed by the governors were put into effect.[5] The change in governance made little difference. Few of the new governors took any interest in the institution, and in 1791 it was revealed in the Irish house of commons that the board's authority had been delegated to the treasurer, who had been bed-ridden for six years.[6]

Regulation of the hackney trade

The Foundling Hospital was to be supported by a tax on property of 6 pence in the pound per annum and an additional 6 pence in the pound for houses 'where beer, spirituous liquors etc. are sold'.[7] The hospital was also to be supported by taxes on coaches, carriages, carts, hearses, hackney cars and sedan chairs. In effect, the act made the governors the regulators of the transport trade, and they were given powers to license and set standards for the owners of coaches, carriages and other forms of transport.[8] The governors also had powers to regulate fares, and they published charts showing the tariffs for journeys from the city centre to locations on the outskirts. Carriages without licences could be seized and held in the Foundling Hospital.[9]

From 1775, only infants under the age of 12 months were to be admitted to the Foundling Hospital.[10] The children were to be raised as Protestants and from this period they wore a badge on their clothing with a seal representing a female with a distaff, symbolising industry, and with the motto 'The diligent hand maketh rich.'[11] The number of children returning to the institution from the homes of their country nurses was beginning to rise. In 1791, the Foundling Hospital was responsible for the welfare of 5,347 children, of whom 4,816 were with nurses in the country.[12]

The English Quaker and reformer John Howard visited the Foundling Hospital in

3.1   The logo of the Foundling Hospital, depicting a girl holding a distaff for spinning. From the title page of W.D. Wodsworth, *A history of the ancient Foundling Hospital of Dublin from the year 1702* (Dublin, 1876).

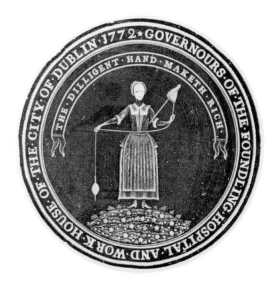

1787 and 1788 and was favourably impressed, describing it as 'a noble institution, if there was more attention to cleanliness and order'. He attributed the latter to 'the loss of Lady Arabella [*sic*] Denny's visits'. Howard recorded that he saw 'many fine children and the girls were neatly clothed but several had eruptions on their hands'. There were fifty-six children in the infirmaries. 'Soap is not allowed here, though absolutely necessary for washing the hands of children, whose parents, being of the lowest class, are in the city generally deficient in cleanliness, and have a tendency to scrophulous disorders.'[13]

The transport of infants from around Ireland

In response to the rising numbers of children cared for in the hospital, the governors appealed to the clergy throughout the country to have deserted children supported locally until they were deemed strong enough to travel. Their appeal fell on deaf ears, and thousands of newborn infants continued to be brought to the Foundling Hospital from all over the country by 'foundling carriers'. These infants were carried in jolting, springless carts, or in a basket or sack on the backs of the carriers. Some of the infants were provided with clothing suitable for the journey to the Foundling Hospital but often the clothing was stolen or sold on the way. The foundling carriers were usually hardened women of ill repute. The writer William Carleton described an encounter with one of these women in his autobiography. He met her when they were both making a pilgrimage to Lough Derg. They stayed in the evening at the same lodgings. Carleton said that he slept soundly but that when he awoke the following morning some of his clothes and all of his money were missing. He later discovered that:

> this woman was notorious throughout most of Ulster and as I discovered afterwards she had been one of those well-known characters who were engaged in carrying illegitimate children up to the Foundling Hospital in Dublin ... she was subsequently prosecuted for robbing a carman and transported.[14]

It was suspected that some babies were either killed or allowed to die, thus saving the carriers the bother of a long journey. The carriers also pocketed the admission fees for the Foundling Hospital that were entrusted to them. In 1818, George Speight, a clergyman in Cavan, wrote to the Foundling Hospital expressing his fears for an infant whom he had sent to the hospital:

> I beg leave to inform you that on the 18th of last month I sent from this town to the Foundling Hospital by a woman whose name is Mary Lawden, a male infant baptized by the name of Wm. Burrowes, and as no account has been received by me of this child's arrival in Dublin, I am induced to suspect that the carrier has been guilty of some foul play towards it. I therefore request you will have the goodness to inform me as soon as possible whether or not this child has been received at the hospital.[15]

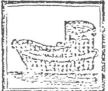

D U B L I N   FOUNDLINGS.

RECEIVED by the Hands of *Alice Muckleboy*
a *Male*   Infant, from the Parifh of *Ahaderg C. of Down*
and admitted into the Foundling-Hofpital, belonging to the Work-Houfe of the
City of Dublin, this   Day of *October 1762*
with the following Clothing, viz.   Biggins ———— Forehead-Cloaths   Caps /
   Shirts /   Waftcoats ————Rockets ——— Clouts ————Flannel / —
   Pilches ————Swathes ————Ribbons —— Bibs ————Frocks ——
   Petticoats. /
                        Tho.ͤ Annefley Porter.

3.2   A receipt signed by the porter and given to an Alice Muckleboy when she delivered an infant boy
to the Foundling Hospital from the parish of Aghaderg in County Down. From J. Sands, 'Pre-Famine
poverty in the parish of Aghaderg', *Before I Forget*, 3 (1989).

Up to ten infants could be carried on a single journey in a kish or creel. The mortality during transit was very high, and many died before or soon after admission to the hospital. William Wodsworth copied 'observations' from the original admissions registry that show clearly why such a small number of infants transported to the Foundling Hospital survived the journey:

- 'This child was injured in carriage' (a frequent entry).
- 'This child is "black"' (frequently).
- 'Died on coming into the house' (often occurs).
- 'These children were brought into the hospital, dying, by the women who were formerly accused of murder.'
- 'Piteous. This child much abused in carriage.'
- 'This child had its arm fractured.'[16]

Rather than consign their infants to this mode of transport, mothers frequently walked more than 100 miles to bring their children to the Foundling Hospital. Comparison of the mortality rates of infants who were brought to the Foundling Hospital from a distance greater than 50 miles compared to those admitted from Dublin city and county revealed a higher mortality in the former.[17] Most of the children brought to the hospital from outside Dublin came from northern counties. In the first decade of the nineteenth century 7,432 babies were admitted to the Foundling Hospital from Dublin city and county, 1,828 from Co. Down, 1,432 from Co. Tyrone, 1,099 from Co. Antrim and 1,057 from Co. Armagh. The numbers were much lower for the southern counties, and Limerick was the only southern county to have a figure (1,167) similar to the northern counties.[18] A number of reasons have been postulated for these low figures, but there can be little doubt that the fear of Catholic mothers that their children might be brought up as Protestants was a major factor.

Surgeons

John Halahan and Philip Woodroffe were surgeons to the Foundling Hospital in the last quarter of the eighteenth century. Halahan was born in Cork in 1753 and was appointed assistant master of the Rotunda Hospital when he was 23 years of age. He was one of the founders, in 1784, of the Royal College of Surgeons in Ireland (RCSI), originally known as the Society of Surgeons. He was a co-founder of the Dublin General Dispensary in Temple Bar in 1785, and he held the chairs of anatomy and midwifery in the RCSI. He was elected to the chair of surgery in 1799 and held this post until his retirement in 1804. He was also professor of anatomy to the Hibernian Society of Artists.

Woodroffe was a barber-surgeon who was appointed assistant surgeon to Dr Steevens' Hospital in 1763. Two years later he was appointed resident surgeon, and he held this post until his death. He was also surgeon to the House of Industry Hospitals and the Hospital for Incurables. He was a founder of the RCSI, and in 1788 he was elected president of the college.

The reforms of Sir John Blaquiere

Despite the general indifference of society, one individual was stirred into action by the situation in the Foundling Hospital. Sir John Blaquiere (later Lord de Blaquiere), the son of an émigré Huguenot bookseller in London, had come to Ireland in 1772 to serve as chief secretary for Ireland when Lord Harcourt was appointed the lord lieutenant. Following the departure of Lord Harcourt in 1777, Blaquiere remained in Ireland to pursue a political career serving in the Irish house of commons for twenty-eight years. He was director of public works in Dublin. In 1791, Blaquiere proposed to the Irish house of commons that the existing laws governing the Foundling Hospital should be changed. He suggested that the number of governors should be reduced to nineteen and that they should have much greater powers. Under the act that had set up the original institution in 1703, the members of Dublin Corporation had been made perpetual governors. They responded angrily to the new bill, and they were supported by a number of influential people, including the Irish politician and patriot Henry Grattan. Blaquiere countered by emphasizing the apathy

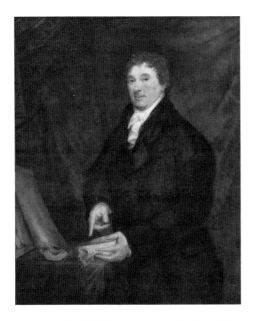

3.3   John Halahan, surgeon to the Foundling Hospital, by Hugh Douglas Hamilton. Photograph: David H. Davison. Reproduced with permission of the Royal College of Surgeons in Ireland.

3.4   John, lord de Blaquiere, by Charles Turner after John James Masquerier. Reproduced by permission of the National Portrait Gallery, London.

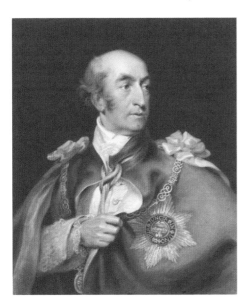

of previous governors and the high mortality within the institution. He pointed out that at six of the ten meetings of the governors during the previous year, only one member of Dublin Corporation had attended and that at three of the meetings there had been no representative from the corporation present. Blaquiere also stated that on one occasion, when 'a dirty little office' was to be filled, as many as fifteen aldermen had attended the meeting. An infuriated Grattan responded by claiming that Blaquiere's charges against the corporation 'did not lessen the city, they lessen him'. Other members claimed that he was exaggerating the state of the conditions in the hospital and that his statements were an 'unfounded libel upon the good name of the country'.[19] Although Blaquiere later withdrew his bill due to lack of support, he began to conduct his own personal investigations into the Foundling Hospital and subsequently brought his findings to the attention of members of the Irish house of commons. Blaquiere portrayed graphically how baskets full of infants were transported around the country and asked his fox-hunting friends whether they would transfer a litter of pups from one of their hunting hounds in such conditions. The house responded by setting up a committee of inquiry in 1792.

The 1792 committee of inquiry

The committee of inquiry began its proceedings by interviewing the staff of the hospital. The matron of the hospital, Alice Hunt, informed the committee that more infants might have survived on admission if there had been a sufficient number of wet nurses available to nurse them. However, the hospital could not recruit wet nurses because the wages were very low and the women were afraid of contracting venereal disease from the infants. Infants who were placed in the infirmary and who were not breastfed had virtually no chance of survival as the general mortality rate for infants who were fed by hand was in the region of 88 per cent. The surgeon, Philip Woodroffe, claimed that in the previous year 788 of the infants admitted to the institution had venereal disease and only one of them survived. He believed that the only way of preventing these deaths was to cure the parents.[20] The committee members found that there were such gross inconsistencies between the facts and figures supplied to them by the different officers of the Foundling Hospital that they could not reach firm conclusions, but decided to 'submit the whole of the said evidence, returns and accounts to the consideration of the house'.[21] Despite the distressing evidence described in the report, it evoked no response from parliament. However, the general public, who saw the children whenever they were marched to church services in the city, were beginning to express concern for their welfare. In 1796, the *Freeman's Journal* described how onlookers at St Thomas's church were horrified by the condition of the children and they vented their fury at the supervisor who rode a horse 'more like a negro-driver than one to take care of the children of charity'.[22]

Blaquiere persists

In 1797 Blaquiere broached the subject again in the Irish house of commons. He stated that he had visited the hospital and found fourteen infants left to die in an upper room.[23] He also claimed that there had been no improvement in the mortality rate within the institution or among children with nurses in the country. Parliament responded in its usual manner by setting up another committee. The committee investigated the period 1790 to 1796 at the hospital and found that there was a very high infant mortality rate. The majority of infants who died had been brought from distant parts of the country. The expectation at the hospital was that all babies sent to the infant infirmary would die.[24]

In the six years under investigation, the physician to the Foundling Hospital, William Harvey, had confined his attention to older children and had never visited the infant infirmary, as he did not consider it part of his duties. Harvey was considered a pillar of the establishment. He had studied medicine at Leiden and was appointed physician to Dr Steevens' Hospital in 1779 and physician general to the army in 1794. He was president of the College of Physicians of Ireland at the time of the inquiry and served in that role for six separate terms. He was elected president on two occasions after the inquiry (1800 and 1802), which suggests that the revelations relating to the Foundling Hospital did not damage his reputation or career.[25] Woodroffe visited twice a week, but he prescribed only for surgical problems. The apothecary to the hospital,

James Shaughnissy, visited the infant infirmary at most once a quarter, but often not even once a year. It was his duty to attend every day and his residence was in the hospital. Shaughnissy maintained that all the infants he sent to the infirmary were suffering from venereal disease. The hospital's returns revealed that 5,216 infants suffering from venereal disease were admitted to the infant infirmary between 1790 and 1796 and only three survived. Over the same six-year period there were 12,786 children admitted to the Foundling Hospital, 7,807 of whom died (61 per cent). This was a large increase on the mortality rate of the previous six years, when 12,566 children were admitted and 3,856 of them died (30 per cent).[26] The matron, Alice Hunt, again claimed that it was very difficult to get wet nurses from the country and also said that there was a great reluctance to take new children because of fear that they would not be paid because of 'the landing of the French', a reference to the French expeditionary forces sent to Ireland by Napoleon to support the United Irishmen. Once again, the poor condition of the infants on their arrival at the hospital was cited as the reason for the high mortality rate.[27] Catherine Maquean, a nurse in the infant infirmary, said that all the infants were given a bottle containing sleeping potion which, no doubt, hastened their deaths.[28]

The committee established a subcommittee to inspect the infant infirmary and they wrote a graphic and damning report:

> In the foundlings' infirmary, a black and gloomy apartment, were eighteen infants, lying three and four together in filthy cradles, and with covering, in the opinion of your committee, insufficient to preserve vital heat in the bodies of infants at an inclement season, and remote from fire. This infirmary exhibits a scene which must excite the most unfeeling to pity – there are only two women to attend this infirmary. Your committee made some observations on the miserable situation of those infants, and were informed by Mrs Hunt (the chief matron) by way of accounting for what your committee considered inhuman neglect – 'that those children were just laid there to die'.[29]

'Weak and prejudiced minds'

The response of the house of commons to the report of the committee was much more appropriate on this occasion. The committee found that there was neglect and demanded the resignation of the physician, surgeon and the resident apothecary. All three resigned and on the recommendation of the committee, Blaquiere introduced a bill for the reform of the hospital. The bill made rapid progress through the commons but it ran into difficulties in the house of lords as it had implications for the Dublin establishment. Most of the governors of the Foundling Hospital were leading figures in Dublin society. There was a major public outcry about the conditions in the Foundling Hospital and efforts were made to defend the governors. Henry Grattan was among those who spoke in defence of the governors in the house of commons. Blaquire responded that he was surprised 'that so eminent a person as Mr Grattan should have become the advocate of abuses which disgraced the society of men'.[30] The governors of the Foundling Hospital continued to argue that the children were so ill on admission that nothing could be done for them.[31]

In the face of this opposition the bill collapsed in the house of lords. One year later, following further complaints about the conditions within the Foundling Hospital, another bill was introduced to reform the institution. It was now proposed that the existing governors should be removed and that the hospital should be put under the control of a selected board for one year so that reform could be initiated. Although Dublin Corporation objected because the bill excluded its members from the board, it was passed quickly through both houses of parliament in 1798.[32] It was a victory for Blaquiere's determination to introduce major reform in the management of the Foundling Hospital. Curiously, Blaquiere was not perceived by his contemporaries as being a highly principled reformer. According to the historian Constantia Maxwell, Blaquiere, when chief secretary of state, entered into an 'unworthy intrigue' with John Hely-Hutchinson to have the latter appointed provost of Trinity College Dublin in 1774.[33] Blaquiere opposed Catholic relief and he was created 1st baron de Blaquiere in 1800 as a reward for his support of the Act of Union. Jonah Barrington, celebrated for his racy memoir, *Personal sketches of his own times*, has left us a vignette of Blaquiere:

> Sir John certainly was a pluralist, enjoying, at one time, the first, the middle, and the last pension on the Irish civil list. He was director of the public works in Dublin; and to his jobbing is that capital indebted for its wide streets, paving, lighting, and convenient fountains. He made as much as he could of these works, it is true; but every farthing he acquired in Ireland he expended in it. If his money came from the public purse, it was distributed to the public benefit: if he received pensions from the crown, butchers, bakers and other tradesmen pocketed every shilling of it. He knew employment to be the best species of charity.[34]

Committee of lady governesses

The new board of governors met for the first time on 12 June 1798 in the Foundling Hospital and not in the Tholsel, which previously had been the location for meetings. There were nine governors and one of them was a doctor named George Renny who was physician to the Royal Hospital Kilmainham. Renny took an active interest in the affairs of the Foundling Hospital. He was particularly focused on the plight of infants who were said to suffer from venereal diseases. Renny encouraged the new surgeon, John Creighton, to examine the infants on admission and to treat them according to the

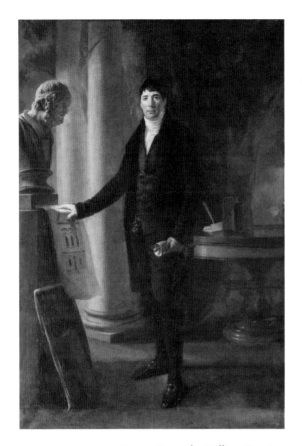

3.5   George Renny by William Cuming. Photograph: David H. Davison. Reproduced with permission of the Royal College of Surgeons in Ireland.

diagnosis in each individual case.[35] Creighton established that approximately one in fourteen of the children was infected with venereal disease. Up to this time, all kinds of eruptions on the skin of the children had been wrongly attributed to venereal disease and, because of this, a large number of children had been sent to the infirmary in error.[36] Creighton, who was born in Athlone, served as surgeon in the Foundling Hospital for thirty years. He lived in Merrion Square West, had a large private practice and attended the family of the duke of Wellington. He was professor of midwifery in the RCSI between 1794 and 1819 and was elected president of the college in 1812 and 1824.[37]

A committee of thirteen lady governesses was established, drawn largely from the aristocracy. They were given responsibility for the internal management of the hospital, which they took in rotation and they worked hard to improve the standards of care for the children. The governesses replaced the filthy cradles, which were 'alive with vermin', and dismissed those officers found wanting in carrying out their duties. The number of wet nurses was increased and a new diet was devised for the children. The 'special' diet recommended by the College of Physicians in 1775 was replaced with a diet 'with plenty of milk, bread, broth and vegetables but no beer'.[38] There was a significant improvement in the mortality rate of the children. In the year ending 1799 a total of 1,471 infants was admitted to the Foundling Hospital and 439 (or one in three) died before they could be boarded out to wet nurses in the country. The manner in which the infants arrived in the hospital was still a significant cause of death and was outside the control of the institution. The governors were very pleased with the work of the lady governesses and contrasted their conduct 'with the frivolous and irrational dissipation of the day'.[39] As a mark of their appreciation the governors ordered 'arm chairs with stuffed bottoms' for the comfort of the lady governesses when at the hospital.[40]

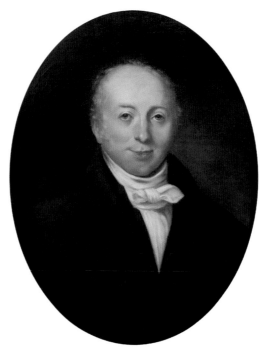

3.6   Abraham Colles, artist unknown. Reproduced by
permission of the Worth Library, Dublin.

Abraham Colles, surgical apprentice

The first record of medical training taking place on the site dates from this bleak period. The renowned surgeon Abraham Colles, who described Colles' fracture of the wrist, was apprenticed to the Foundling Hospital surgeon, Woodroffe, between 1790 and 1795. The medical historian Sir Charles Cameron wrote that Colles 'worked hard under his master at Steevens' and the Foundling Hospital – the latter having a good opportunity of becoming acquainted with the diseases of childhood ...'[41] The young Colles would have examined and treated children in the three-storey Georgian infirmary that still survives opposite the main entrance to the Trinity Centre for Health Sciences. Colles was appointed to the chair of anatomy and physiology and to the chair of surgery in the College of Surgeons in 1804. He was elected president of the college when he was 28 years old.

Inoculation against smallpox

Infectious diseases swept through the Foundling Hospital from time to time. For instance, the media reported in 1815 that 500 children had measles at the same time in the hospital and that almost all of them recovered.[42] Smallpox was a major cause of death and disfiguration in this period, and between 1661 and 1745 it accounted for 20 per cent of all deaths recorded in the Dublin bills of mortality. An English physician, Edward Jenner, who introduced vaccination against smallpox, had observed that milkmaids did not get the disease. He hypothesized that this was because they developed immunity to the smallpox virus from the cowpox they had contracted from cows. In 1796, Jenner vaccinated a young boy with scrapings taken from a cowpox lesion on the finger of a dairymaid in Gloucestershire. Cowpox was a harmless virus endemic among dairymaids. Two months later Jenner found that the boy was immune to smallpox despite his repeated attempts to infect the child by injection with the smallpox virus. Jenner published his observations in 1798.

John Creighton, surgeon to the Foundling Hospital, was among the first to introduce smallpox vaccination to Ireland in 1800, and in the same year he persuade the governors of the Foundling Hospital to establish, in Clarendon Street, the Dispensary for Infant Poor and Cow-Pock Inoculation.[43] Not all doctors shared Creighton's enthusiasm for the new technique and they claimed that any protection acquired from vaccination was temporary. This worried Creighton as he did not want parents to stop having their children vaccinated. In 1804, with the permission of the board of guardians, Creighton asked the surgeon general, George Stewart, to try to inject with smallpox nine children in the Foundling Hospital whom he had vaccinated. He had vaccinated the children between December 1800 and July 1801. None of the children developed smallpox. Despite this success, a vocal group led by a surgeon named William Goldson in Portsmouth opposed smallpox vaccination and continued to assert that the vaccination only gave protection for three years at the most. In order to refute these assertions Creighton and Stewart's experiment in the Foundling Hospital was repeated on the same nine children in 1809 together with ten others who had been vaccinated by Creighton between July 1801 and August 1802. Again, none of the children developed smallpox.[44] Two of Creighton's own children, John and Richard, were among the nineteen inoculated.[45] Creighton became an enthusiastic follower of Edward Jenner and his method of vaccination. The demand for inoculation became so great that Creighton in 1804 established the Cow-Pock Institution at 1 North Cope Street in Dublin. He worked there 'without fee or reward'. Over 12,000 patients were successfully vaccinated at the institution in the first five years of its existence. In a letter which Jenner wrote in 1809 he expressed his delight at the progress made in Dublin:

> It is with the greatest pleasure I perceive the rapid increase of vaccination in your metropolis, and the uninterrupted success that has attended the practice, at once a proof of zeal, industry and attention of the medical officers, for which I beg leave to make my most grateful acknowledgements.[46]

Creighton was succeeded as surgeon to the Foundling Hospital by his eldest son, John, who continued his father's work in the Cow-Pock Institution.

Additional buildings

A significant building phase began at the beginning of the nineteenth century, when Francis Johnston was employed as the architect. Johnston was born in 1760 in Armagh, where his father was an architect. He studied architecture and subsequently based his practice in Armagh before moving to Dublin in 1793. Johnston became one of Ireland's most distinguished architects, and the work on the Foundling Hospital was his first significant commission in Dublin.

In 1803, he remodelled the front of the original building, adding a crenellated parapet and a cupola to the dining hall, and changing the blind gables of the east and west ranges, giving the façade of the hospital a classical appearance. He rebuilt the mid-eighteenth-century dormitory range, known as the 'foundling range', adding a third floor in the process. He also designed a new three-storey children's infirmary, which survives and is currently known as Hospital 1. This was built immediately south of the foundling

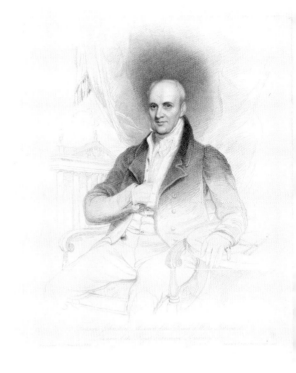

3.7   Francis Johnston, architect. Engraving by Henry Hoppner Meyer. Reproduced with permission of the National Portrait Gallery, London.

range and was finished in 1810. The wards faced south and commanded 'a cheerful view over a beautifully wooded and richly cultivated country, terminating in the Wicklow mountains'.[47] Johnston replaced the mid-eighteenth-century chapel with a new chapel, which had a north-south axis and was perpendicular to the foundling range.[48] The new chapel had a central aisle 70 feet long and 15 feet wide. The roof was supported by Gothic pillars that also supported galleries. There was a large Gothic window over the altar. Girls sat in the galleries of the church and boys sat below in the main aisle. Over the vestibule in the northern side of the church there was a special seat appropriated to the governors and governesses, and above this there was an upper gallery communicating with the nurseries for the use of the nurses and other female servants of the hospital.[49]

Additional accommodation was made available to provide space for the manufacture of camlet, flannel, baize and livery cloths and employed about 180 boys and girls.[50] The factory was very productive, with 15,624 yards of calico and 1,606 pairs of

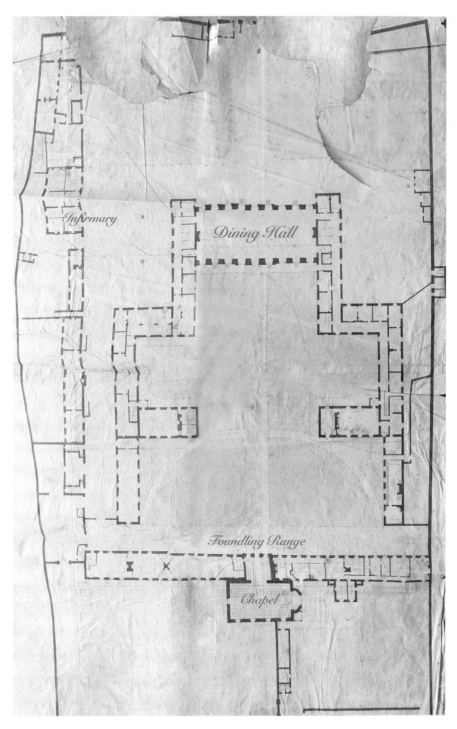

Infirmary

Dining Hall

Foundling Range

Chapel

3.8 Ground-floor plan of the Foundling Hospital as it was in 1803, showing the sizes and uses of the rooms before Johnston's alterations. Drawing from the office of Francis Johnston. Reproduced from the RIAI Murray Collection with permission of the Irish Architectural Archive.

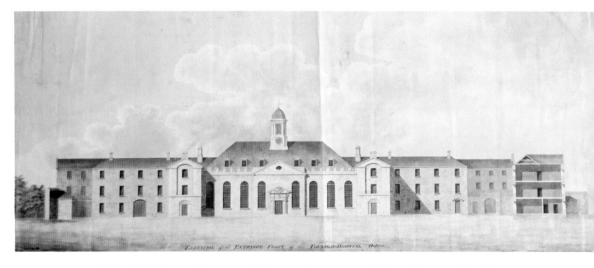

3.9   The façade of the Foundling Hospital, showing Johnston's remodelling of the original building. Reproduced from the RIAI Murray Collection with permission of the Irish Architectural Archive.

3.10   Proposed façade of the Foundling Hospital range (below), and with a flap lifted to reveal the mid-eighteenth-century dormitory range that it replaced (above). Reproduced from the RIAI Murray Collection with permission of the Irish Architectural Archive.

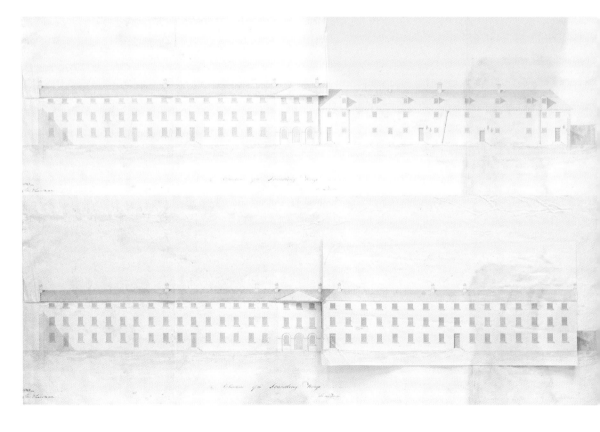

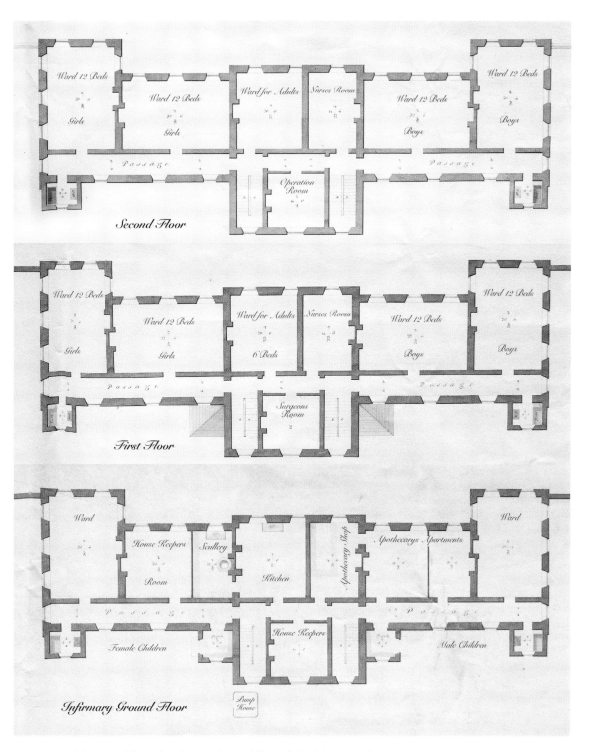

3.11   Plans of the ground floor, first floor and second floor of the children's infirmary (now Hospital 1). Reproduced from the RIAI Murray Collection with permission of the Irish Architectural Archive.

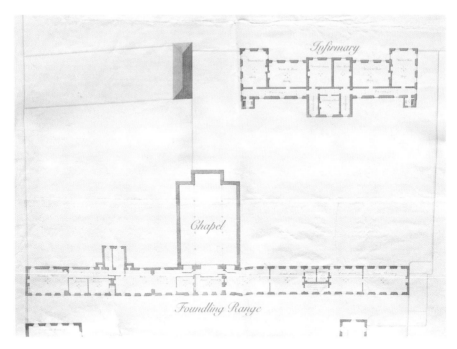

3.12 Plan of Foundling Hospital, showing the positions of the chapel and infirmary (now Hospital 1). Reproduced from the RIAI Murray Collection with permission of the Irish Architectural Archive.

3.13 The interior of Johnston's church in the 1950s not long before its demolition. Private collection.

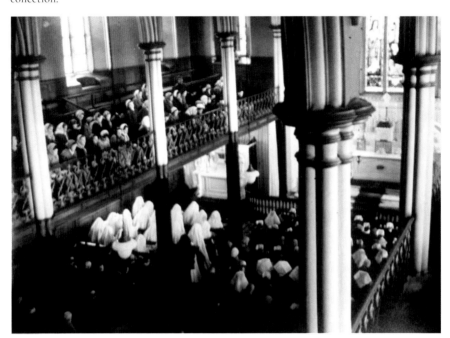

stockings being manufactured in one year.[51] Johnston went on to design the Chapel Royal and the Record Tower in Dublin Castle, Nelson's Pillar and the General Post Office in Sackville Street (O'Connell Street).[52]

Reform of spiritual care

The new governors did not limit their concerns to the physical well-being of the children, they also set out to reform their spiritual care. Towards the end of the eighteenth century some of the anti-Catholic laws in the country had been relaxed and there was increased religious tolerance. However, after the 1798 rebellion the atmosphere changed. The Protestant ruling class felt threatened, and this resulted in increased hostility towards Catholics. The Protestant evangelical movement was also beginning to shape public opinion and policies. The new governors formed the opinion that the children were spending too long with their Catholic nurses. They therefore decreed that the children were to be returned to the Foundling Hospital when they reached the age of 7 and they would then spend at least three years undergoing religious instruction in the Protestant faith.

Educational reforms in the hospital were led by the chaplain, Revd Henry Murray who, according to a report of the commissioner of the board of education in 1810, introduced many of the concepts of Alexander Bell and Joseph Lancaster, educational pioneers of the time. The method they advocated was known as the 'monitorial' system, and was based on the use of the brighter students to assist the teacher. Murray is described by Wright in his *Guide to Dublin* as a man 'whose abilities and general information are universally acknowledged, and who is deservedly esteemed as a theological writer'.[53] There were sixteen schools at the Foundling Hospital at this time, twelve for girls

3.14 Title page of Mrs Trimmer's *An abridgement of the New Testament*. Private Collection.

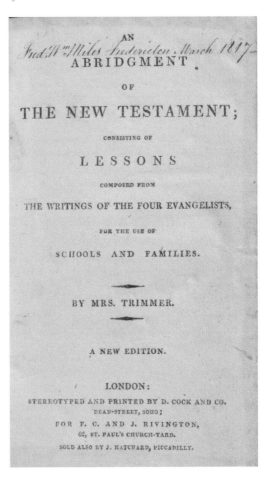

and four for boys, and many of the teachers were recruited from the brighter students who had been educated in the institution. The education of the girls was overseen by 'a prudent superintendent mistress'. The education of the boys was directed by Murray.[54] Each school mistress was allotted a dormitory, where she slept with the children under her care. She also had a schoolroom and a small apartment of her own. New rules were drawn up for the education of the children in the Foundling Hospital. From April to September the girls rose at 5 a.m. and individually recited the Lord's Prayer to the mistress in charge. School began at 6 a.m. and there was a break at 8 a.m. for a service in the chapel. After this the children had breakfast. The children then read the collect for the following Sunday, this was followed by a spelling lesson and then each child stood in turn and read a lesson from Mrs Trimmer's *An abridgement of the New Testament*. The children spent most of the rest of the day reading psalms, praying and learning how to spell and went to bed at 8 p.m.[55] They were taught to say the following prayer:

> O Great and Eternal Jehovah, who has vouchsafed to say in Thy most blessed and holy Word, that when our fathers and mothers should forsake us, Thou, O Lord, didst not forget us. May we return our most humble and hearty thanks for the performance of those gracious promises. We are living monuments of their fulfilment. We were orphans; many of us were exposed to perish but for Thy preserving hand. Thou, in Thy great and tender mercy, didst raise up friends for us even the great and noble of the land. He caused them to become our nursing fathers and nursing mothers, and placed us where we wanted no good thing ...[56]

Visitors to the Foundling Hospital

In 1806 the government appointed six prominent commissioners of the board of education to investigate the educational institutions in the country. The commissioners of education included the provost of Trinity College, the primate of all Ireland and Richard Lovell Edgeworth, father of the novelist Maria Edgeworth. The commissioners visited the Foundling Hospital, and their subsequent report of 1810 praised the institution and noted that the commissioners were 'struck with the order and regularity which every where prevailed, as well as with the neatness and healthy appearance of the children in the schools and work-rooms'.[57] The mortality rate of infants admitted to the institution had improved but it was still very high among the children who were boarded out. The commissioners estimated that one in five of the children entering the institution would survive to the age of ten. It was difficult to find apprenticeships outside the institution for the children who survived, as employers were reluctant to accept them, and this factor contributed to the rising number of children being maintained in the Foundling Hospital. There were tax concessions to encourage members of the upper class to take apprentices, but the children were to be sent exclusively to Protestant masters and mistresses. A premium of £10 for every child apprenticed was introduced in 1802, and those who hired their staff from the Foundling Hospital were exempted from a tax on servants.[58]

An English visitor who toured Ireland in 1804 was very impressed by the Foundling Hospital, describing it as a 'delightful place'. He wrote that the children looked healthy and were 'well clad':

> The whole of this institution (the Orphan-school) is conducted on a plan from which our best public charities in England would do well to borrow many useful hints. –A houseboy (that is, a boy who has been two years in the school) is appointed to sleep with one of the younger children, to be his tutor and companion; to teach him, and to hear him say his prayers; to wash and comb him; for all which he is responsible to the master ...
>
> The principal school-books are four different expositions of the catechisms, each plainer than the latter; and the children are gradually brought forward from the more easy to the more difficult ...[59]

Another visitor, John Carr, who visited the institution in 1805, was informed that many infants were shipped across from Scotland and were then being slipped into the Foundling Hospital despite the disapproval of the governors.[60] This trafficking of children was eventually controlled by changing the method of accepting the infants. Rather than placing them in the cradle, the person bearing the infant had to 'knock at the door and deliver the child; and though it is received without any question being asked, yet the bearer being obliged to show him- or herself, has been found a very great check upon the former illicit practice'.[61] Carr had a number of criticisms and suggestions for improvement, but his overall impression was favourable and he observed that the institution 'appeared to be very humanely conducted'. He also commented that the dormitories were 'remarkably' clean and that the children were well fed.[62]

Edward Wakefield visited the Foundling Hospital in 1812 and wrote a description of it as part of a general account of social conditions in Ireland. The institution did not make a favourable impression on him. All the wet nurses were responsible for more than two infants each, and he was told that during periods when many infants were admitted, a single nurse could be feeding up to five babies. Wakefield saw children who had just returned from their wet nurses in the country and most of these were in a miserable condition. He condemned the practice of proselytising in the institution, which still insisted that all children should be raised in the Protestant faith, and he argued that the system had failed in its purpose. 'Even in this institution', he wrote, 'the demon of religious discord shews his cloven foot, and interferes to excite jealousy and suspicion. This evil, this destroying influence on Irish prosperity and Irish happiness, cannot be too much execrated.'[63]

The Foundling Hospital in 1813

The historian John Warburton has left us a detailed description of the Foundling Hospital in 1813. Some of the original fourteen acres had been lost when the Grand Canal Company constructed a canal running through the southern part of the grounds of the hospital. The remaining land on the south of the canal became useless to the hospital. The institution had a frontage of nearly 400 feet on James's Street, one quarter of which was occupied by a prison or bridewell for vagrants. Warburton described this bridewell as 'a troublesome nuisance, which should be removed'.[64] The remaining frontage on James's Street was 'secured by a lofty substantial wall, through which is the principal entrance by a large park gate contiguous to which is a doorway and a neat porters' lodge'. When one entered the front gate there was a large gravel area in front of the hospital. The main door of the hospital led directly into the dining hall which, according to Warburton:

> possesses a noble simplicity which, added to the beautiful proportion of its parts, strikes the eye of the most incurious, and entitles it to rank with the finest rooms in the British empire: the floor is of an excellent stone brought from Cumberland, of a reddish tinge, fine grain, and well laid; the walls are wainscoted to the height of nearly 6 feet, and at each end is a large fireplace encompassed by a semicircular iron grating ... The hall is at present furnished with 40 tables with necessary forms, and as each table is sufficient to accommodate 20 children without crowding, 1,000 may with ease and comfort sit down to their meal at once, leaving an uninterrupted avenue of 15 feet wide through the centre of the hall, a space often occupied by visitors who come hither to contemplate one of the most gratifying of all human exhibitions ... In favourable weather the boys are paraded in front of the hall immediately before the hour of dinner; the girls, at the same time, assemble in the interior court, and the children of the various schools, distinguished by their appropriate badges, and conducted by their respective masters and mistresses, enter the hall ...[65]

Rising costs

Following the major scandals unearthed towards the end of the eighteenth century, considerable attention had been devoted to the welfare of the infants in the infirmary:

> As the governesses pay the most unremitting attention to the infant nursery, it is scarce necessary to add, that in the apartments appropriated to this department, which are spacious, well ventilated, cheerful and comfortable, there prevails such a degree of neatness and cleanliness, such an attention to the comfort of the helpless objects of the charity, as never fails to excite sensations of heart-felt delight in the visitors: here four dry and sixteen wet nurses are in constant attendance; and as each

of these, with the assistance of a double cradle, can manage two infants, this number is at present found sufficient.[66]

Thomas Cromwell recorded favourable impressions of the Foundling Hospital in his book, *Excursions through Ireland*, which was published in 1820: 'The happiest changes have ... taken place in the conduct of this hospital, and the children appear clean, contented and happy.'[67]

Impact of reforms

As a consequence of the reforms, greater numbers of infants survived and were sent out to the country to be nursed.[68] In 1802, a total of £8,143 was spent on wet nurses in the country, but by 1810, this had doubled to £16,110. The cost of this success began to cause alarm. Over 26,000 children were admitted between 1800 and 1811, but of these only 7,432 came from Dublin. The funding, amounting to approximately £8,000 per annum, came from local taxes and was insufficient to support the activity of the hospital. As a consequence

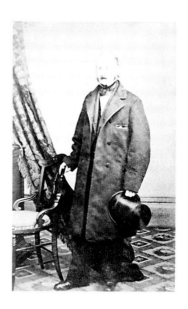

3.15   John Pigott, who was tax collector for the Foundling Hospital in 1818. This photograph was taken in New York in 1863, when Pigott was aged 67. Courtesy of Christopher Pigott.

large parliamentary grants were necessary and had to be regularly increased in the early years of the nineteenth century, from £17,500 in 1802 to £30,250 in 1812.[69] Of 51,527 children admitted to the hospital between 1798 and 1831, over 12,100 died while waiting to be sent out to nurse, 700 were returned to their parents and the remaining 38,600 children were sent out to nurses. Sixty per cent of the infants sent to nurses survived beyond two years. This was a remarkable improvement, and these figures were, at the time, among the best of those reported by foundling hospitals in Europe.[70]

Hard lives of apprentices

The number of children apprenticed throughout the country was also a source of concern to the governors of the Foundling Hospital. There were over 2,500 children dispersed as apprentices all over Ireland and it was impossible for the governors to ensure their welfare. As a consequence, some children suffered through neglect and ill-treatment. Children were sent out when they were just over 12 years of age and a single employer might take as many as six children at a time. The life of an apprentice involved very hard work and long hours. Conditions for some children were so harsh that they fled from their employers without permission (described at the time as 'elopement') as the following entries, taken from the apprentices register during the period 1824 to 1833, reveal:

Jane Barker	was seduced.
Mary Templeton	eloped and turned prostitute.
Mary Page	eloped in consequence of her mistress having accused her of improper intercourse with her master and went to live with Abraham Black, ever since she has conducted herself with great propriety.
William Beckett	beat continually by his master without any fault on his part.
Rose Carter	eloped, said she did not like to be a Protestant.
Anne Cayley	eloped in consequence of ill-treatment and bad food.
Ann Gannon	eloped, owing to her master's violent temper.
Mary Dutchman	complained of having been beaten 'too often'.
Catherine Drew	left owing to inhumane treatment from her mistress.[71]

The anguish of mothers

Many mothers sent their infants to the Foundling Hospital only as a last resort when they could not care for them. The anguish of some of these mothers is apparent in letters about their children written to the Foundling Hospital and reproduced in Wodsworth's history of the institution. The letters also reveal that infants were sometimes admitted against the wishes or knowledge of the mothers, as is shown in the following letter:[72]

To:
The Right Honourable and Honourable the Governors and Governesses of the Foundling Hospital.

The humble petition of ROSE TRENCH most humbly sheweth –
That your petitioner had the misfortune to be seduced by a person of the name of Thomas Stockdale under a promise of marriage during the time petitioner did live in the Phoenix Park in the service of her Grace the Duchess of Richmond – That said child which petitioner bore to said Stockdale was sent to nurse, where he remained for a considerable time till the nurse demanded her wages when he the said Stockdale took the child and under an assumed name of John Johnson sent him to the Foundling Hospital, tho' very well able to keep said child.
May it therefore please this honourable board to take petitioner's case into consideration and grant said child to her, and petitioner faithfully promises that she will take all the motherly care in her power of the child, and petitioner will for ever pray.

ROSE TRENCH

Malthus condemns foundling hospitals

At the beginning of the nineteenth century the whole concept of foundling hospitals came under scrutiny. The English political economist, Thomas Malthus, condemned such hospitals in his famous *Essay on the principle of population*. Malthus wrote that foundling hospitals increased mortality, destroyed parental feelings and contributed to vice.[73] The chaplain of the Foundling Hospital, Henry Murray, wrote a seven-page rejoinder entitled *A short defence of the Foundling Hospital in Dublin*. Murray argued that Malthus had taken the Foundling Hospital at St Petersburg as the example to justify his arguments. St Petersburg's Foundling Hospital laboured under even more difficult conditions than the Dublin hospital and had a far higher death rate, as infants were brought to St Petersburg from different parts of Russia in dreadful weather conditions.[74] Despite Murray's enthusiasm for the benefits of foundling hospitals, the governors of the Dublin Foundling Hospital discouraged proposals to build similar hospitals around the country and instead advocated a campaign of instruction that they believed would have the effect of 'correcting the dissipation of the lower orders'.[75]

The restriction of admissions

The population of Dublin had increased significantly, from 60,000 residents in 1700 to 224,000 in 1821.[76] This population increase and the decline of the weaving trade in the city led to considerable hardship. The number of orphans increased due to the frequency of epidemics and the deaths of fathers in the Napoleonic wars.[77] In 1820 as many as 8,740 children were supported by the governors, with well over 2,000 being admitted annually at this time.

The Foundling Hospital began to restrict admissions from the country during the winter months in order to discourage the transport of infants in inclement weather conditions.[78] Dublin Corporation objected to the new regulation, claiming that it encouraged infanticide, but the hospital governors argued that they were actually saving lives by stopping the transportation of infants during the harsh winter months. The governors again decided to discontinue the use of the cradle at the front gate as they had done ten years previously to check the trafficking of infants from Scotland. However, it was not removed immediately, as the novelist Charles Lever saw it when he was a medical student at nearby Dr Steevens' Hospital in the early 1820s. He described it as 'a large cradle hewn out of stone and neatly chiselled, which hung in front of the Foundling Hospital ...'[79] By stopping the use of the cradle, anonymity was removed and anyone bringing a baby to the hospital from then on was questioned about the parents and the reasons for their inability to maintain the child.[80] The new arrangements reduced the number of admissions and had a marked effect on the mortality rate. In 1819, only 201 infants died out of 1,788 admitted, a reduction of mortality of over 50 per cent.[81] The Foundling Hospital was visited around this time by John

Griscom, professor of chemistry and natural philosophy in the New York Institution, who later recorded his impressions:

> We went into the schools and workshops, and candour obliges me to confess, that I consider the institution, in general, as under very enlightened and judicious management. In the girls' school were 400 pupils, and in the boys' 300, taught principally on Bell's system. We heard some of the classes read in the Scriptures, and answer questions on what they had read, dictated by the monitors and both questions and answers afforded evidence of superior mental training. The employments consist chiefly of carding, spinning, weaving, and tayloring, and shoemaking. The clothes and shoes used in the hospital, are all made in the shops of the establishment. Some of the boys, about 12 years old, were weaving broadcloth. To encourage them in habits of industry, they are allowed to possess one-sixth of their earnings, and some of them by this means have on hand more than £6. The chapel of the institution may be called elegant. The refectory is large, convenient, and clean. When assembled at their meals, a boy mounts into a pulpit, and says grace, after which about twenty of them sing a short hymn. The kitchen is kept in very cleanly order, and the pea soup destined for dinner was of an excellent quality. The girls were mostly employed in spinning stocking yarn. The nursery is very clean, the cradles are made with a double head, to accommodate each two infants, and a clock is kept in the apartment ...[82]

In a further attempt to control the numbers being admitted, the governors introduced a new rule in 1822 requesting £5 from the parish from which each child was being sent. Of all the rules, regulations and laws introduced over the previous one hundred years, this was the one that had the most effect. Almost immediately the annual admission rate fell to less than 500, with 418 being admitted in 1822 compared to 1,602 four years earlier.

Parliament orders the closure of the Foundling Hospital

A parliamentary committee concluded in 1829 that there were sufficient alternative charitable outlets for abandoned children and that it was no longer necessary to keep the Foundling Hospital open. They concluded that no matter how well-intentioned individual reformers might be, there were inherent problems within the system that justified its termination. Parliament agreed and ordered the closure of the institution. The governors reluctantly acquiesced after pointing out that there was a real danger that infanticide would increase again.

There were a number of reasons for the decision to close the hospital in addition to the increasing number of facilities being developed by voluntary bodies for the care of orphaned and abandoned children. The passing of the Roman Catholic Relief Act in 1829 changed the religious atmosphere and undermined the religious goals of the

Foundling Hospital. However, there is no doubt that the financial cost of maintaining the foundling children was a major consideration. In April 1831 the lord lieutenant issued a decree that the hospital should be closed.[83]

'A void in the heart'

Although the Foundling Hospital was now closed to new admissions, the governors maintained responsibility for the large number of children already admitted. In 1839, there were 3,855 individuals still under the care of the governors:[84]

a.	Children at nurse in the country	1,503
b.	Children in the course of being apprenticed or under medical treatment in the hospital	46
c.	Adults on the invalid list	210
d.	Apprentices	2,096

The invalid adults were foundlings who did not leave the hospital because of some significant disability. When the institution was in the process of closing, all of these adults were boarded out in the country so that of the 3,855 individuals only the forty-six children of category (b) were resident in the Foundling Hospital. In March 1840, these children were transferred to a building at 49 Cork Street, and the officers and servants still on the staff were transferred with them.[85] The number of foundling children receiving government support gradually dwindled over the remainder of the century. The first historian of the Foundling Hospital, William Dudley Wodsworth, served as the honorary inspector of invalid foundlings. One of his responsibilities was to make sure that they were receiving adequate care:

> During my travels in discharge of the duties of the honorary office of 'inspector of invalid foundlings' amongst the few remaining individuals thus to some extent under my care, I was much struck by the feeling of painful wonderment and anxiety existing with many of them as to whom their parents might possibly have been. There seemed to be a void in the heart upon the subject, aching to be filled.[86]

The local government board reported that sixteen of the foundling invalids were still receiving government support in 1895. Some of these survived into the twentieth century, the last dying in 1911.

The buildings did not remain vacant for very long, as they were requisitioned by the poor law commissioners who were charged with implementing the government policy of introducing a network of over 100 workhouses throughout Ireland. The buildings of the Foundling Hospital were used to accommodate the workhouse of the South Dublin Union.

4

The South Dublin Union Workhouse

Irish property should support Irish poverty[1]

Under the Elizabethan poor law each parish in England had to provide for its poor. The assistance, in the form of money, food, clothing or goods, was usually provided through a system of 'outdoor relief', which, as the name implies, did not require the recipient to enter an institution. A similar system was not introduced in Ireland. In the early nineteenth century the English poor law was reviewed and much harsher measures were introduced to ensure that people would apply for relief only in the direst circumstances. The new poor law, introduced in 1834, developed the workhouse system in England. Edwin Chadwick devised the principles under which the poor law in England should function and these became known as the 'workhouse test'. The first principle, known as the 'all or nothing' principle, dictated that an individual would receive total provision for himself and his family in the workhouse or nothing at all. The second principle, known as the principle of 'less eligibility', ensured that conditions within the work-house were worse than the living conditions of the poorest paid worker in the outside community. The English poor law was administered by a three-man commission and the country was divided into unions, so called because several parishes were united for administrative purposes. Each union supported its own workhouse.

The condition of the poorer classes in Ireland

The philosophy behind the English workhouse system was to make relief so harsh that only those unable to work would avail of it. This approach could not be applied in Ireland as there was no work available for the destitute. In 1833, a royal commission of inquiry was established to examine the condition of the poor in Ireland. Richard Whately, Church of Ireland archbishop of Dublin, was appointed chairman of the commission. He was a very scholarly man who had formerly held the chair of political

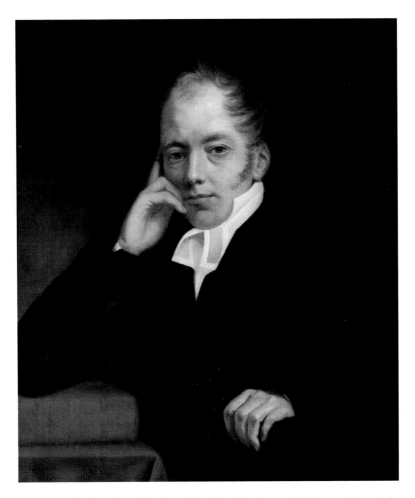

4.1   Richard Whately, archbishop of Dublin, by Thomas Phillips and his circle.
By permission of the Provost and Fellows of Oriel College, Oxford.

economy at Oxford. Whately believed in the separation of church and state, supported Catholic emancipation and was a very strong opponent of slavery. He recognized that much of the poverty in Ireland was related to economic circumstances and one of his first acts in Dublin was to establish a chair of economics at Trinity College, which is still known as the Whately Chair of Political Economy.

From the beginning Whately and his commission were under political pressure to promote the establishment of the English workhouse system throughout Ireland. However, Whately was not in favour of a quick fix and instead produced three detailed reports on poverty in Ireland and its causes. The commissioners found that labourers in Ireland lived under appalling conditions, receiving about a quarter of the pay of their counterparts in England. They also identified an oversupply of agricultural

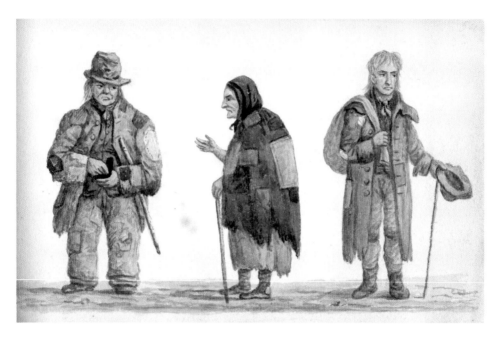

4.2   Three paupers dressed in patched clothing, painted around 1824 by Sampson Towgood Roch. © National Museums Northern Ireland.

labour, with families of agricultural labourers representing about a quarter of the population in Great Britain and about two-thirds of the population in Ireland:

> Their habitations are wretched hovels, several of a family sleep together upon straw, or upon the bare ground, sometimes with a blanket, sometimes even without so much to cover them; their food commonly consists of dry potatoes, and with these they are at times so scantily supplied, as to be obliged to stint themselves to one spare meal in the day ... Some go in search of employment to Great Britain during the harvest, others wander through Ireland with the same view. The wives and children of many are occasionally obliged to beg, but they do so reluctantly and with shame, and in general go to a distance from home, that they may not be known. Mendicity too is the sole resource of the aged and impotent of the poorer classes in general, when children or relatives are unable to support them.[2]

The commissioners were shocked by some of the scenes of destitution that they encountered in Dublin. There was no staircase in one house in the Coombe and they had to climb to the first floor with the help of logs of wood. There, in a dingy room, they found an emaciated mother and two daughters, another woman, who was too ill to move, with her two daughters, an old woman lying on a heap of straw and 'two other equally wretched objects'.[3] The commissioners calculated that there were at least 2,385,000 persons in Ireland who were destitute for at least thirty weeks in the year. They found that nine out of every ten beggars were women, including young widows or deserted wives with children, and old women without resources.

The commission rejected the English workhouse system in its report and instead proposed a plan to develop the country's resources and economy. It proposed that provision should be made for the sick and infirm and for destitute children, financed by local taxes. The commissioners' solution to the problem of the able-bodied unemployed was an extensive programme of public works with projects such as the reclamation of waste land, improvements in the standard of housing and the development of industries such as fishing and mining. The commissioners also advocated a policy of assisted emigration and were not in favour of providing relief for the able-bodied poor. This decision was unrealistic because this group formed a very significant number of those who relied on begging for survival and it gave ammunition to those who wished to undermine the report.[4] The British cabinet rejected the recommendations on the grounds that the commission had gone beyond its remit, which was to deter pauperism. The government was under pressure to stem the numbers of poor people emigrating to Britain from Ireland, as they were regarded as a burden on the poor rates. It was generally believed in England that pauperism was caused by the recklessness and barbarism of the native population. The home secretary, Sir John Russell, believed that the workhouse system would deliver significant results in the short term, and he decided to push ahead with its implementation.

George Nicholls and his tour of Ireland

Russell asked George Nicholls, one of the three English poor law commissioners, to investigate whether the machinery of the English poor law could be established in Ireland. Nicholls was a former sea captain with the East India Company who had subsequently worked as a banker.[5] He did not believe in outdoor relief and was confident that pauperism would be best reduced by the workhouse test, and he also knew what Russell expected of him. He travelled to Ireland in August 1836 and embarked on a six-week tour of the country. He witnessed many scenes of poverty and destitution but his observations were dispassionate and lacking in empathy:

> One of the circumstances that first arrests attention in Ireland, is the almost universal prevalence of mendicancy ... To assume the semblance of misery, in all its most revolting varieties, is the business of the mendicant. His success depends upon the skill with which he exercises deception. A mass of filth, nakedness, and misery, is constantly moving about, entering every house, addressing itself to every eye, and soliciting from every hand: and much of the dirty and indolent habits observable in the cabins, clothing, and general conduct of the peasantry, may probably be traced to this source: and I doubt even if those above the class of labourers altogether escape the taint.[6]

Nicholls calculated that about 100 workhouses, each capable of accommodating 800 inmates, would be adequate for the country. The number of workhouses required was increased to 130 in the early 1840s. Nicholls supported the concept of the workhouse test but he realized that it would tax even his ingenuity to operate it effectively in Ireland. He pointed out, in his first report, that to implement the workhouse test it was essential that workhouse inmates should be worse clothed, worse fed and worse accommodated than the poorest independent labourers of a neighbourhood. However, he noted that it would be virtually impossible to devise accommodation, diet and clothing for the inmates of a workhouse inferior to those of the Irish peasantry. Further, while the Irish poor law, like its English equivalent, forbade relief outside the workhouses, English boards of guardians circumvented these rules to supply

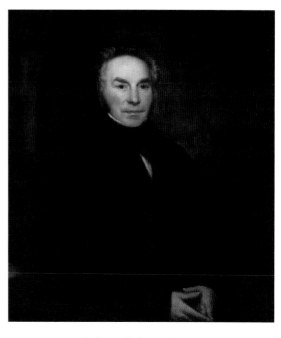

4.3   George Nicholls, English poor law commissioner, by Richard Ramsay Reinagle. Reproduced with permission of the National Portrait Gallery, London.

some outdoor relief to widows, orphans and deserted wives. The same rules were strictly imposed in Irish workhouses, with few exceptions, so that relief could only be given in the workhouse. As a result many of the inmates of the workhouses in Ireland were women and children.

Russell was happy with Nicholls' report, the cabinet formally adopted it and asked Nicholls to prepare a bill, based on his report, to present to parliament.[7] Archbishop Whately, who realized that his commission had been sidelined, was infuriated by Nicholls' proposals and was highly critical of them. In the face of strong opposition, the Poor Relief (Ireland) Bill was placed before the house of commons in 1838. As many as eighty-six petitions with over 31,000 signatures were presented against the bill and only four petitions with approximately 600 signatures were presented in its favour. Daniel O'Connell described Nicholls as a man who 'calculated everything and was accurate in nothing'.[8] O'Connell and Lord Castlereagh were on the same side in the house of commons for the first time, both opposing the bill. However, it was to no avail as the cabinet was determined to introduce a workhouse system modelled upon the English system. The Poor Relief (Ireland) Act was passed in July 1838.

Architect of the workhouses

Under the Poor Relief (Ireland) Act, Ireland was divided into unions, with a board of guardians elected in each union to supervise the poor law. The board was elected by the ratepayers, who were local property owners responsible for supporting the union. Voting qualifications were based on the valuation of an individual's property. Votes were distributed on a sliding scale with those paying high rates receiving more votes than those paying modest rates. Many of the elected members were local magistrates and justices of the peace. The guardians had to levy a rate in each union to support the poor law and they were also responsible for the running of the union's workhouse.

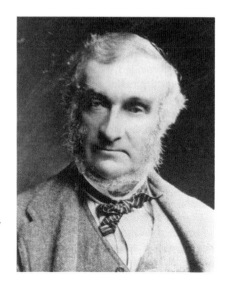

4.4   George Wilkinson, workhouse architect. Reproduced with permission of the Irish Architectural Archive.

The 1838 act obliged the guardians in each union to relieve destitution as far as the resources of the workhouse permitted. It did not give the destitute a right to relief, but this right was added to the law in 1847 during the Famine.[9] The government decided that the poor law commissioners for England and Wales should implement the Irish poor law, and they appointed Nicholls as resident commissioner in Ireland. Nicholls arrived in Ireland in September 1838, accompanied by four assistant commissioners who were experienced in the English poor law system but had no experience of Ireland. One of these, Richard Earle, was placed in charge of the Dublin region and Denis Phelan, a doctor working in Clonmel, was appointed to assist him.[10]

The South Dublin Union covered an area of 69 square miles. It was divided into eight electoral divisions and each division could elect a certain number of guardians depending on its size. The electoral divisions in the South Dublin Union included South City, Donnybrook, Rathmines, Rathfarnham, Whitechurch, Tallaght, Clondalkin and Palmerstown, and covered a population of over 180,000 people. There were forty-four guardians on the board; the electoral divisions elected thirty-three of these and there were also eleven *ex officio* members.

An English architect named George Wilkinson, who was practising at the time in Oxford and who had already designed a number of English workhouses, was appointed to supervise the construction of the workhouses throughout Ireland. The new workhouses were planned to accommodate different groups such as the old and infirm, vagrants, 'lunatics' and 'idiots' and were surrounded by high walls similar to those of a prison. Wilkinson was a tireless worker and by 1843 he had supervised the building of 112 workhouses around the country and seventeen others were nearly completed.[11]

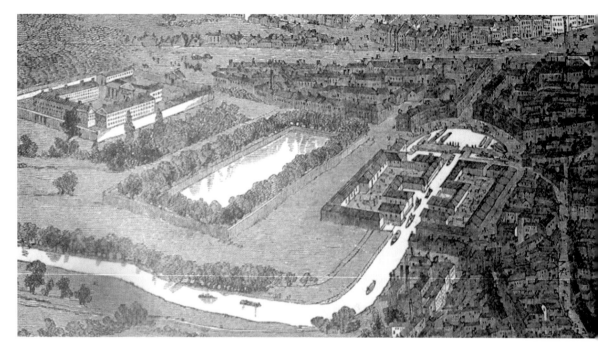

4.5   The workhouse of the South Dublin Union (left), the City Basin (centre) and Grand Canal Harbour (right) in 1846. *Illustrated London News*, 6 June 1846.

The Foundling Hospital becomes the South Dublin Union Workhouse

The buildings of the Foundling Hospital were transferred to the poor law commissioners in 1839 to be developed into a workhouse for the South Dublin Union. The House of Industry, North Brunswick Street, became the North Dublin Union Workhouse. The South Dublin Union Workhouse was situated in a grim area of the city, which was reflected in the names of the streets in its immediate vicinity. Cut-throat Lane ran along the west wall of the workhouse, Pigtown Lane was on its eastern side and Murdering Lane almost faced the entrance. The names Cromwell's Quarters and Roundhead Row were substituted for Murdering Lane and Cut-throat Lane by Dublin Corporation in 1876.[12]

Wilkinson supervised a number of alterations to the Foundling Hospital buildings. The plan was to develop a workhouse to accommodate 2,000 paupers with provision for further buildings to house 600 more. Wilkinson was also asked to design an entrance building on James's Street, which would contain a boardroom and clerical offices.[13] The board of guardians of the South Dublin Union borrowed £7,000 for the construction of the new buildings and for alterations to the old. The workhouse was declared suitable for 'the reception of paupers' on 25 March 1840.[14] It presented a grey and forbidding façade on the streetscape, with access through an arched entrance, the doors of which were shut at night.[15] On 16 December 1840, Christopher Maguire was appointed as first master of the workhouse, and three days later Jane Dollard was appointed as matron.

Attention to detail

The administrative structure devised to run the unions was highly centralized. The local board of guardians had to report regularly to the poor law commissioners, who were based in London. The board had to operate within very strict guidelines that specified how often it met, the order of business, the keeping of minutes, the reports of the masters and matrons of the unions, and the duties of all the staff, from the medical officer to the porter.

Nicholls gave particular attention to the workhouse diet. He sent his assistants to carry out surveys of the diet of Irish labourers and of the inmates of jails and hospitals. They reported that the poor survived on potatoes and milk, which they had for breakfast and for dinner, with an occasional egg or a herring. Based on this information, Nicholls devised the diet for the workhouse, which consisted of two meals, a breakfast of eight ounces of stirabout (oatmeal boiled in water) and half a pint of milk, and a dinner that consisted of three and a half pounds of potatoes and one pint of skimmed milk. Children aged 9 to 14 were given three meals a day, which included six ounces of bread for supper. Younger children could have rice or bread instead of oatmeal or potatoes.[16]

The administration of the workhouse

The position of guardian was unpaid even though it demanded a considerable time commitment. The board met every Thursday, and on Mondays the guardians met 'to admit paupers'. The guardians also served on several board subcommittees. These included subcommittees for provisions, clothing, finance and building, and two visiting committees. Eight to eleven guardians served on each committee. The beginning of each meeting of the board was devoted largely to financial affairs, and the collection of rates and the books of the rate collectors were examined closely. The governors had to deal with constant complaints by individuals that their property was being overvalued, as rates were a new form of tax that were bitterly resented by those on whom they were levied.

The meetings of the board of guardians took place in the workhouse of the South Dublin Union. Over time the workhouse itself became known as 'the South Dublin Union' or 'the Union' and its affairs were always major items on the agenda of the board meetings. A 'medical want book', listing any medical items required, was read at the weekly meetings of the guardians and orders were made for the various articles required. The guardians examined the 'establishment accounts' in detail, which included items as varied as stationery, mops, tin ware, pigs and a metal stove. Members of visiting committees appointed by the board of guardians inspected the union workhouse on a regular basis and reported to the board. They could be quite critical in their observations. A visiting committee that reported to the board of guardians on 18 January 1844 drew attention to the poor ventilation in the nursery, to dirt on the stairs and in the ward for boys, and to the condition of the footwear and clothing of the boys.[17]

Admission to the workhouse

Paupers were admitted to the workhouse by order of a guardian, a warden or the master. On admission to the workhouse, paupers were divided into five basic groups: males over 15; females over 15; boys between 2 and 15; girls between 2 and 15; and children under 2. Each group was sent to a different area of the workhouse, apart from children under the age of 2, who were allowed to stay with their mothers. The breaking up of families was very distressing for those being admitted. Parents were allowed access to their children on Sundays and only by special request at other times. On Sundays the children often did not eat their bread at the dinner hour but saved it so they could eat it later with their parents. Even though much of the justification for establishing the workhouse system centred on setting 'able-bodied males' to work, there were twice as many 'able-bodied females' (and sometimes three times as many) in the workhouse.[18] Children were not admitted without their parents unless orphaned or deserted and a man or woman, if married, could not be admitted without his or her spouse. Likewise, an individual could not be discharged without his or her entire family.

The paupers' clothes were taken on admission, fumigated and placed in a store. The paupers were washed and then dressed in workhouse attire. Men were issued with a cap, shirt, jacket and trousers of grey frieze or corduroy. Women were given a cap, petticoat, gown, shift, apron and shoes. Children also had to wear workhouse clothing. All those admitted were then placed in a probationary ward and examined by the medical officer. If they were too sick to work they were placed in the infirmary. Those who were considered well were placed in spartan accommodation and subjected to the workhouse regulations with regard to work. Those workhouses designed by Wilkinson on greenfield sites had a separate area for each type of inmate. He achieved a similar effect in the workhouse of the South Dublin Union by the use of high walls so that the different categories of inmate were well segregated from each other. The wall in the women's yard was about 36 feet long and 8 feet high to prevent communication with the men.[19]

First admissions

On 24 April 1840, Patrick Gill became the first person to be admitted to the workhouse of the South Dublin Union. He was a 60-year-old unmarried Catholic shoemaker who had become blind. According to the admission and discharge register, he was in very poor health. John Field, an unemployed clerk, and his wife Catherine, whose health was described as indifferent, were the next entries on the register. There were seventy-three admissions on the first day and they ranged in age from 2 to 90 years. From the register it is clear that from the very first day the South Dublin Union admitted significant numbers of sick, disabled and elderly poor and not just the able-bodied men and women as envisaged by the advocates of the workhouse system.[20] About 50 per cent of those admitted suffered from an identifiable illness or disability. The workhouse was immediately placed under great pressure, with up to 500 admitted in one week and 1,473 admitted in the first month. Most of the admissions came from the Dublin Mendicity Institution in order to facilitate its closure. The poor law commissioners were pleased with the transfer, despite the inexperience of the guardians and their lack of training. The commissioners decided that this success 'may be regarded as a proof of the soundness of the workhouse principle'.[21]

The workhouse of the South Dublin Union housed the largest number of destitute poor in the country. On 4 August 1840 there were 1,624 inmates in the workhouse: 454 men, 745 women, 199 boys, 204 girls and 22 infants.[22] This was a very significant number of admissions in a short period of time. In the first twelve months, 3,252 people were admitted. Some of these stayed for short periods. However, the number of inmates in the workhouse on 25 March 1841 had risen to 2,080.[23] Under the admission rule, known as the 'all or nothing' principle, entire families would have to be admitted if the father sought relief. On some occasions, when they thought it appropriate, the board of guardians did not strictly enforce the workhouse rules. For instance, on 26 June 1845, permission was given to one of the pauper women to leave the workhouse 'for the purpose of getting a situation' and to leave her child in the workhouse for three months.[24] From the early years, unscrupulous people used the workhouse to abandon relatives – usually parents or children. Efforts were made to track down these family members and make them contribute to the cost of maintaining their relatives. In August 1845, legal action was initiated against a number of individuals for abandoning their wives in the workhouse. These men were not paupers but men with trades such as scrivener, cabinetmaker, fish porter, letter carrier, whitesmith and shoemaker.[25] In one case, taken in 1844, Peter Harrington was sentenced to two months' imprisonment with hard labour for desertion of his wife, an inmate of the workhouse. Proceedings were also taken against individuals who deserted their children or parents.

The staff of the workhouse

The staff of the workhouse consisted of a master, matron, clerk, chaplain, schoolmaster, medical officer, porters and other staff as required. The master was seen as a servant of the board of guardians and, during meetings of the board, he sat in an adjacent room and was summoned by a bell when required. The master was responsible for keeping a register of everyone admitted to the workhouse and had to ensure that all those who were capable of employment were not idle at any time. He also read prayers to the inmates before breakfast and after supper each day. The matron had specific duties relating to the moral conduct and behaviour of the female inmates and children, and she had to ensure that the children were given some training that would make them suitable for employment in the future. The chaplain conducted a religious service every Sunday, preached to the inmates and at least once a month had 'to examine and catechise' the children.

Chaplains were appointed from the main religions, and from the beginning a deliberate attempt was made to reduce the possibility of proselytism, which had caused difficulties in the Foundling Hospital. The bell in the cupola over the great dining hall tolled at intervals during the day to summon inmates to prayer. No one was obliged to attend a religious service that might be contrary to his or her religious principles, and children were to be educated in the religion of their parents or guardians.[26] In spite of these rules, there were allegations of proselytism against staff, and the board of guardians received many acrimonious letters on the subject, which often resulted in equally

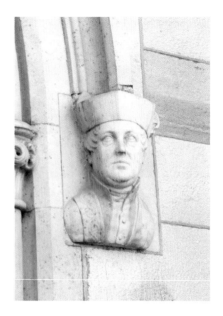

4.6   Corbel head of Revd George Canavan on the entrance door of St James's church in James's Street. Canavan, who was the second chaplain to the South Dublin Union, was the driving force behind the construction of the church, but the Great Famine stopped the work, and he did not live to see the building completed. With permission of Fr John Collins, moderator of St James's parish. Photograph: Anthony Edwards.

acrimonious debates. In 1841, the board of the South Dublin Union was informed that eight boys who were being brought up as Protestants were refusing to go to service on Sundays. The boys said that they wanted to conform to the Catholic faith, and they denied that they had been under any pressure to change their religion. They were reprimanded for demanding the right to choose their own religion. They were punished by solitary confinement for four hours each day for two days, and they were to receive half rations.[27] The Revd Thomas Kingston, rector of St James's parish, was appointed as the first Church of Ireland chaplain in 1840. In the same year, Revd Patrick Mooney from St James's parish was appointed as the first Catholic curate; he was succeeded by Revd George Canavan in 1842.[28]

The schoolmaster and schoolmistress were responsible for the education of the children in the workhouse. The girls were taught sewing and were employed in the domestic work of the institution, including the laundry. The boys were taught tailoring, shoemaking and carpentry, and some worked in the garden.[29] A master shoemaker was appointed in 1845 and his hours of work were fixed at 6 a.m. to 7 p.m. in summer and from 7 a.m. to 7 p.m. in winter.[30] The porter, apart from his portering duties, was also charged 'to prevent the admission of any spirituous or fermented liquors, or any article of food not provided for the inmates in the workhouse'.[31]

Times for visiting the workhouse were very limited. In the early years, visitors were only admitted between 11 a.m. and 1 p.m. on the first and third Mondays of each month. From the beginning the South Dublin Union Workhouse was recognized as one of the principal workhouses in the country, and staff were sent there from other unions for training.

A day in the workhouse

The inmates' day started at 6 a.m., when they were awakened by a bell. They then assembled in the dining hall, where the master read the morning prayers and they were inspected. Breakfast was eaten in silence and usually consisted of the stipulated milk and stirabout. After breakfast the able-bodied men worked in the fields or broke stones, the women did housework or looked after the ill, and the children went to the workhouse school. Older and frailer people spent their time mending clothes, spinning wool or unpicking old ropes to obtain oakum, which was sold to shipbuilders, who mixed it with tar and used it as a sealing material.

Dinner typically consisted of potatoes and skimmed milk. Each person's potatoes were placed in a net, weighed and then boiled in the net. Like breakfast, the meal was eaten in silence. At a meeting on 3 September 1840 the governors ruled that water could be placed on the tables during dinner. After dinner the inmates were expected to continue working, and they retired to bed after evening prayers, with lights out at 9 p.m. The inmates were forbidden to enter the dormitories until bedtime and were not allowed to have beer or tobacco or to play cards.[32]

Appointing medical staff

One of the first tasks to which the guardians of the South Dublin Union devoted their energies was the appointment of a physician, a surgeon and a resident apothecary. At a meeting on 9 January 1840, they debated whether the physician and surgeon should be paid £60 or £100 per annum, however the poor law commissioners imposed a salary of £60. The first medical staff appointed to these posts were Cathcart Lees, Peter Shannon and James F. Grant, as physician, surgeon and apothecary, respectively. Grant was appointed at a salary of £60 a year 'with apartments, coals, candles, and a sufficient quantity of the provisions used in the establishment'.[33] The board of guardians passed a resolution in June 1841 proposing that the salaries of the physician and surgeon should be increased to £100 per annum. The poor law commissioners were opposed to any such increase:

The commissioners do not consider it just towards the ratepayers that the guardians should testify their approval of the services of an officer by raising his salary; the true principle is to adjust the amount of remuneration to the extent of duty to be performed, and to see that the duty is performed by any one who undertakes it at the fixed rate of remuneration.[34]

The guardians were not to be frustrated so early in their aims, and the poor law commissioners agreed to send their medical assistant commissioner, Denis Phelan, to investigate the medical workload in the North Dublin Union and South Dublin Union. His report reveals that there was a busy 'hospital' or 'medical' component to the workload of the South Dublin Union Workhouse from its inception. Between April 1840, when the workhouse opened, and August 1841, the physician and surgeon treated 5,750 cases and the mortality rate was 9 per cent. On the day of Phelan's inspection, the South Dublin Union contained 126 patients in wards designated as hospital wards and there were seventy-eight patients in the sick and infirm wards.

The physician and surgeon visited the sick every day in the hospital wards and in the sick and infirm wards, and they also saw other inmates who were reported ill. The duties of the apothecary were to prepare and dispense the medicines as directed by the physician and surgeon and to 'regulate' the diet books. He was also required to give medical attention to those who became ill when the physician and surgeon were not in the hospital.

Phelan suggested that the resident apothecary should be given greater responsibility for routine care and that the physician and surgeon should confine themselves to more complex cases. This would obviate the need for increasing their salaries. The board of guardians countered by inviting the eminent doctors Sir Henry Marsh, physician-in-ordinary to the queen in Ireland, and James W. Cusack, surgeon to Dr Steevens' Hospital, to visit the South Dublin Union to assess the workload of the doctors in October 1841. They were unequivocal in their support for an increase in remuneration, declaring that the current salaries did not 'by any means adequately remunerate a perfectly qualified physician or surgeon for the labour, time, and care essential to the due discharge of the responsible duties devolving upon them'.[35] The poor law commissioners eventually agreed, in February 1842, to withdraw their opposition to the proposed salary increases.

Peter Shannon, the first surgeon, lived at 207 Great Brunswick Street (now Pearse Street). He studied at the RCSI, qualifying in 1835. He was awarded an MD by Glasgow University in 1840 and became a fellow of the RCSI in 1844. Shannon was a member of the Dublin Pathological Society and he contributed case reports to the *Dublin Quarterly Journal of Medicine*.

John Cathcart Lees was the first physician to the South Dublin Union. He was born in 1811, the son of a lawyer, John Cathcart Lees, and Mary Lees, who was the daughter of Sir Robert Shaw of Bushy Park, Co. Dublin. Lees studied medicine at the RCSI and Trinity College Dublin, graduating from Trinity College in 1837. As his original intention was to become a surgeon, in 1830 he was indentured to Rawdon Mac-namara, surgeon at the Meath Hospital. He decided to abandon surgery in favour of medicine and he became a licentiate of the College of Physicians in 1842 and a fellow in 1845. Lees was also physician to the Institution for Diseases of Children in Pitt Street, the first children's hospital in the British Isles. He wrote a number of papers for the *Dublin Journal of Medical Science* during his time in the South Dublin Union. These included 'An account of an epidemic of ophthalmia which prevailed among the children of the South Dublin Union during the summer and autumn of 1840', 'Observations on hypertrophy of the brain in children' (1842), and 'Cases and observations on the dropsy following scarlet fever' (1843). He was elected physician to the Meath Hospital in 1843. He resigned from the South Dublin Union in 1845 and was succeeded as physician by Robert Mayne.[36] The poor law commissioners established an inquiry when it was alleged that there had been a monetary arrangement between Lees and Mayne under which Lees was to be paid £300 by Mayne: £100 on his resignation and a further £200 when Mayne was later elected to the office, on the understanding that Lees would use his influence to support Mayne's candidature.

The practice of buying posts was one of the standard ways of being appointed to the staff of voluntary hospitals at the time. No remuneration was given to doctors who worked in the voluntary hospitals; they earned their living from the fees charged to private patients. The hospital appointments were prestigious and helped their private practices. However, the position Lees sold was a salaried poor law post. Despite the fact that both physicians confirmed the substance of the allegations, the poor law commissioners ignored the findings of their inquiry and confirmed the appointment of Mayne.[37] The commissioners subsequently issued a recommendation to all boards of guardians throughout the country 'to fix salaries at so low a rate that they shall not be worth selling'.[38]

Robert Crawford Mayne was born in Allenstown, Co. Meath in 1811 and educated in the Drogheda Grammar School. He subsequently received some medical instruction from Dr Robert Pentland in the Drogheda Infirmary before beginning studies in Dublin at Trinity College and the RCSI.[39] After graduation he taught anatomy in the Richmond School of Medicine, where he acquired a reputation as an excellent lecturer. He obtained the fellowships of both the RCSI and the College of Physicians but he practised as a physician. Mayne read papers regularly to the Dublin Pathological Society based on his work in the South Dublin Union. He also published in the *Dublin Journal of Medical Science* on a range of topics, including cerebrospinal meningitis, dysentery, aneurysms and patent foramen ovale. His paper on pericarditis in the *Dublin Journal of Medical Science*, which was written when he was still a student, was translated into French and German.[40] William Stokes referred to Mayne's work on pericarditis several times in his book, *The diseases of the heart and the aorta*, which is generally acknowledged as the first textbook of cardiology.[41] Stokes also referenced Mayne's work on rheumatic carditis and varicose aneurysms. He described Mayne's clinical observations as 'afford-

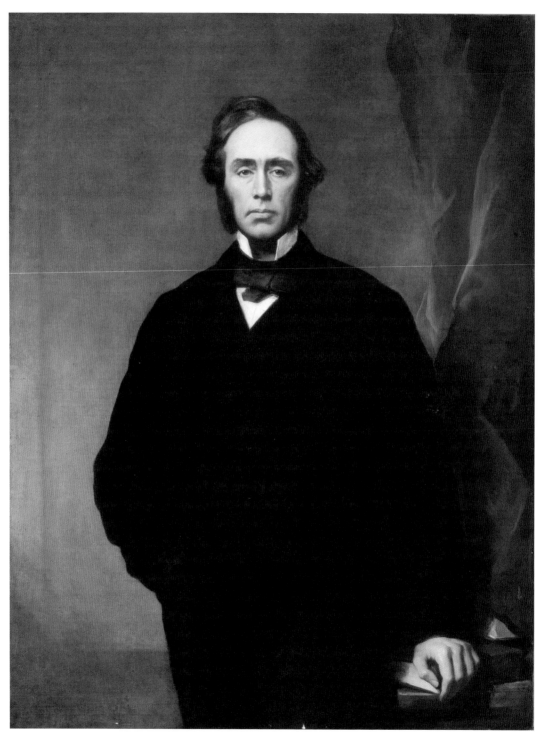

4.7   Robert Mayne, physician to the South Dublin Union, artist unknown. Reproduced with permission of the Royal
College of Physicians of Ireland.

ing an example of the accuracy of observation and logical deduction which distinguish the various memoirs with which Dr Mayne has enriched our science'.[42] Mayne also contributed to *Todd's cyclopaedia of anatomy*, one of the major publications on anatomy at that time. In 1853, Mayne succeeded Dominic Corrigan as lecturer on the practice of medicine in the Carmichael School of Medicine. He was elected physician to the Adelaide Hospital in 1859.

Doctors as advocates

From the beginning, the medical officers took an independent stand, frequently criticizing the board over conditions in the South Dublin Union Workhouse. They were particularly critical of the overcrowded dormitories, where sometimes as many as five children shared a bed. In 1844, Robert Mayne sent a paper to the board of guardians outlining the appropriate amount of space that should be available for each child in the workhouse. He advocated that 400 cubic feet of air should be allowed for each infant and each nurse in their sleeping wards in the nursery, 300 cubic feet of air should be allowed for each healthy child in the Children's House and 400 cubic feet per patient in the sick wards. He made a detailed submission giving the dimensions and cubic feet of each ward and the number of nurses and children. He also listed the number of beds in each ward and it is apparent from his figures that the ratio of children to beds was approximately 2:1. There were wards for sick boys, sick girls, boys with sore heads, children with measles, children with 'itch' and sick infants, and two wards for children with sore eyes. There were also three wards to accommodate forty-one healthy infants and their wet nurses.[43]

There were no professional nurses in the early nineteenth century in Ireland. According to Florence Nightingale, in this period nursing was left to women 'who were too old, too weak, too drunken, too stupid or too bad to do anything else'.[44] Washing and feeding sick men and women who were not related to them was considered immodest and demeaning for young, unmarried, well-bred women.[45] The guardians supplemented the untrained women that they employed as nurses with inmates whom they referred to as 'pauper nurses'. Some of these nurses, although lacking training, were caring and compassionate individuals. One nurse is reported to have worked for twelve consecutive nights caring for a sick child in March 1844.[46] Nursing in the South Dublin Union was very demanding work, and in addition to their nursing duties, the matron had the authority to roster nurses to work in the laundry for up to three hours each day.[47]

Visitations of the Sisters of Mercy

Catherine McAuley, who founded the religious order of the Sisters of Mercy in 1831, began her visitations to the sick by visiting the poor in their homes, and in public hospitals and institutions in Dublin. The Sisters of Mercy began visiting the South Dublin

Union in 1840, but the master of the workhouse opposed the visits and they ceased for a time.

The difficulties the sisters encountered in gaining access to the South Dublin Union Workhouse were discussed at meetings of the board of guardians in July and August 1841, when it was denied that any attempt was being made to stop the sisters. On 13 August 1841, C.P. Shannon, one of the Catholic guardians on the board, wrote to Catherine McAuley informing her 'that no prohibition exists against their visiting the South Dublin Union Workhouse' and inviting the sisters to resume their visitations.[48] However, this invitation proved premature as, at a meeting of the board of guardians two weeks later, the master made it clear that the nuns could not be admitted without a resolution from the board. A motion was then proposed by C.P. Shannon, and passed by the guardians, which gave the nuns access to

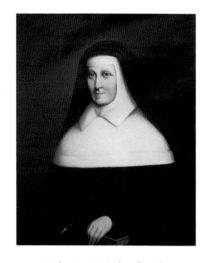

4.8   Catherine McAuley, founder of the Mercy order. Photograph: David Knight. Courtesy of the Mercy International Association.

the institution 'at all hours allowed visitors in order to visit such sick persons of their persuasion as may desire to see them'.[49] The sisters resumed visitation to the sick on the wards, primarily on Sundays, but in March 1842 their request for permission to give religious instruction to children in the workhouse was refused.

The board minutes of the South Dublin Union show that voting on motions frequently revealed political and religious bias among the guardians. Disputes over the baptism of children, rows between the chaplains regarding the use of the chapel and other issues, and conflict between the Protestant and Catholic schoolchildren, were often ultimately brought before the guardians for resolution. The deliberations on these subjects could frequently become acrimonious and on one occasion it was suggested that a constable should attend meetings of the board 'in order to preserve peace and prevent the boardroom being made the scene of violence and assaults'.[50]

Conditions for infants and children

The care of destitute children was entrusted to the boards of guardians under section 41 of the Poor Relief (Ireland) Act 1838. The number of children under 15 in workhouses across Ireland was 76,724 in 1853.[51] Most of these children lived in appalling conditions. During the rest of the nineteenth century, a succession of acts of parliament made it progressively easier to board children out, so that by 1900 the number of children in the South Dublin Union had fallen significantly.[52] The board of guardians wrote to the poor law commissioners in 1844 requesting that the commissioners should apply to parliament for permission to place infants with wet nurses in the country. The guardians argued that evidence had shown that metropolitan workhouses were inappropriate places to care for infant children, as the mortality rate was very high.[53]

Permission from the poor law commissioners was required if the board of guardians wished to make even minor improvements in the diet of the inmates, including the children. Frequently, requests from the board were ignored and the resulting annoyance and frustration was often vented at board meetings.[54]

Criticism of workhouse system

The implementation of the workhouse system at first led to a fall in the number of beggars on the streets but the impact was short lived, as George Nicholls reported:

> Many of the beggars had in fact entered the workhouses, and thus the public were relieved from their solicitations; but the relief was short-lived, for others soon flocked in from the neighbouring districts, and many who had entered the workhouses experimentally as it were, or through fear that their vocation might be suddenly put a stop to, again left them and resumed their former practice of begging; and thus after a time, the streets and suburbs of Dublin were as full of beggars as before.[55]

The guardians were forthright when expressing their opinions on policies relating to the poor. Some of the guardians were highly critical of the workhouse system in general. They viewed it as a very expensive way of giving relief to only a fraction of those in need. They pointed out that the commissioners of the poor law inquiry calculated that there were 2 million paupers in the country and that the 130 workhouses could only give relief to a maximum of 40,000. It was argued that this was unfair to both the paupers and the ratepayers. The subject was discussed at a board meeting in 1844 and the guardians decided to send a petition to both houses of parliament at Westminster. The detailed submission was highly critical of the poor law and the workhouse system. It stated that Nicholls, who introduced the system, was 'totally unacquainted with the wants and wishes of the people of Ireland'.[56] It detailed the cost of the workhouses in Ireland and claimed that this was excessive and that, despite all the expenditure, 'the establishment of the poor law has not given any additional employment to the able-bodied labourer, the waste lands of Ireland remain un-reclaimed, her coast fisheries neglected and her mineral wealth unexplored'.[57] The submission pointed out that the basis for distress and destitution in Ireland was traceable to the absence of employment for the country's able-bodied population and that investment should focus on developing employment rather than maintaining an expensive workhouse system.[58] The board sought the support of several MPs at Westminster including Daniel O'Connell. However, the guardians' efforts were in vain and the workhouse system continued unchanged.

Discipline in the workhouse

During the first year of the workhouse, concerns were raised at the board meetings that the master of the workhouse and the schoolmaster were 'illegally beating and ill-treating pauper children'. As a consequence, the master was required to keep a punishment book to record 'every case of punishment inflicted in the house', specifying the offence, the punishment, by whom it was awarded and the name and age of the offender.[59] Children who absconded from the workhouse were dealt with severely by prosecution. Two children who absconded in August 1844 were imprisoned for one week.[60] Later that month the board of guardians received a report on two absconding brothers:

> The master reported that No. 7611 John Murray aged 12 years and his brother Arthur No. 6475 aged 9 years absconded on Tuesday 13th instant with the house clothing – last Tuesday evening Mr Burke schoolmaster met the former mentioned boy in James Street and brought him back to the workhouse. He had exchanged his trousers and got his jacket dyed a dark colour to prevent it being recognised.[61]

The boys sometimes used diversionary tactics in their attempts to escape. In May 1845, a boy named John Eustace threw stones at one of the men overseeing the boys' yard in order to allow other boys an opportunity to climb the boundary wall. Eustace was brought before the board where it was decided that he should be punished.[62] Such misbehaviour was typically punished by beating with a birch rod by the schoolmaster.[63] Boys who were considered 'refractory' could be assigned to chop blocks of wood.

Minor infringements of discipline by adult inmates were dealt with in-house by the guardians. On one occasion, eight men who were refusing to work were ordered to break three bushels of stones each day and their dinner was held back until they had completed the task.[64] A woman caught selling bread to buy snuff was reprimanded and placed on a half rations for a week.[65] More serious misdemeanours were reported to the police; a pauper, Michael Kavanagh, was prosecuted for taking lead from the roof of the workhouse.[66]

In May 1845, the board decided to review all pauper inmates and children of six months standing in the workhouse in an endeavour to reduce the numbers.[67] This move did not receive the support of all the board members. At a meeting on 29 May 1845, a member of the board, Captain Nowlan, was highly critical of these reviews, pointing out that most of the inmates were admitted because of destitution:

> therefore to dismiss a destitute inmate without providing work for him may prove a cruel exercise of power and in the case of destitute children may throw on this board the responsibility of cutting short their lives.[68]

The board members were unaware that within a short period the numbers being admitted to the South Dublin Union Workhouse would not fall but would soar to unprecedented levels as famine gripped the country.

5

The Great Famine

There, day after day, numbers of people, wasted by famine and consumed by fever, could be seen lying on the footpaths and roads waiting for the chance of admission.[1]

The population of Ireland increased dramatically in the second half of the eighteenth century, rising from 2.5 million in 1750 to 5 million in 1800 and continued to grow, reaching 8.2 million by 1841. Until the middle of the eighteenth century the Irish diet consisted of oatmeal and dairy products supplemented by potatoes. This changed to a diet that depended mainly on the potato, and as the potato was a good source of nutrition, the health of the population improved and the mortality rate fell, especially among children. Better health led to earlier marriages and a rising birth rate. When a disease attacked the potato crop in the autumn of 1845, it was a portent of major disaster.[2]

The potato blight was caused by a fungus, *Phytophthora infestans*, which attacks the leaves and the stalk and then penetrates beneath the soil to destroy the tuber. The eastern regions of the country bore the brunt of the crop failure in 1845. The full impact of the blight did not become apparent until it was found that apparently good potatoes, which had been stored in pits after they had been harvested, were rotten. The famine that followed over the next five years had a devastating impact leading to the death of around 1 million people from starvation and epidemic disease and to the emigration of another 2 million within a decade. The response of the government at Westminster was hopelessly inadequate and the workhouses throughout the country became the last refuges of the starving and dying.[3]

As a result of the failure of the potato crop, the guardians of the South Dublin Union received a letter from the poor law commissioners on 6 November 1845 authorizing them to change the dietary regime of the workhouse.[4] Copies of a report from the three commissioners appointed by the government to advise on ways of preserving the crop were distributed at the meeting. Two of the three were English scientists, Lyon Playfair and John Lindley. The chairman of the group was Robert Kane, a medical graduate, who had studied under the famous Irish physicians Robert Graves

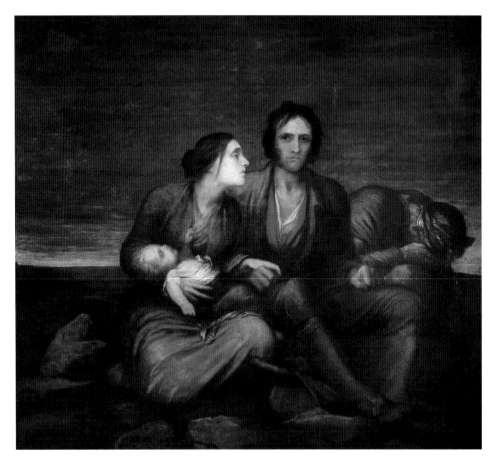

5.1 *The Irish Famine* (1850), by George Frederic Watts. Reproduced with permission of the Watts Gallery Trust, UK.

and William Stokes, and who would later become the first president of Queen's College Cork. Lyon Playfair was a highly respected chemist and a friend of the prime minister, Sir Robert Peel. John Lindley was the first professor of botany in the University of London and was responsible for making Kew Gardens the centre of botanical science for the British empire.

The scientists recommended a complicated procedure to make use of the affected potatoes, which involved pulping them to get rid of the diseased part and subsequently making bread from the residue. In November 1845, the guardians of the South Dublin Union were asked if they would facilitate a trial of the process proposed by the commissioners to convert diseased potatoes into 'wholesome food'.[5] Robert Kane visited the workhouse in December and selected the 'able-bodied men's yard' as the site in which to erect the equipment necessary for the trial. The experiment was not successful and the cost of the drying apparatus would have made the process imprac-

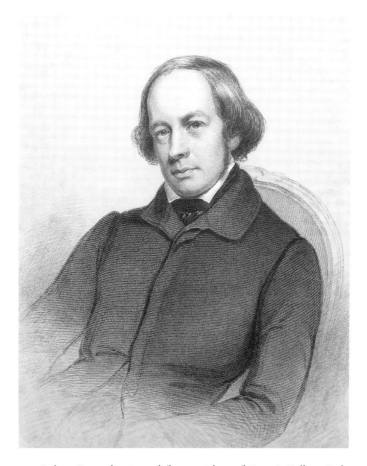

5.2   Robert Kane, chemist and first president of Queen's College Cork. Reproduced with permission of the Royal College of Physicians of Ireland.

tical on a large scale. As a consequence, it was abandoned.[6] This was the first scientific experiment carried out on the site.

Changes in workhouse diet

At the close of 1845, the South Dublin Union was experiencing a gradual increase in demand for admissions to the workhouse. On 8 November there were 1,579 inmates and within a month the number had increased by 200.[7] The total capacity of the workhouse was estimated to be around 2,000, and this figure was reached in February 1846. The master reported in January that he would have to dispose of four tons of waste potatoes, and the use of potatoes was discontinued altogether in March. A substitute bread was given on Tuesdays, Thursdays, Saturdays and Sundays, and oatmeal made into stirabout on the other days.[8] Three weeks later, the medical officer reported that there had been

SOUTH DUBLIN UNION.

RETURN of Paupers who were admitted into, or Discharged from, the Workhouse; and of the number of Sick, and the number Born, or who died therein, during the Week ended SATURDAY, *24* day of *May* 184*5*

	ADMITTED.							DISCHARGED.						DIED.					
	Males, aged 15 and upwrds.	Females, aged 15 and upwrds.	Boys under 15.	Girls under 15.	Children under 2.	BORN. Males.	Females.	TOTAL.	Males, aged 15 and upwrds.	Females, aged 15 and upwrds.	Boys under 15.	Girls under 15.	Children under 2.	TOTAL.	Males, aged 15 and upwrds.	Females, aged 15 and upwrds.	Boys under 15.	Girls under 15.	Children under 2.	TOTAL.
During the Week, ended as above.	12	29	5	4	1	„	„	51	21	18	4	4	1	48	1	„	„	„	1	2
Remaining on the previous Saturday, as per last Return.	450	735	216	207	30	„	„	1638	RETURN OF SICK AND LUNATIC PAUPERS.											
TOTAL,	462	764	221	211	31	„	„	1689	No. in Hospital on the above date. In W. House	No. in Lunatic and Idiot Wards on the above date. In Sep. Wards	OBSERVATIONS in case of any unusual number of these classes of Paupers.									
									421	53										
Deduct Discharged and Died, during the Week ending as above.	22	18	4	4	2	„	„	50	In Fever Hospital	In Mc'with otherinmate										
REMAINING ON THE ABOVE DATE.	440	746	217	207	29	„	„	1639	5	23										

Number of Inmates that the Workhouse is calculated to contain, 2000.

NEXT MEETING to be held on *Thurs* day, the *5* day of *June* 184*5*

5.3 This table shows that in the week ending 24 May 1845 there were 51 admissions, 48 discharges and 2 deaths, leaving 1,639 inmates in the workhouse, 426 of whom were sick. This would have been the pattern on most weeks before the onset of the Famine. Minutes of the meeting of the board guardians of the South Dublin, 29 May 1845.

'a great increase of bowel complaints', and this was blamed on the stirabout.[9] Maize was purchased in April, but it was not well received by the inmates, most of whom refused to eat it. The medical officers reported that bowel complaints 'to an unprecedented extent continue to prevail amongst the aged and infirm inmates'.[10]

Famine fever

In May 1846, due to the increasing number of acutely ill inmates, it was proposed that females suffering from fever should be removed from the infirmary to the infirm wards. The visiting medical officers strongly objected to the proposal:

it has always appeared to them an object of paramount importance to have the power of separating at the very first accession of illness, those who labour under infectious

SOUTH DUBLIN UNION.

RETURN of PAUPERS who were admitted into, or Discharged from, the Workhouse; and of the number of Sick, and the number Born, or who died therein, during the Week ended SATURDAY,   5ᵗʰ day of *December* 1846

	ADMITTED.								DISCHARGED.						DIED.					
	Males, aged 15 and upwrds.	Females aged 15 and upwrds.	Boys under 15.	Girls under 15.	Children under 2.	BORN. Males.	BORN. Females.	TOTAL.	Males, aged 15 and upwrds.	Females aged 15 and upwrds.	Boys under 15.	Girls under 15.	Children under 2.	TOTAL.	Males, aged 15 and upwrds.	Females aged 15 and upwrds.	Boys under 15.	Girls under 15.	Children under 2.	TOTAL.
During the Week, ended as above.	19	31	2	7	3	..	..	62	6	19	9	4	1	39	5	19	4	4	11	43
Remaining on the previous Saturday, as per last Return.	1480	312	287	244	62	..	..	1885												
TOTAL,	1499	343	289	251	65	..	..	1947												
Deduct Discharged and Died, during the Week ending as above.	11	38	13	8	12	..	..	82												
REMAINING ON THE ABOVE DATE.	1488	305	276	243	53	..	..	1865												

RETURN OF SICK AND LUNATIC PAUPERS.

	No. in Hospital on the above date.	No. in Lunatic and Idiot Wards on the above date.	OBSERVATIONS in case of any unusual number of these classes of Paupers.
In Work House.	} 759	In separate Wards. } 53	
In Fever Hospital.	} 11	In Wards with other Inmates. } 23	
TOTAL	770	TOTAL 76	

Number of Inmates that the Workhouse is calculated to contain, 2000.

NEXT MEETING to be held on , *Thurs*-day, the 17ᵗʰ day of *December* 1846

5.4   This table shows that in the week ending 5 Dec. 1846 there were 62 admissions, 39 discharges and 43 deaths, leaving 1,865 inmates in the workhouse, 770 of whom were sick. During December there was a severe outbreak of dysentery in the South Dublin Union, and this is reflected in the mortality rate. Minutes of the meeting of the board guardians of the South Dublin Union, 10 Dec. 1846.

disorders from the other inmates of the workhouse and this can only be accomplished by having an hospital detached from the chronic and infirm department.[11]

The institution was assuming the role of an acute hospital and the resident medical officer was under great pressure because of the increasing numbers of acutely ill inmates, many of whom were malnourished on admission. The board of guardians recognized this and increased the resident medical officer's salary from £60 to £80 per annum.[12] With the onset of the winter of 1846, the numbers seeking refuge in the workhouse began to rise rapidly. While workhouses provided shelter for the destitute and the starving throughout the Famine when all other doors were shut to them, the fatality rate of inmates was high. Infectious diseases were spread by overcrowding and poor sanitation, and the workhouse of the South Dublin Union was no different from other workhouses in this regard.[13] There were almost 900 patients receiving medical treatment in the workhouse in December 1846.[14] This rise in numbers was a cause for concern as many were suffering from 'famine fever', caused by two diseases – typhus and relapsing fever – both of which were spread by lice. Dysentery was also a major cause of serious illness, accounting for 268 cases in December 1846. The medical officers, at the request of the board of guardians, invited Dominic Corrigan, a distinguished physician, and Philip Crampton, a well-known surgeon, to visit the workhouse to advise on the factors responsible for the high rates of mortality from infectious diseases. Corrigan and Crampton visited the South Dublin Union on the 29 December. They delivered a prompt report in which they attributed the propagation of diseases to two major factors:

> 1st. To the circumstance that for some months past, a large proportion of those admitted into the workhouse have been persons broken down in constitution; and many of them as already noticed, labouring under dysentery.
>
> 2nd. To the circumstance, that in the workhouse itself the wards are so crowded, and the ventilation so defective, that disease, no matter how caused at first, must soon acquire and maintain a highly contagious character; and, as universally the case under such circumstances, will also assume a fatal form, bidding defiance to the effects of the best medical skill.[15]

They advised the guardians to make more accommodation available and to improve the ventilation in the existing wards. However, as soon as any extra space was created it was filled immediately by starving and sick people because of the high number seeking admission. Corrigan and Crampton also drew the attention of the board to the impossible workload of the medical officers:

> We must observe that the labour your medical officers at present undergo is more than we think they can continue to endure, and a failure of their energies in the present trying circumstances will be productive of injury to the poor as well as themselves. Each of the medical officers has now under his care about 270 patients; allowing only five minutes on an average for seeing each patient, 22 hours would be required to go through the whole number; or supposing that only half the number require to be seen daily, the duty to be yet done is far beyond what your present staff of medical officers can efficiently perform.[16]

The physician Robert Mayne wrote a description of the epidemic of dysentery in the South Dublin Union. His figures were drawn from the male wards, for which he had clinical responsibility. His colleague Peter Shannon looked after patients in the female wards, where, Mayne confirmed, 'the disease prevailed with equal severity'.[17] The epidemic was at its most virulent in the autumn of 1847, with 75 newly admitted male patients in September alone. In an attempt to limit the spread of the disease the 'dysentery' wards were 'all in their turn cleared, fumigated with chlorine, scoured, painted and then furnished with new bedding; the entire process occupying about a week'.[18] Typhus, relapsing fever and dysentery were much more virulent and more lethal in a population greatly weakened by starvation.[19] Although 1,533 people died from epidemic and contagious diseases in the South Dublin Union during the Famine, the mortality was much lower than that of workhouses in other urban areas such as Cork, where 5,745 died, and Belfast, where 2,399 died.[20]

At the South Dublin Union doctors struggled to cope with the growing number of patients and also acted as advocates for the sick when challenged by the guardians, who were anxious to keep the overall costs down. In July 1847, a subcommittee of the board questioned the apothecary James Grant, who also served as a resident medical officer, and the surgeon Peter Shannon, on the level of the patients' consumption of wine, spirits, chicken, eggs and the produce of the garden. They justified the use of the items mentioned on the basis that those seeking admission to the workhouse were in a very poor state.[21] The apothecary also supplied porter as nourishment.

Selected healthy inmates nursed the sick under the supervision of a nurse named Haydon, who was the only nurse employed in the workhouse. The medical officer reported that the task of attending so many sick people was so great that Nurse Haydon was 'altogether overpowered by fatigue'. He requested more support for her and an assistant nurse was subsequently appointed at 10 shillings per week 'with rations'.

The graveyard of the workhouse was located on ground now occupied by Hospital 2, and on some of the surrounding area. At the time, inmates who died were buried in the workhouse cemetery. The number of deaths in the workhouse was increasing and burial space was becoming a problem. In November 1847 the guardians expressed their disapproval of the practice of burying paupers 'in the garden attached to the workhouse', and they recommended that 'a contract be entered into with some of the cemeteries in the neighbourhood of the city'.[22] At the next meeting they ordered that 'no pauper from this day forth be buried within the precincts of this workhouse' and decided to send all deceased paupers to Glasnevin Cemetery.[23]

Uncompromising government policy

When the poor law was introduced in 1838, George Nicholls emphasized that the only situation with which a properly implemented poor law could not cope was a general famine.[24] It was a prophetic insight. Within a few years the British government's insistence on responding to the emerging famine only through the poor law had disastrous results. According to official government policy, the cost of all relief should be borne by local rates. Yet many of the property owners, because of the prevailing hardship, could not pay the rates. The guardians of the South Dublin Union accepted that the rate of 1s. 6d. in the pound 'could not be collected at present from the pauperised class of small farmers'.[25] Property owners in urban areas were under similar pressure. The guardians made significant reductions in the rates, hoping to increase the flow

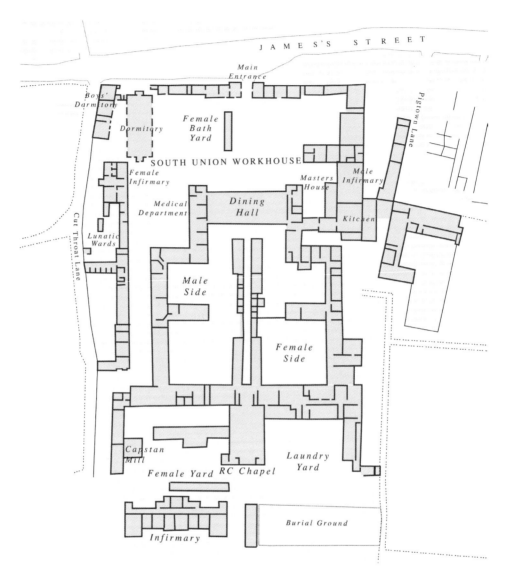

5.5 Map of the South Dublin Union, showing the Famine cemetery. Drawing by Anthony Edwards based on Valuation Office collection, sheet 19, 1854.

of income. They knew that the country was experiencing an unprecedented crisis and that local measures were not sufficient to meet the demand. They expressed these concerns in a plea to the government and the prime minister, and they asked them to suspend all legislation impeding the importation of food to feed the starving population.[26] In 1847, the guardians were worried about the possible forced return of Irish emigrants in England, particularly those in Liverpool. It was calculated at the time

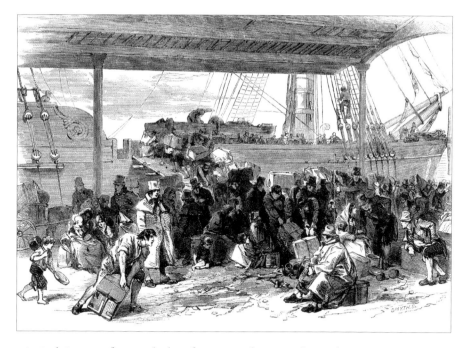

5.6   Irish Famine refugees embarking for America from Waterloo Docks in Liverpool. *Illustrated London News*, 6 July 1850.

that approximately 40,000 destitute Irish had emigrated to Liverpool, largely from the southern and western parts of the country. If all these people were returned to Ireland by the British authorities they would arrive in Dublin and become the responsibility of the city. The guardians decided to make every effort to protect the Dublin ratepayers by attempting to stop the deportation of Irish paupers from England. The appeals of the guardians fell on deaf ears, and around 15,000 men and women were returned to Ireland from Liverpool in 1847.[27]

Starvation in Dublin

Most contemporary accounts of the Famine describe conditions in rural Ireland and there are few accounts of conditions in the cities. The starvation rate was lower in Dublin than in other parts of Ireland and this led many hungry and destitute people to migrate to Dublin seeking food. On arrival they mingled with the large number of beggars already in the city, with a resultant steep rise in deaths due to dysentery and fever in Dublin in 1847.[28] In her book, *Annals of the Famine in Ireland*, an American visitor, Asenath Nicholson, has left graphic descriptions of the poverty and hardship which she witnessed in Dublin during the early months of 1847. Many of the starving people she encountered would have died without her assistance:

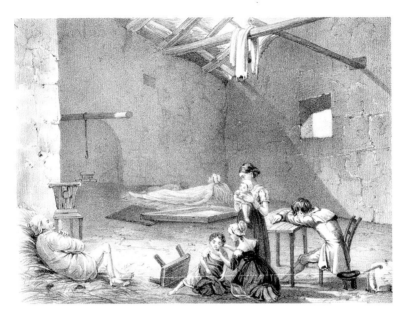

5.7 Contemporary Famine scene. Lithograph drawn by A.S.G. Stopford. Image courtesy of the National Library of Ireland.

One of these miserable families was that of a widow. I found her creeping upon the street one cold night, when snow was upon the ground. Her pitiful posture, bent over, leaning upon two sticks, with a little boy and girl behind her crying with the cold, induced me to inquire, and I found that she was actually lame, her legs much swollen, and her story proved to be a true one. She had been turned from the hospital as a hopeless case, and a poor, sick, starving friend had taken her in, and she had crawled out with a few boxes of matches to see if she could sell them, for she told me she could not yet bring herself to beg ...[29]

A dispensary doctor, Lombe Atthill, who worked in Dublin during the winter of 1847, described similar experiences in his book, *Recollections of an Irish doctor*:

The tenement houses in which the poor lived were crowded from attic to cellar. I have known four families, each consisting of several individuals, living in one small room, a corner allotted to each family, without a stick of furniture amongst them. One instance I never shall forget. I narrate it to give some idea of the hopelessness of the task devolving on the medical man at this sad period. My district embraced the low-lying slums contiguous to the river Liffey. One day I received a ticket directing me to visit a woman in one of these streets, not of the worst class. Calling at the address given, I was told that the patient lived in the 'kitchen', and as there was no communication between the house proper and the so-called kitchen I had to go out of the front door and down into the area to gain entrance. There I found the woman in a veritable cellar, into which neither air nor light could enter, save through the door. Her case was one of typhus fever, so I gave her an order for admission to the fever hospital.[30]

The Revd Thomas Willis, writing in 1845, described appalling conditions in St Michan's parish, which was the poorest in Dublin. The parish was 'wretched and pestiferous', with more than 23,197 families living in single rooms, often sublet to lodgers in order to pay the rent.[31] 'Nothing marks their poverty', he wrote, 'more than when congregating around the public fountain, struggling to have their little supply. There are many lanes and courts in which a tumbler of water could not be had safe for drinking.'[32]

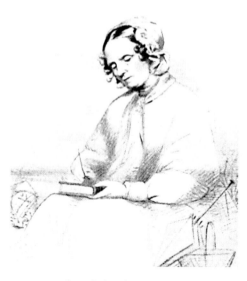

5.8   Asenath Nicholson by Anna Maria Howitt. *The Bookman*, Nov. 1926

5.9   Lombe Atthill. Frontispiece from L. Atthill, *Recollections of an Irish doctor* (London, 1911).

Admission crisis

As the crisis escalated, accommodation in the South Dublin Union became hopelessly inadequate. There were over two thousand inmates in the workhouse and there was relentless pressure to admit an ever increasing number of destitute and starving people. At a meeting in January 1847, the guardians decided that they needed more room to cope with 'the present awful visitation'.[33] They asked the poor law commissioners to instruct their architect, George Wilkinson, to prepare a plan for a substantial building in the workhouse of the South Dublin Union to accommodate an additional one thousand paupers.

The shortage of fever beds in Dublin in 1847 was attributed in part to an administrative decision, made on financial grounds, to close almost three hundred beds at the government-funded Fever Hospital in Cork Street. To support additional fever beds,

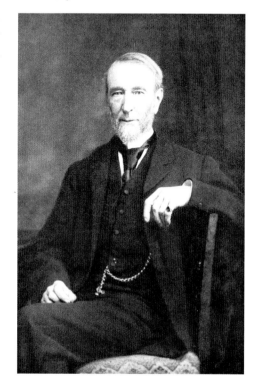

the guardians requested central funds but the treasury rejected their petition because it would show an 'indulgence' to the South Dublin Union that it would not be able to grant to other places where fever might be equally prevalent.[34] In another attempt to increase space for admissions the guardians offered an allowance, not exceeding 1s. 6d. per week, to infirm adults who would volunteer to leave the workhouse. It was hoped that as many as a thousand places might become available. However, this offer was available only to single people or to married couples without children.[35]

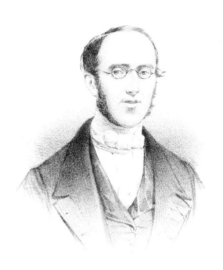

5.10   John Oliver Curran. Image courtesy of the National Library of Ireland.

In March 1847, the board of guardians was informed that there was a significant increase in the number of patients suffering with fever in the South Dublin Union. The Cork Street Fever Hospital could not accept the patients so the guardians decided to establish their own fever hospital in the Tenter House on Cork Street. The Tenter House was used originally by the wool handweavers of the Liberties to dry cloth, but in 1847 the building was vacant.[36] Patients were also admitted to temporary 'fever sheds' in Kilmainham, separated from the workhouse by a number of fields. The sheds were situated on the South Circular Road at the Rialto end of the modern St James's Hospital campus. Even with these facilities there was not enough capacity to cope with the sick and dying and, by the autumn of 1847, the fever hospitals in Dublin and the South Dublin Union were overwhelmed. In a letter to a Dublin newspaper, one doctor described patients lying in the gutter and on the pathway outside the temporary fever sheds at Kilmainham, with their mouths open, 'their black and parched tongues and encrusted teeth visible even from a distance'.[37] The well-known surgeon and author William Wilde also witnessed these scenes of great hardship outside the fever sheds:

> There, day after day, numbers of people, wasted by famine and consumed by fever, could be seen lying on the footpaths and roads waiting for the chance of admission; and when they were fortunate enough to be received, their places were soon filled by other victims of suffering and disease.[38]

John Oliver Curran, a young doctor on the teaching staff of the Apothecaries' Hall, campaigned against the inadequacies of the fever services and, in particular, the conditions in the overcrowded sheds at Kilmainham. His agitation led the French government to send two medical commissioners to Dublin to investigate the famine conditions. One of the commissioners developed typhus and was cared for by Curran, who in the process developed the disease himself and died in October 1847, aged 28. Curran had been an outstanding pupil of the renowned Irish physician William Stokes. Stokes treated Curran and he was very distressed when he could not save his life. Curran's friends and colleagues were incensed by his death and they wrote an angry letter to the lord lieutenant decrying the paltry support given to doctors dealing with fever patients.[39]

Soup kitchens

The government first responded to the growing crisis in Ireland by a policy of relief through public works, but by the beginning of 1847 they realized that this policy was not working and that a system of direct relief funded from the treasury was required. The Temporary Relief Act 1847 empowered government agencies to use soup kitchens to feed the starving and was the first act to introduce a policy of outdoor relief in Ireland. Three relieving officers were appointed for the southern part of the city by the guardians of the South Dublin Union. As the situation deteriorated, the government also decided that the poor law commission, which was based in London, was too remote to respond rapidly to events in Ireland. A separate poor law commission, which reported to the lord lieutenant, was established in Dublin in 1847. Edward Twistleton, an Englishman, was its first chief commissioner, and he was joined by Sir William Somerville and Thomas Reddington.

'Nourishing soup'

In 1847, at the invitation of the lord lieutenant, Alexis Benoit Soyer, the French chef of the London Reform Club, opened his 'new model kitchen' in front of the Royal Barracks (now the National Museum of Ireland, Collins Barracks). He claimed that he had developed a nourishing soup for the poor that cost only three farthings a quart. He had placed the soup on the à la carte menu for the patrons of the Reform Club and it was declared excellent.[40] There were two recipes. The first was composed of 1/4 pound of leg of beef, 2 gallons of water, 2 ounces of dripping, two onions, and other vegetables including the peelings of two turnips, 1/2 pound of flour, 1/2 pound of pearl barley, 3 ounces of salt and 1/2 ounce of brown sugar. The second recipe used 'legs or clods of beef, with a portion of cow-heels', and was even cheaper than the first, as 100 gallons could be made for £1.[41] Soyer claimed that a bowl of his soup once a day, together with a biscuit, would sustain the strength of a healthy man, but contemporary analysis of the soup cast major doubt on its nutrient content.[42] Not surprisingly there was considerable scepticism among the poor about the nourishing value of the soup. At around this time the physician William Stokes was stopped by a woman begging on the street. She informed Stokes that she was very weak from starvation. He asked her why she did not go to the soup kitchen for some soup. 'Soup, is it, your honour,' she replied, 'sure it isn't soup at all ... but a quart of water boiled down to a pint to make it strong.'[43]

Soyer was invited to address the guardians of the South Dublin Union in March 1847. The minutes of the meeting record:

> The valuable information afforded by him to promote the preparation of cheap and nourishing articles of diet for the poor, entitle him to the thanks of the board, for his attention to the cooking department of this workhouse.[44]

While Soyer's motives were honourable and he was genuinely concerned about feeding the starving, he was politically naïve. The British government used the publicity surrounding Soyer and his model soup kitchen as propaganda to counter critics who claimed that the

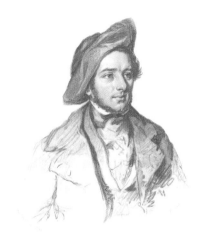

5.11 Alexis Benoit Soyer by Elizabeth Soyer. Reproduced with permission of the National Portrait Gallery, London.

5.12 Soyer's 'model soup kitchen'. *Illustrated London News*, 17 Apr. 1847.

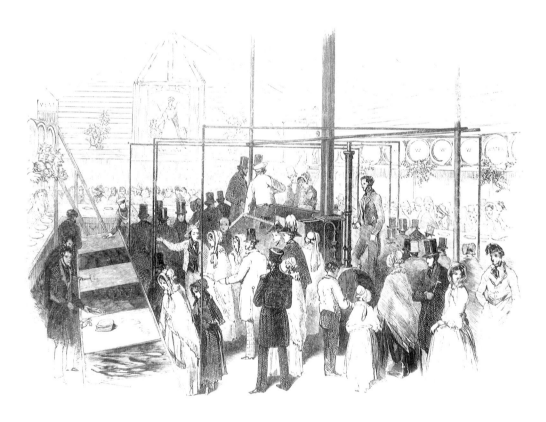

government's inactivity was responsible for the death of thousands of people.[45] The 'new model kitchen' was a wooden building about 40 feet long and 30 feet wide with a door at each end. There was a 300 gallon soup boiler in the centre of the structure and beside it a very large oven capable of baking 100 kilograms of bread at a time. It also housed three long tables, each with a row of 100 holes, just big enough to hold a white enamel bowl with a metal spoon attached by a fine chain. The starving people queued outside and were admitted at the sound of a bell, 100 at a time. As many as 8,750 people drank soup and received a portion of bread each day.[46]

In December 1847, the guardians purchased the model kitchen and moved it to the workhouse. The patent oven was designed to bake about 8,000 pounds of bread per day; it was bought for £150 and cost £200 to install. The model kitchen was used to cook and bake food for the workhouse and to bake the bread used for outdoor relief. It was anticipated that there would be a significant savings in fuel with the new system, as the existing consumption of coal in the kitchen of the workhouse was 1 ton per day, whereas the new model kitchen used 2 tons per week.[47] The model kitchen was later moved to Dolphin's Barn, where it was used to make soup for large numbers of infirm poor.[48]

Outdoor relief

The outdoor relief established by the Temporary Relief Act 1847 was extended by the Irish Poor Relief Extension Act later in the year. This act empowered the guardians of the unions to give outdoor relief at their own discretion to the aged, infirm, sick poor and widows with two or more dependent children. Although the act legitimized outdoor relief, the strict selection criteria for those entitled to relief had the effect of reducing the overall number receiving assistance in the south Dublin area.[49] In August 1847, the board of guardians began to plan arrangements to feed a thousand qualifying paupers daily with rations of porridge and bread, which would be distributed from three or four rented depots in south Dublin. Destitute patients, who were being discharged from the fever sheds, would receive an allowance of milk and bread daily for ten days after discharge.[50] These plans were designed to keep the poor from starving and to reduce demands for admission to the workhouse. Some members of the board seemed more concerned that paupers might barter their rations for items such as snuff and tobacco, and argued that only porridge should be used for outdoor relief as this could be bartered less easily than bread.[51]

Increased accommodation

In December 1847, George Wilkinson was asked to design galleries for the dining hall to provide extra accommodation.[52] The guardians also decided to proceed with their plans, first proposed in January, to build new accommodation in the workhouse for 1,300 additional paupers. The funds for construction had to be borrowed, as the

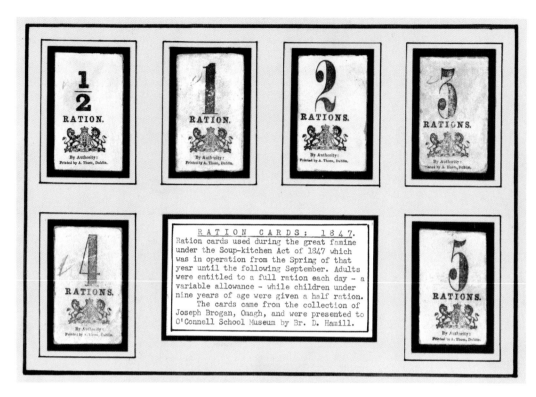

5.13 Ration cards issued by the relief commissioners, who were appointed in 1845 to administer temporary relief. The half ration was for children under the age of 9. Brother Allen Collection. Courtesy of the Military Archives, Ireland.

board was not awarded a grant by the government for the project. At a meeting at the beginning of January 1848, they instructed that advertisements should be inserted in the newspapers, inviting proposals:

> from one or more persons to lend to the guardians of this union a sum of £8,000, in sums of not less than £500 from each person, at 6 per cent per annum or less, said loan being required for the enlargement of the workhouse, the repayment thereof to be secured by sanction of the poor law commissioners upon the rates of the Union.[53]

The new buildings were designed by Wilkinson. The guardians were constantly seeking means of creating new space within the workhouse by adapting existing accommodation for ward use and by sending as many inmates as possible out on outdoor relief. A large square building in an enclosed yard was acquired at Island-bridge in January 1848 and the guardians had this fitted out for immediate occupation by children aged between 2 and 7 years.[54] The guardians also used a building in Dolphin's Barn as an auxiliary workhouse and school for children.

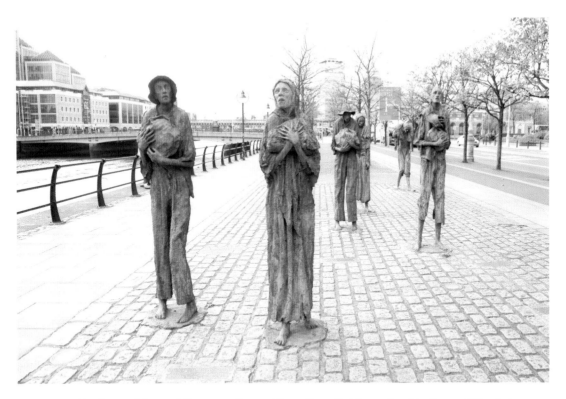

5.14   The Famine Memorial figures on Custom House Quay, Dublin, sculpted by Rowan Gillespie in 1997. Photograph: Anthony Edwards.

Rural paupers

In January 1848, the poor law commissioners sought to limit the number of inmates in the workhouse to 2,225 at any one time.[55] The board of guardians found it impossible to comply with this rule as there were already approximately 2,500 people in the workhouse and the numbers applying for admission from rural areas were increasing. Some of the guardians believed that paupers did not enter their local workhouse because of the 'the superior treatment allowed to paupers' in the South Dublin Union.[56] In an attempt to change this, the board of guardians wrote to the poor law commissioners asking them if they would, as far as possible, seek uniformity in the diet and treatment of paupers in the different workhouses throughout the country. However, others among the guardians attributed the problem, not to variations in diet, but to absentee landlords who were not doing their duty.[57] It is also likely that many paupers preferred the anonymity offered by the Dublin workhouse to the perceived indignity of admission to a local institution.

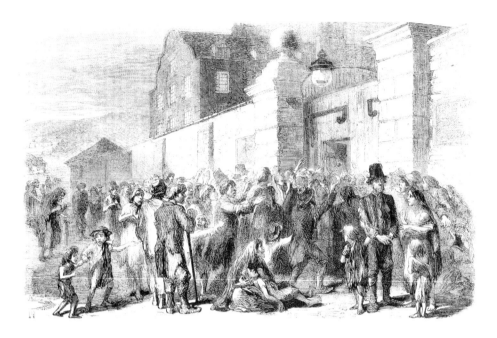

5.15   The Irish Famine: starving peasants at a workhouse gate. From Robert Wilson, *The life and times of Queen Victoria* (London, 1887).

Increase in numbers

By March 1848, the number of inmates had risen to 3,434 and there was a very significant increase in the numbers of able-bodied men (593) and women (1,025). Most of the inmates (2,225) were accommodated in the main workhouse buildings and in the fever sheds (734). The rest were accommodated in auxiliary and temporary buildings in the grounds of the workhouse and in two off-site locations, Dolphin's Barn Lane and the Tenter House. In the first week of March 1848 the South Dublin Union also distributed outdoor relief to 5,898 people.[58]

The greatly increased number of people being admitted to the South Dublin Union during the Famine (a total of 6,717 in 1848) led to a very significant rise in the costs of running the institution, from £13,232 in 1844 to £49,865 in 1848.[59] The 'family test' (or 'all-or-nothing' principle) was not applied with any degree of rigour during the Famine years, and 70 per cent of those admitted were without any other member of their family. There was a dramatic difference in the age profile of those admitted in 1840, which was the first year of the South Dublin Union, and of those admitted in 1848. Only 32 per cent of the inmates were under the age of 41 in 1840, whereas 77 per cent were in 1848. This reflects the severity of the Famine, as hunger and illness pushed more and more young people into the workhouse.[60]

Unrest among the inmates

There is evidence that from the beginning of 1846, the increasing number of inmates made it more difficult to maintain order in the workhouse. The guardians discussed the problem of discipline but they also stressed the importance of continued vigilance to ensure that officers did not abuse their power. They decided that in extreme and urgent cases, the matron was to be empowered 'to confine refractory girls' for a maximum of six hours in any individual case.[61] These measures were later considered insufficient and the matron was given the power to employ 'refractory girls' in breaking up two bushels of stones a day, and food was to be withheld until the work was done.[62] At a meeting on the 1 April 1847 the master reported to the board:

> that there are more than 70 male adults from 15 to 22 years of age in the house, many of whom are incorrigible idlers and ill-conducted. He begged to suggest to the board the necessity of appointing an overseer for the purpose of keeping them constantly employed at stone-breaking.[63]

A special meeting of the board of guardians was called in February 1848 because of the 'alarming insubordination' which had spread throughout the workhouse in the previous thirty-six hours. A number of people were discharged for insubordination at this meeting and others were sent before the magistrates. At the same meeting the guardians received the following letter from the inmates:

> Gentlemen of the Board,
>
> Painful and starving necessity obliges us to address you with these few lines regarding our food. We have waited patiently, time after time, expecting a change. We can subsist no longer for we are in a state of starvation. We want nothing unreasonable. All we want is our own country meal for breakfast, and white bread for dinner. A quart of water rice is no substitute for dinner for girls to work hard on. We cannot nor wont. It is not sufficient to support nature. Gentlemen, when our own meal and flour was dear we got better stirabout for breakfast and white bread, and now it is so reasonable we leave it to your own kind considerations.
>
> Gentlemen of the Board of Charity, if you be so kind as to grant this our petition we will be for ever in duty bound to pray for your welfare.
>
> We the inmates of the workhouse.[64]

The following May there was a mass escape of thirty-five boys. Several of them made their way out into the country but most were subsequently apprehended. As a consequence, the schoolmaster was dismissed and the grim buildings of the workhouse became more prison-like as iron bars were placed on the windows of the boys' dormitory.[65] The problem of offenders who were being repeatedly sent to the magistrates' court because of misbehaviour was discussed at a meeting of the board in November. The guardians suspected that these repeat offenders almost certainly had an ulterior motive:

> it being ascertained that the diet supplied in the city prisons to the refractory inmates of this workhouse is preferred to the workhouse diet, wherefore the same persons have been repeatedly imprisoned, and those persons have encouraged others to transgress as a means to attain what they regard as more indulgent treatment.[66]

In response, one might have expected that the guardians would seek to improve the meals in their own institution. Instead they wrote to the master of prisons, asking him 'if the law so permits, to order bread and water or an inferior diet for the paupers sentenced to imprisonment for refractory conduct'.[67]

The prevailing social chaos was also reflected in the growing number of robberies in the workhouse.[68] The situation did not improve over the following year, and in September 1848 the guardians asked the commissioner of police to send two police constables to patrol the workhouse every night.[69] Officers of the workhouse were subject to physical attacks both inside and outside the institution. The master was attacked by two sisters when returning from the city centre and sought refuge in a shop on James's Street.[70] Captain Nowlan, one of the most diligent members of the board, was assaulted by a female applicant, who struck him on the head with a large stone when he was presiding at an admission board.[71] On another occasion three young women inmates smashed the windows of the board room during a meeting of the admission board.[72]

The search for suitable work

The able-bodied were supposed to work six days a week in the workhouse, but the absence of suitable work was a constant problem. A special subcommittee was set up by the board of guardians in October 1847 to make suggestions about the work that might be undertaken. The subcommittee reported back later in the same month suggesting that all work undertaken should support and clothe the paupers in the workhouse. They proposed that the guardians should lease land 'for the cultivation of produce in accordance with the established dietary, and of flax on which to employ the women in the several operations of scotching, hackling, spinning, and weaving'. They also recommended 'that another hand-mill be purchased, in order that the whole of the wheaten meal required for the institution be ground by the paupers'. They did not recommend 'the breaking of stones, except as a punishment for the refractory adult males'.[73]

Captain Nowlan condemned the inefficient management of the workhouse by the board of guardians at a meeting in September 1848. He emphasized the importance of giving able-bodied inmates constructive work, otherwise they would rapidly become institutionalized, or without skills, they might steal to survive on discharge, 'so that those who begin in being inmates of the house end by becoming inmates of a jail'.[74] He noted that expensive equipment for spinning and weaving had been allowed to fall into disrepair and that the board was regularly spending money hiring masons and carpenters and other workers to carry out tasks that could be completed by inmates. He pointed out that nearly £3,500 per annum was spent on salaries and rations for the staff, and carpets were supplied for the sitting rooms of the officers:

> even the subordinate officers in the house are furnished profusely with every article of furniture – to take an instance, a nurse receives as her weekly rations eight pounds of the best mutton, sixteen pounds of the best bread, seven quarts of new milk with as much coals, candles, soap etc. as she can use, and for the support of a destitute widow with six children, to whom we give no clothing, no shelter, no fire, no light, we, the guardians of the poor, assign the pittance of three pounds of bread daily.[75]

Cholera epidemic – the final straw

The beginning of 1849 saw a further increase in the numbers seeking admission to the South Dublin Union. Weak and starving, the population was struggling to recover from the Famine and had little resistance to the epidemic of cholera that now spread throughout the country. Cholera is contracted by drinking water or eating food that has been contaminated with faeces spread through the seepage of infected sewage into the water supply. There had been a previous epidemic in 1832, but this one was far more destructive. The epidemic started in Afghanistan in 1845 and slowly made its way through the Middle East to Europe.[76]

In December 1848, the board of guardians received a letter from the Dublin Sanitary Association enclosing a copy of a report on strategies to be undertaken should cholera revisit the country.[77] The guardians instructed the apothecary to immediately prepare two fifty-bed hospitals to accommodate patients suffering from cholera and other epidemic diseases. The master of the workhouse was also asked to prepare one hundred beds with bedding. A subcommittee established by the board reported one week later. It recommended that accommodation should be acquired in south Dublin to serve as a temporary cholera hospital, and that the fever sheds at the Kilmainham end of the South Dublin Union should also be used for patients with cholera. As a result, a temporary hospital was established in Brunswick Street (Pearse Street).[78] The committee also recommended that a medical officer should be appointed to each parish with the purpose of 'promptly attending outdoor patients attacked with cholera and transmitting same to hospital, if necessary, without delay'.[79] Placards were posted 'directing all poor attacked with bowel complaints to apply where they may be properly attended'.[80] Overcrowding in the wards of the South Dublin Union was still a major problem and exposed the inmates to virulent infections. Around this time the matron warned the board that 'pestilence' would be the result of the crowded state of the female healthy wards: 'There are 136 beds with three in each and in the nursery there are four persons in each bed ... additional dormitories, day rooms are greatly required.'[81]

The arrival and spread of the epidemic

The first cases of cholera in Ireland were reported in Belfast towards the end of 1848. At a meeting of the South Dublin Union's cholera committee that was held at the hospital in Brunswick Street on the 13 February 1849, William Moss, the medical officer for that area, reported five deaths out of the six cases of Asiatic cholera he had treated within the previous week. There were many cases with 'premonitory symptoms' of cholera that had been treated with good results.[82]

In mid May the board received a report from the physician in charge of the Kilmainham sheds stating that patients were being admitted in an advanced state of cholera because of inattention to premonitory symptoms. The board decided to make representations to the Roman Catholic clergy to urge their congregations to seek medical attention at the first sign of symptoms. The number of people infected was beginning to rise and the epidemic was obviously spreading. At the same board meeting it was reported that there were 11 cases of cholera in the Brunswick Street Hospital, 31 cases in the Kilmainham sheds, and Moss indicated that on district visitation they had identified 36 cases. The board responded by intensifying medical visitation in the areas from which the patients originated. Doctors were recruited as assistants on a week-to-week basis to carry out the inspections.[83] By the end of the month, numbers had escalated to 30 cases in the Brunswick Street Hospital and 77 cases in the Kilmainham sheds, 31 of whom had died in the previous week. Increasing numbers were also being found at the district inspections. The total number of admissions to the Kilmainham fever sheds and Brunswick Street Hospital in the six months from the start of the epidemic was 458 patients, 199 of whom had died, while 72 were still in hospital.[84]

Two Irish poets die from cholera

James Clarence Mangan, author of the beautiful lyric poem, 'Dark Rosaleen', developed cholera towards the end of May 1849. He was admitted to the Kilmainham sheds in early June. Mangan's general health was very poor and he was addicted to alcohol and opium. He had already spent time in the South Dublin Union, having been admitted to the fever sheds in the spring of 1848. Mangan was considerably weakened by the cholera and remained for some days in the Kilmainham fever sheds. After leaving the sheds he took refuge in a 'miserable garret in Bride Street' where he deteriorated rapidly.[85] In mid June he was admitted to the Meath Hospital under the care of Dr William Stokes. He died a week after admission on 20 June 1849, aged 46. His last

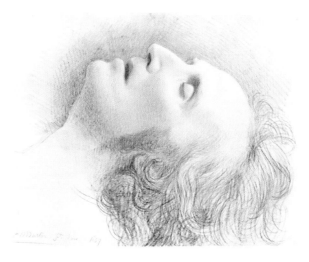

5.16 James Clarence Mangan. A sketch of the poet's head drawn shortly after his death by Sir Frederic Burton. Reproduced with permission of the National Gallery of Ireland.

poem was published in *The Irishman* shortly before his admission to the fever sheds in Kilmainham. It was a cry from the heart entitled 'The Famine':

> Despair? Yes! For a blight fell on the land
> The soil, heaven-blasted, yielded food no more
> The Irish serf became a Being banned
> Life-exiled as none ever was before.
> The old man died beside his hovel's hearth,
> The young man stretched himself along the earth,
> And perished, stricken to the core![86]

Another poet of the period, John Keegan, who like Mangan had contributed poems to *The Nation* and other publications throughout the 1840s, was also a victim of cholera. Keegan was born near Abbeyleix, Co. Laois, in 1809. He worked as a clerk to a relief committee during the Famine. His poetry reflected his concern for those affected by the ravages of the Famine. He moved to Dublin in May 1847 where he found cheap lodgings at 8 Lower Bridge Street. Keegan was depressed and in poor health when the cholera epidemic swept across the country in 1849. One of his last poems was entitled 'To the Cholera', and opened with the verse:

> Oh! thou, who comest, like a midnight thief,
> Uncounted, seeking whom thou may'st destroy;
> Rupturing anew the half-closed wounds of grief,
> And sealing up each new-born spring of joy.[87]

Keegan contracted cholera in June 1849 soon after writing the poem and was admitted to the fever sheds at Kilmainham, where he died shortly after admission. The editor of *The Irishman* newspaper announced the news of his death:

> Another son of genius is gone. Death is becoming an epicure and selects the choicest victims. It is not many weeks since we closed the grave over James Clarence Mangan; his friend and fellow poet, John Keegan, did not tarry long behind him ... There were no legends, familiar to the peasantry, with which he was not acquainted. His poems were thoroughly idiomatic, and racy of the soil. They were the Irish heart translated and set to music. They touched us more than the polished lines of drawing-room bards, because they did not consecrate affection, but showed us ourselves.[88]

An anthology of his writings was published in 1907.[89]

Death of medical officer and the end of the epidemic

By the end of June 1849 there were signs that the epidemic was abating. Tragically, it was at this time that Gordon Jackson, medical officer to the Kilmainham fever sheds, contracted cholera and died a few hours after the first symptoms appeared.[90] He had worked continuously and tirelessly at the fever sheds, sleeping on the premises. Jackson was a talented doctor with great potential and he was a lecturer in the School of Practical Medicine and Surgery in Meath Street.[91]

The Brunswick Street Hospital was closed in September 1849 and two months later a decision was made to close the Kilmainham sheds in the South Dublin Union.[92] Even though the cholera epidemic and the potato blight were no longer major issues by the end of 1849, the mortality rate did not fall significantly for a further two years. Despite the persistent high mortality figures there was a political eagerness to declare that the crisis had been resolved.

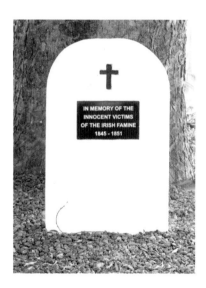

5.17 Memorial to the victims of the Irish Famine situated near the site of the Famine burial ground in St James's Hospital. The memorial was erected by the Committee for the Commemoration of Irish Famine Victims. It was unveiled by Lord Mayor of Dublin, Christy Burke, on 27 July 2014. Photograph: Anthony Edwards.

6

A vast hospital

This institution is now a vast hospital containing a larger number of cases of acute and chronic medical and surgical diseases than has ever before been collected within the walls of a Dublin hospital.[1]

Although conditions throughout the country improved gradually after the Famine, this was not reflected in the level of admissions to the South Dublin Union Workhouse.[2] The influx of impoverished people from the country had resulted in a very significant increase in the population of Dublin. During this period, many of the former Georgian mansions of the upper class gradually became the tenements of the poor.[3] Throughout the Famine the South Dublin Union Workhouse had been a last refuge for the starving, and with scarce resources and overstretched capacity it had provided food and medical care for the destitute. This experience would shape the role of the workhouse of the South Dublin Union in developing services for the sick poor throughout the second half of the nineteenth century.

Growth of medical cases

At the beginning of 1851 there were approximately 3,000 inmates in the South Dublin Union. The medical officers wrote to the board in February, calling attention to the large number of patients. They gave several reasons for this. One was the gradual withdrawal of government grants from some of the Dublin hospitals, and particularly the Lock Hospital, where patients with syphilis were treated. The medical officers attributed some of the rise in numbers to the growing reputation of the workhouse infirmary among the poor for treating disease and to the admission of significant numbers of sick paupers from rural areas of the country.[4] They estimated that there were 1,195 patients in the workhouse needing treatment. The diseases from which they suffered included dysentery, fever, syphilis, ophthalmia, chest infections and influenza. In response to a request by the medical officers, an additional physician and apothecary were employed on a temporary basis to help with the workload.[5] There was keen competition for these posts. Lombe Atthill, who later became a distinguished master of the Rotunda Hospital, was one of the candidates for the post of physician. He described the process of election in his memoirs, *Recollections of an Irish doctor*:

> In this instance, as, indeed, in all others in Ireland, religion and politics played an important part in the election. There were some twenty or more candidates, and there were consequently several rounds of voting, those candidates who obtained the fewest votes being on each occasion thrown out, till their number was reduced to three, namely, a Roman Catholic gentleman, a Nonconformist, and myself. Hitherto, I had on each occasion headed the list, and did so on the semi-final round, when the Roman Catholic, having obtained the fewest votes, was thrown out; and I, turning to him asked, 'Who will your friends now vote for?' He replied, 'Against you, as you are the Conservative candidate,' which, in truth, I was not, the result being that I was defeated by just one vote.[6]

At the same meeting that appointed the extra medical officer the board discussed the expenditure on medication. In order to control this expenditure they decided to draw up a dispensary or formulary for the use of the workhouse and ordered 'that no medicine but those entered in this dispensary be allowed, except on special requisition of one of the medical officers to the board stating the disease and why the medicine is required'.[7] This was the first hospital formulary to be used in the workhouse infirmary.

Emigration

The board of guardians had been giving financial assistance to those wishing to emigrate from the country since 1844 and in 1848, in common with other workhouses, they began to promote the emigration of healthy inmates. In the same year, emigration was encouraged by new regulations jointly agreed between the poor law commissioners and the emigration commissioners. The assistant master was asked to draw up a list of 200 able-bodied female paupers between the ages of 16 and 26 who might be suitable for emigration.[8] Under the scheme, orphaned girls were recruited from all the workhouses in Ireland between May 1848 and April 1850. In the first two years, 4,175 girls left Ireland in twenty ships for Australia, the majority disembarking at Sydney, Port Philip and Adelaide.[9] Fifty-six of these girls were selected from the South Dublin Union.[10]

A growing number of the male and female inmates in the South Dublin Union began to see emigration to the United States, Canada or Australia as the best chance of starting a new life. The board of guardians was prepared to fund the passage of selected inmates and in 1851 they appointed an emigration committee to oversee the selection process. This committee examined 776 inmates who had applied to emigrate and of these they considered 377 suitable. These consisted of 148 male emigrants for New York and Quebec, 50 young females for Australia and 179 females for New York

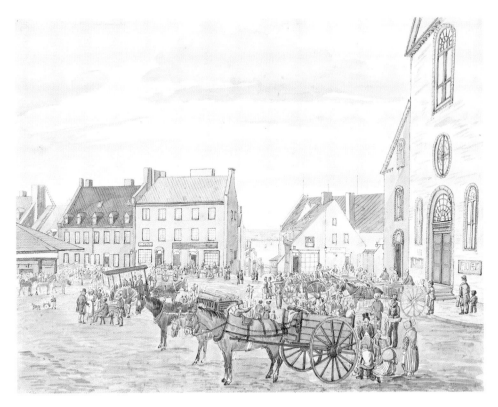

6.1 'Quebec Market Place, 26 June 1829', by James Pattison Cockburn. Library and Archives Canada, Peter Winkworth Collection of Canadiana, e000756729. Courtesy of the National Archives of Canada.

and Quebec.[11] Some of those who were not selected decided to opt for drastic measures to achieve their aims. In June 1852, a wardmaster, on seeing smoke, found four women setting fire to a sheet, and to a bedtick and bolster, which were filled with straw. The women had planned to set fire to part of the workhouse in order to precipitate their arrest and transportation.[12]

Another 200 healthy females were sent to Canada in the summer of 1854. Further group emigrations were arranged during the decades that followed although the numbers selected were smaller. The great majority were female and they were sent to Canada.[13] Most of these women had to accept menial and badly paid positions as maids.[14] A group of specially selected women were sent out in 1866, and these fared better. Alexander Buchanan, the chief emigrant agent at Quebec, wrote:

Thirteen servant maids arrived here that had been sent out by the South Dublin Union; they were disposed of at once, most advantageously. They seemed to be, and have proved themselves, a most respectable lot of girls, and as they were accustomed to the general duties of house service, they had no difficulty in procuring ready employment. If you can aid in obtaining a further supply of such girls for next season, you would confer a favor on the inhabitants of this city.[15]

Between 1871 and 1874, 40 women were sent to Canada from the South Dublin Union and in the early 1880s, when the economic situation deteriorated in Ireland, another 147 women and 77 men were also sent to Canada. They were very carefully selected by a committee of the guardians, aided by the doctors and chaplains, and all found employment as soon as they arrived in Canada.[16] Mr Bryan, the master's clerk, accompanied one group on the journey in 1882, and he sent a letter to the board on his arrival in Canada:

> Just arrived here, all well, any amount of men wanted. One looking for 200 railway workers – our boys, except Keegan, are going to Peterboro for some work at one dollar, forty cents per day and a guarantee of winter work or a forfeit of one hundred dollars to each man.[17]

When Bryan returned to Dublin, his report on the journey to the board of guardians was equally enthusiastic and he stressed the potential of Canada as a land of opportunity for emigrants.[18] A number of those who emigrated left children behind them in the workhouse with the intention of sending for them later when they were established in an occupation. Some parents sent the full fare for tickets for their children while others sent less and appealed to the guardians for a supplement, which was usually granted.[19]

'A vast hospital'

Emigration made very little impact on the numbers in the South Dublin Union, and the places vacated were soon filled. By February 1852, there were 3,500 inmates and the wards and dormitories were overcrowded, with two women sharing each bed in the sick wards and three sharing a bed in the healthy wards.[20] However, when the medical officers requested that the employment of William Moss, who was assisting them on a temporary basis, should be continued for another month, the request was refused. The doctors appealed the decision, stating:

> This institution is now a vast hospital containing a larger number of cases of acute and chronic medical and surgical diseases than has ever before been collected within the walls of a Dublin hospital.[21]

They pointed out that in Dublin voluntary hospitals, such as the Meath, Dr Steevens' and the Richmond, the number of patients under the care of an individual medical officer varied from twenty-six to sixty and that these hospitals also had resident pupils, clinical clerks and paid nurses to assist the physicians and surgeons. They further reported that the former prejudice against the workhouse had ceased among poor people and that many now entered the institution 'for the sole purpose of obtaining hospital relief'.

The board was unmoved by their appeal and instead inquired into the number of hours that the physician and surgeon were spending in the hospital. They found that Mayne spent 15 hours and 15 minutes each week in the hospital, according to the porter's book, and Shannon spent 12 hours and 15 minutes. The guardians again refused to appoint more medical staff and stipulated that the average daily attendance of medical officers, Sundays included, should be above 6 hours.[22] The doctors responded:

> The labour of investigating disease soon exhausts the energies of the most diligent physician – to treat it successfully the symptoms must be traced to their source – and to do this effectively requires a vigorous exercise of the mind – the true criteria of a physician's labour is the nature and the number of cases to which he applies his mind ...[23]

The medical officers approached the board again a few months later, drawing attention to their ever-increasing workload:

> The workhouse has become a monster hospital. Many of the patients labour under diseases which demand the closest attention – and public opinion requires to be satisfied that this attention is paid to them. During the past winter the medical officers were examined on oath as to the treatment of three patients who had long before passed from under their observation – and at the present, an enquiry is pending touching the particulars of others. To such enquiries the physician has no just reason to object but he cannot be prepared to answer them should too many patients be committed to his charge.[24]

Support for voluntary hospitals

During the eighteenth century a number of voluntary hospitals were established in Dublin to care for the poor. These relied largely on donations and were independent of government control, although they received some financial support from the government in the form of grants. In the early 1850s, the government declared its intent to withdraw parliamentary grants gradually from the voluntary hospitals and to place them under the jurisdiction of the poor law commissioners. The guardians of the workhouse realized that this could put extra pressure on them to provide for the sick poor so they involved themselves, together with the voluntary hospitals, in intense political lobbying to reverse the government's position.[25] There was also a threat to close the Royal Hospital Kilmainham, which provided accommodation for old soldiers. Again the guardians realized that the closure of this hospital would place increasing demands on the workhouse, so they petitioned parliament to keep the hospital open and the petition was successful.[26]

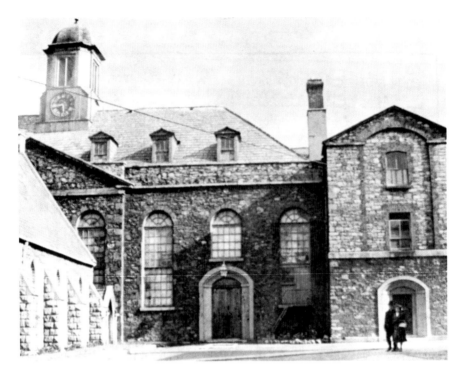

6.2   The front of the dining hall, with the Church of Ireland chapel that was built onto the façade on the left. Photograph c.1940s. Private collection.

Sectarian system

The workhouse of the South Dublin Union was run along strict sectarian lines at this time. There was separate accommodation for Catholics and Protestants, with separate hospitals and wards, and separate workrooms in the schools.[27] Over subsequent years there were regular disputes, often over trivial matters, between the Roman Catholic and the Church of Ireland chaplains, and they frequently wrote to the board of guardians complaining about each other's activities. The use of the church, designed by Francis Johnston, was also a source of great dispute between the chaplains. In 1863, it was decided that a new church for the Church of Ireland would be built in front of the dining hall and connected to it at the main entrance. This was an act of architectural vandalism as it effectively destroyed the façade of the dining hall.[28]

Clogs and straw mattresses

The inmates wore clogs as part of an economy measure. The medical officers objected to their use by infirm and weak patients, as they claimed that they caused many accidents. As a result the use of clogs was discontinued for this group.[29] Straw or coconut fibre was used as bedding and was usually infested with fleas. In the healthy wards the straw was changed every three months, in the sick and infirm wards it was changed more frequently and it was also changed following usage by patients suffering from infectious diseases and after all deaths.[30] Some armchairs were acquired in 1857 'for the paralytic and otherwise disabled patients so that they may be occasionally refreshed by being enabled to sit up from bed'.[31]

The erection of a ship's mast

During 1853, three independent assessments of the South Dublin Union were carried out by external visitors. These reports commented favourably on the management and cleanliness of the workhouse. The most significant visit was the one undertaken by George Nicholls in September 1853. Nicholls, who wrote the initial blueprint for the workhouse system in Ireland, carried out an exacting inspection and afterwards expressed satisfaction with what he saw. He suggested that more of the able-bodied young men and women in the workhouse should be considered for emigration. He also suggested that a ship's mast should be erected in the grounds of the South Dublin Union to provide some of the boys with sailing skills. The guardians were enthusiastic about the latter suggestion and they ordered the erection of a mast.[32] A career at sea or enlistment in the army were options for the male inmates, and recruiting agents visited the Union from time to time.[33] The guardians leased a farm in Inchicore so that boys could be trained in agriculture.[34]

Further plans for expansion

There was great pressure on space in the workhouse because of the social distress and poverty that followed the Famine and the number of inmates climbed steadily, exceeding 4,000 for the first time in early 1854.[35] The children's wards were greatly overcrowded. There was a total of 120 beds to accommodate 192 sick children, and 17 nurses and wardmaids.[36] One of the measures taken to alleviate the overcrowding was to convert Johnston's infirmary (now Hospital 1), which was being used as a general infirmary, back to its original purpose as a hospital for children. At the beginning of 1854, the dining hall of the workhouse was converted into a dormitory as a temporary measure, with two tiers of beds accommodating 292 inmates.[37] A special committee was set up to consider extending accommodation within the workhouse and it reported in January 1854. Among the committee's proposals was the erection of a general hospital, distinct from the other buildings and capable of accommodating 800 patients. This was the first proposal to build a general hospital in the grounds. The committee also proposed extending the accommodation for the inmates of the workhouse, including the children.[38] George Wilkinson, the architect, was asked to draw up plans for buildings that would be suitable for the accommodation of 800 to

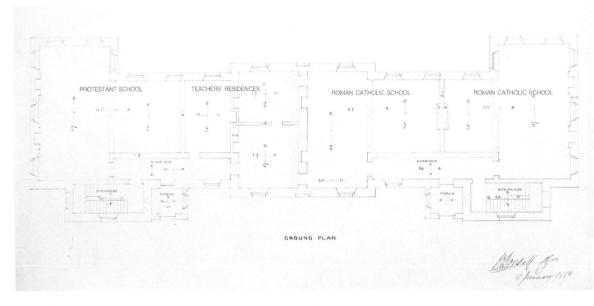

PROTESTANT SCHOOL TEACHERS' RESIDENCES ROMAN CATHOLIC SCHOOL ROMAN CATHOLIC SCHOOL

GROUND PLAN

6.3   Ground-floor plan of the school that was opened in 1860 (now Hospital 2). Reproduced from the RIAI Murray Collection with permission of the Irish Architectural Archive.

1,000 extra inmates. Wilkinson presented his plans to the building committee of the board of guardians in early April. His design for a building in stone with a lining of brick allowed for the accommodation of 500 infirm paupers or 800 to 1,000 healthy paupers.[39] These buildings were erected on the southern grounds of the workhouse and have since been demolished.

In 1857, the board acquired five acres of land adjacent to the South Dublin Union, known as the 'orchard ground', for the purpose of building an auxiliary workhouse. Work began on the erection of new school buildings for the children in 1859. One of these school buildings is still extant on the grounds of St James's Hospital and is currently known as Hospital 2. It was built on the workhouse burial ground, which was located directly east of the infirmary, and was opened in 1862. It provided class-room faculties for Catholic and Protestant children of both sexes on the ground floor, together with dormitory accommodation on the first and second floors. Mornings in the new schools were devoted to study and the afternoons to industrial pursuits and exercise.[40] Boys were trained as shoemakers, weavers, tailors, carpenters and bakers, and girls received training in embroidery, knitting and domestic duties.

The capstan mill

The South Dublin Union, in common with a number of other Irish workhouses, installed a capstan mill for grinding corn. The mill was modelled on a ship's capstan

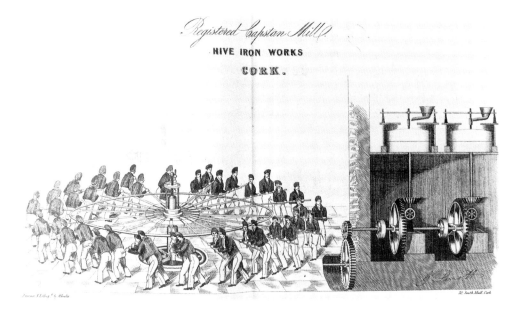

6.4   A capstan mill. These human-powered mills were used to grind corn. Poor law commissioners, letters to James Burke, 1848. Courtesy of the National Archives of Ireland.

for winding the cable of the anchor and could employ as many as one hundred people at one time. The inmates walked around in a circle for hours pushing the wheel that worked the mill. The work was very monotonous and dangerous and if someone fell they could be trampled on. The mill was designed to provide repetitive and tedious work for able-bodied males but in the workhouse of the South Dublin Union it was also worked by females. This practice created adverse publicity for the guardians and they were accused in *The Nation* in April 1851 of having 'eight hundred fine young women in the South Dublin Union, for whom they had nothing better to do than turn a capstan, or great horse-mill which grinds their corn ...'[41] The issue was also raised in the house of commons by an Irish MP, Francis Scully, who said that working a capstan mill was 'a kind of employment on which it was disgraceful to have women employed, one that tended to make them lose all self-respect and correct moral feeling'.[42] James Kavanagh, chief inspector with the board of national education, objected strongly to the use of women and children to drive these mills:

> In the South Dublin Union the master brought me into the capstan room, and working the mill were some 150 women, many of whom, he stated, were girls of the town, and these mixed up between the same spokes for hours with, doubtless, many virtuous females.[43]

The poor law inspector for the South Dublin Union responded by claiming that only females of 'bad character' worked on the capstan mill.[44] In spite of this defence, Kava-

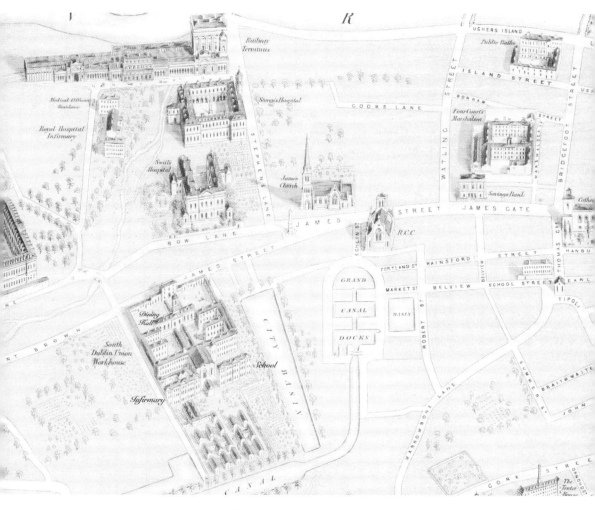

6.5 Section of the 1861 map of Dublin by the land surveyor Daniel Heffernan, showing the South Dublin Union. Annotations have been added to indicate the positions of the dining hall, the infirmary (now Hospital 1) and the school (now Hospital 2). Reproduced, with permission, from N. Marnham, 'Daniel Edward Heffernan's map of Dublin 1861', *Architecture Ireland*, 18 June 2016.

nagh's criticism appears to have hit home, as the capstan mill was abandoned in workhouses after 1855.

The problem of women of 'bad character' mixing with young adolescent girls was raised by concerned individuals from time to time. It was claimed that pressure was being exerted on the young women to become prostitutes, and an inquiry by the poor law commissioners in 1855 found some evidence that girls in the South Dublin Union were being encouraged to take up prostitution by women of 'bad character'.[45]

Inmate insubordination

Disorderly behavior, particularly among the female inmates, was a recurrent problem for the authorities at this time. On one occasion four women dressed themselves in male attire having obtained the clothes from the tailor by force. They then found a way out onto the roof of the day rooms and smashed a great quantity of slates by dancing on them.[46] Shortly after this event there was a major riot when twenty female inmates climbed onto a roof and it took a combined force of workhouse officers and eight policemen to get them down. As with previous episodes, the guardians attributed the gross misbehaviour to a desire to be convicted and transported to the colonies where they might have a better life.

Desperate to find a solution to the unruly behaviour, in 1857 the guardians acquired a large building, formerly Boylan's Factory, which adjoined the national schools under the care of the Sisters of Mercy in Baggot Street. It was to be used as an auxiliary workhouse for females under the supervision of the Sisters of Mercy, who would be accountable to the board of guardians.[47] The nuns wished to take girls from the workhouse whom they believed had a reasonable chance of reforming, but the guardians insisted on sending them the most refractory girls. The nuns could not control their charges and as a result the girls managed to destroy the Baggot Street clothing stock. It was apparent to all that the experiment was not a success, so the auxiliary workhouse in Baggot Street, which had opened in 1857, was closed in 1860, and the girls were readmitted to the South Dublin Union.[48]

Episodes of arson in the South Dublin Union in the early 1860s led to the purchase of a fire engine, and the open fireplaces in many of the wards and dormitories were replaced by hot-air pipes.[49] In an attempt to control disruptive behaviour, the most disorderly women were isolated in a dormitory of their own. This measure was not successful, and there were further outbreaks of fire in the main dormitories. The board of guardians appealed to the police commissioners for assistance. They responded by placing six constables and a sergeant in the grounds of the workhouse each night to preserve order. The master was also empowered by the board of guardians to employ six or more night watchmen.[50] Arsonists who were apprehended were treated severely: three young girls who were caught trying to set fire to their beds in 1859 were sentenced to penal servitude for three years.[51] Two men were sentenced in 1863 to four years penal servitude for setting fire to their dormitory.[52]

A parliamentary committee in 1861 found that a total of 495 young girls from the South Dublin Union had been sentenced to imprisonment between January 1850 and May 1861. The offences listed included riotous behaviour, damaging property, stealing and arson.[53] The superintendent of Mountjoy Female Convict Prison observed that the most difficult prisoners that she had to cope with were women who had been reared in the workhouse of the South Dublin Union:

[T]hey seem to be amenable to no persuasion, advice or punishment. When they are corrected, even in the mildest manner, for any breach of regulations, they seem to lose all control of reason – they break the windows of their cells, tear up their bedding ... Their language, while in this state of excitement, is absolutely shocking. They are not at all deficient in intelligence or capacity for better things. They learn quite as quickly, perhaps more quickly than the average prisoners, and when in school are generally very attentive.[54]

A riot in the dining hall

A riot in the dining hall of the South Dublin Union in April 1860 attracted considerable publicity. The matron of the workhouse, Jane Dollard, suspected that some of the young women were stealing clothes from the laundry, so she instructed the female officers to search the women as they left the dining hall after breakfast. She left the hall and the master and assistant master supervised the search. The young women objected to being searched in front of men, and matters soon escalated from vocal to physical resistance. The master later gave his version of what ensued in a report to the board of guardians:

> On the search having been gone through for a few minutes by the female officers, the junior girls commenced yelling, cheering and using threatening language. I ordered one to be removed from the hall, for violent disorderly conduct, but she having resisted, and the others having shown a riotous disposition, I was obliged to send for all the officers of the house to keep order. Immediately when they entered, a soda water bottle was thrown at me, and platters and stirabout at the other officers ...[55]

The master reported that he sent for the police and that seven girls were arrested and charged with disorderly behaviour.

The Catholic chaplain, Revd Prideaux Fox, gave a different version of the events when the girls appeared before a magistrate. Fox was a member of the Oblate order and had been appointed chaplain to the workhouse in May 1858 by the archbishop of Dublin, Paul Cullen. He said that he saw everything that happened from a window in the room of James Grant, the medical officer, which overlooked the dining hall. He claimed the male officers behaved disgracefully, searching women and lifting up their clothes, and Grant, who was watching with him, said it was scandalous. Fox described in detail what he saw:

> When I looked out of the window I saw a great many female inmates, most of whom appeared to be in the greatest possible confusion ... Several younger female inmates were in the body of the hall, and were being chased in all directions by several of the male officers – the master standing in the midst of all. Immediately after I first looked out of the window, I saw two females down on the ground. One of them I saw thrown down, but I did not see by whom. One of these girls had

three male officers engaged in searching her ...
I saw them throw her clothes completely over
her head, and turn them down again one by
one. The turning up of the clothes caused a
complete exposure of the person.[56]

Fox's account of the incident was consistent
with the evidence given by the girls who nevertheless were all sent to jail; three of them for
fourteen days and the others for forty-eight
hours. They would have received much harsher
sentences had Fox not testified on their behalf.
The poor law commissioners did not approve of
the priest's behaviour. They subsequently claimed
that he had undermined the authority of the
master and wrote to him demanding his resignation as chaplain to the South Dublin Union.
Archbishop Cullen gave Fox his full support and,
surprisingly, the board of guardians was also supportive, acknowledging that Fox was a diligent
chaplain. However, the poor law commissioners

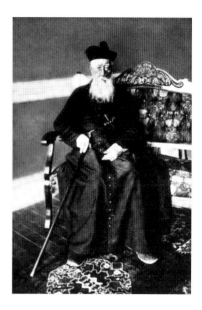

6.6   Revd Prideaux Fox, shortly
before his death in 1905 at the Oblate
Novitiate in Tewksbury, MA, US.
Donahoe's Magazine 53 (1905).

proceeded with his dismissal. Cullen refused to replace him and the priest continued
to visit patients in the workhouse in an unofficial capacity. This infuriated the master
and, despite their earlier support, the board of guardians issued an order preventing
Fox from carrying out any priestly function in the institution. The treatment of Fox
now became a public and political issue. In August 1860 it was the subject of debate
in the house of commons in Westminster when several Irish members, including Isaac
Butt, strongly supported the chaplain.[57] The lord lieutenant was forced to intervene
and Fox was reinstated as chaplain.

Fox continued to serve in the post until October 1861. He was subsequently based
at the Glencree Reformatory in the Wicklow mountains, which was run by the Oblate
order. There he was befriended by Jane Wilde (Speranza), who was holidaying in the
Glencree valley with her sons Oscar and William. She asked Fox to baptise her two
sons as Catholics, and he consented. In later life, Oscar Wilde told friends that he had
a clear recollection of being baptised a Catholic when he was a child.[58]

Fox was replaced in the South Dublin Union by Revd John Carr, a Carmelite from
Whitefriar Street. This was the beginning of the Carmelite ministry to the institution, which lasted until 2001.[59] Carr was to give twenty-two years of service as chaplain. During this time he 'was the uncompromising advocate of the poor and fought
constantly against the physical and moral degradation to which the inmates were
exposed'.[60]

Changing patterns of admission

From the mid 1850s, the numbers of healthy men and women inmates in the South Dublin Union began to fall gradually.[61] The total number of inmates had fallen to 2,155 by December 1859 and the turnover was fairly rapid. This was a result of improved conditions throughout the country and of continuing emigration after the Famine. In 1861, one-third left within two weeks of admission and a little over two-thirds spent less than two months in the workhouse.[62] There was, however, a significant rate of readmission. The 'family test' was never implemented with great enthusiasm in the South Dublin Union and in 1860 the poor law commissioners admitted that the test was a mistaken policy. They went on to state that when the head of a household or any of his dependents needed hospitalization in the workhouse hospital there was no need for other members of the family to be admitted to the workhouse as well. This ruling undermined the 'family test' even further.

About 11 per cent of the women under the age of 50 living in the workhouse of the South Dublin Union on 1 January 1854 were unmarried mothers. Under the provisions of the Irish Poor Relief Act 1838, the mother was responsible for the support of any illegitimate children up to the age of 15. The natural father had no responsibility to contribute to the upkeep of the child. The lack of support for unmarried mothers and the social ostracism meant that many of them went into workhouses to have their children.

Compulsory repatriation of Irish paupers from England

Many of the inmates of the South Dublin Union had been repatriated from England and Scotland to Ireland. Legislation in England and Scotland empowered the authorities to send Irish-born paupers back to Ireland if they applied for relief. Between 1854 and 1858 nearly 6,000 paupers who had been born in Ireland were transferred from England and Scotland to Ireland.[63] Many of these were in very poor physical health when they arrived in Dublin and they were admitted to the South Dublin Union. This was a source of great annoyance to the board of guardians and they made several appeals to parliament to have the process stopped. In 1861, the legislation that empowered this activity was amended and Irish paupers who had been living within an English union for three years could not be removed from that union and were entitled to relief there. However, this law was not strictly adhered to and significant numbers were still transferred, largely from London and Liverpool.

Expanding role of the workhouse hospital

The Medical Charities Act (1851) provided for a greatly increased number of dispensaries and dispensary doctors throughout Ireland. The management of these dispensaries was placed under the aegis of the poor law and a medical commissioner, John

McDonnell, was added to the poor law commissioners. McDonnell is remembered in medical history as the surgeon who performed the first operation under anaesthesia in Ireland in 1847.[64] Each union was divided into dispensary districts and a doctor was appointed to each dispensary. There were fifteen doctors in the dispensary districts of the South Dublin Union at the close of 1851. From 1859, midwives were also appointed to dispensary areas.[65]

Following the establishment of the dispensary system, dispensary doctors began to admit poor, but not necessarily destitute, acutely ill patients to the workhouse infirmaries. This was recognized in 1854 when the poor law commissioners opened the workhouse hospitals to the 'sick poor', the constabulary and domestic servants. This policy was enshrined in law in the Poor Law Amendment Act of 1862. These developments signalled very clearly that the state was moving away from a laissez-faire policy to direct involvement in the provision of health services. This was a very significant landmark in the country's social and medical history, but it has received scant notice in most medical histories of the country.

During the 1860s the number of inmates in the workhouse began to climb again and a census carried out in February 1865 showed that of 3,585 inmates in the workhouse, 2,050 were sick, while only 448 were classified as able-bodied. There were nearly 700 children, 252 infirm and older people, and 168 mentally ill.[66] Although there was separate provision for the mentally ill in Dublin institutions such as the Richmond Asylum and St Patrick's Hospital, some of these patients were still housed in the South Dublin Union.

The physician Robert Mayne and the surgeon Peter Shannon wrote a long letter to the board in June 1861 about the increasing number of patients in the institution. The letter is of particular interest as it describes how the doctors organized their work:

All the acute cases are placed in the hospital wards. These latter are visited by us, daily, so that all the acute cases are seen, and if need be, prescribed for every day. We sometimes even return to the workhouse in the evening, should a particular case require a second visit.

Of the chronic and incurable cases, the most serious are placed in wards which are also visited by us daily. Such of the chronic and incurable cases as require daily attendance, are thus prescribed for daily ...

The infirm patients occupy wards which are visited by us at different intervals ... Should any of these patients however become unwell in the intervals between our visits they are either immediately transferred to the hospital wards, or to the chronic wards, or they are visited by the resident apothecary should the physician or surgeon be absent, or by ourselves should we be on the premises at the time ...

To ensure the proper classification of the patients the surgeon or the physician, at their morning visit inspect every pauper admitted into the workhouse during the preceding 24 hours, and order them to the proper departments; they also hold a dispensary, at which any new cases of sickness arising amongst the inmates are disposed of, and, if necessary, prescribed for ...[67]

Death of Robert Mayne

Mayne resigned in November 1861 and the guardians at their meeting of 14 November 1861 paid the following tribute to him:

> Upon a review of his connexion of nearly 17 years with this board we unanimously testify that his services have been uniformly marked by efficient and kind attention to the sick, and that we cannot refer to a single instance in the official connexion of Dr Mayne with this workhouse except honourable to him and satisfactory to the Board.[68]

Mayne did not live long after his resignation from the South Dublin Union. He died from typhus fever in 1864, aged 53. He was president of the Pathological Society of Dublin at the time of his death. Mayne was very unassuming and, according to the author of his obituary notice in the *Dublin Journal of Medical Science*, 'he had withal a modesty which shrunk from any display, and, in all probability, he was himself the only one in the profession who did not clearly see how really eminent he had become'.[69] He was the first doctor with a significant academic reputation to work on the St James's Hospital site.[70] His portrait hangs in the Royal College of Physicians of Ireland and there is a monument to his memory in St Patrick's cathedral. The Robert Mayne Day Hospital, which was built as part of the first phase of St James's Hospital in the 1980s, is named in his honour.

Mayne was succeeded as visiting physician by Wensley Bond Jennings. Jennings was born in Rosscarbery, Co. Cork, in 1822. He graduated BA from Trinity College in 1845 and was subsequently awarded an MD. He studied medicine at the Carmichael School and was awarded licentiates by the College of Physicians and by the RCSI. He was subsequently elected fellow of the College of Physicians in 1861. He was a member of the Dublin Pathological Society and presented cases to the society. Throughout his career Jennings contributed papers on obstetrical subjects to the *Dublin Journal of Medical Science*. He was appointed lecturer in midwifery to the Carmichael School in 1862. He had a practice, first in Gardiner Place and then in Merrion Square.[71]

The impact of the medical officers

The medical officers wrote again to the board of guardians outlining their considerable workload in September 1865. They pointed out that the workhouse hospital, which combined medical, surgical and midwifery work, was a hospital in the 'full and true acceptance of the term'. They said that this had occurred because:

daily experience has disabused the minds of the poor of many of the prejudices that once existed against these institutions, and while formerly none, save the aged, decrepit and dying applied for admission, at present on the contrary, cases of the most acute and urgent nature, daily here seek relief with the view of returning when convalescent, to their various employments.[72]

The board of guardians finally agreed to a third medical officer on a permanent basis in October 1866 and appointed Joseph Byrne.[73] The three medical officers, Shannon, Jennings and Byrne, divided the care of the wards, as well as the male and female dispensaries in the workhouse, between them.[74] Shannon, the first surgeon to be appointed to the South Dublin Union, continued to work in the institution until 1878, when he resigned on grounds of ill health after thirty-nine years of service.[75]

A special commission of guardians was appointed in May 1870 to report on the duties of the medical officers. They found that the wards were clean and well ventilated and that the patients were happy with the medical care which they received. They found that 'the infirm in body or mind of each sex are properly attended to and more particularly the male and female lunatic departments which are kept in a state of great order and cleanliness'.[76] At this time there were 1,336 sick patients under the care of the three medical officers. Their report concluded that the medical officers 'are kind, humane and most skilful in the discharge of their duties'.[77] They also observed that the medical officers were prompt in their attendance when patients became acutely ill at night.

This praise of the conditions in the workhouse is supported by entries in the visitors' book at the workhouse between the years 1864–6, as the following selection exemplifies:

> **Dr Rochel: (September 23rd, 1864)** I received much attention from the Master of this establishment, which is admirably arranged in its various departments, and it is with much pleasure that I inspected it. (Petersburg)
>
> **David Greig: (May 20th, 1865)** All the departments of the house extremely clean, neat, and orderly. (One of the Acting Committee of Cuthbert's Workhouse, Edinburgh)
>
> **Maria S. Rye: (September 17th, 1866)** Have visited the female wards of this union, and am much pleased with the cleanliness of the whole, the quality of the food, but especially with the garden and wards belonging to the lunatics. I have seen nothing like it in any of my visits anywhere. (London)[78]

The hospitals, wards and schools were visited by some members of the board each week. They also made unscheduled visits to make sure that the standards were maintained at all times.

Towards the end of 1877 the doctors were asked to prepare a report for the board of guardians on the use of 'stimulants' in the hospitals. Shannon pointed out that

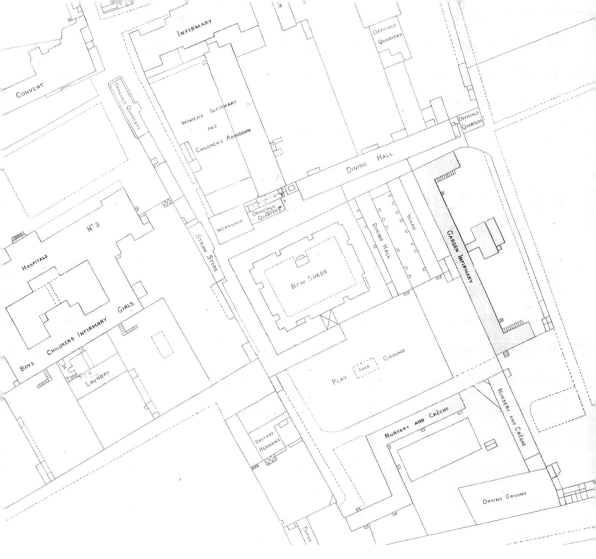

6.7 A section of the map made by the architect J.J. Inglis in 1911, showing the position of the Garden Infirmary (later known as Hospital 4) in the south-east section of the workhouse. Photograph: Anthony Edwards. Reproduced with permission of St James's Hospital.

porter was the only stimulant whose usage was increasing. They attributed this to the greater numbers of chronic and convalescent patients under their care. Byrne agreed and also gave reasons for the increase:

> the asthenic character of the diseases render[s] the administration of more stimulants necessary for the recovery of the patients and ... it would not be desirable in the treatment of the sick and infirm to be restrained with reference to the prescribing of stimulants where he deems it necessary to save or prolong human life.[79]

The guardians were very zealous in controlling the number of visitors to the institution, and at a meeting in February 1875 the following order was given:

That in future no persons (visitors) be admitted on Sundays and on other days, no passes be admitted containing more than the name of one person as visitor. No person shall be admitted at any time upon a pass unless same shall be signed in the genuine and proper handwriting of a guardian. This order not to prohibit the master from admitting a visitor to see any inmate upon any sudden or urgent necessity.[80]

In the mid 1870s, new structures were erected for 'probationary wards', dormitories, officers' apartments and an administrative area fronting James's Street. The development included a new arched entrance. These buildings would remain in place until they were demolished in the mid 1950s as part of the development of St Kevin's Hospital. A building was also erected around 1880 in the 'garden' to provide dormitories and this structure, currently named Hospital 4, became known as the 'Garden Infirmary'.

The challenge of epidemic diseases

Epidemic diseases remained a constant threat throughout the nineteenth century. The Poor Law Amendment Act of 1862 extended the powers of the guardians so that they could treat fever patients who were not destitute in workhouse hospitals. There was another epidemic of cholera in the summer of 1866. Additional sheds were erected adjoining the auxiliary workhouse at Kilmainham, and a doctor was appointed to look after the cholera victims in these sheds. The board of guardians also began negotiations with the voluntary hospitals, seeking their help. Sir Patrick Dun's Hospital agreed to take about twenty patients, and it received two shillings per day for each patient from the board of guardians.[81] The Meath Hospital, the Mater Hospital and the Hardwicke Hospital also agreed to take cholera patients.[82] It was six months before the epidemic abated and in that time there were almost a thousand deaths in Dublin.[83]

The cholera epidemic was followed five years later by an epidemic of smallpox in the city. As in the case of the cholera epidemic, the victims were housed in the sheds near the auxiliary workhouse.[84] Initially the smallpox unit housed twenty-seven patients but it had to be expanded as the epidemic continued into the winter of 1871. Two doctors were appointed to care for the patients as the number of cases increased, rising to over a hundred in January 1872. The fever sheds proved to be inadequate for the numbers of patients and in March part of the chapel was used as additional accommodation. There were more than 12,000 cases of smallpox in the city with nearly 1,100 fatalities.[85] There was another outbreak of smallpox in 1878 but the epidemic affected fewer people and the fever sheds were used to accommodate victims. Isolation was not strictly enforced and there were complaints that patients with smallpox were frequently seen drinking whiskey and porter in nearby fields. They were also seen going out into the streets and returning later in the evening. The guardians responded to these complaints by erecting a twelve-foot-high fence and employing a watchman.[86] There were ninety-two cases of smallpox in the fever sheds in February 1879, but a year later the number had dropped to forty.[87] The smallpox unit was closed in December 1880 as it was estimated that the fever hospitals could cope with any further cases arising in the city.[88] This was the last major epidemic of smallpox in Ireland.

Fever patients were under the care of the physician Edward Byrne, a brother of the medical officer, Joseph Byrne. The patients were nursed by pauper inmates, who were at great risk of potentially fatal infection. Alcohol was used as a stimulant for the fever patients and the medical officers also prescribed dry tea and sugar so that fresh tea could be made for them rather than the pre-made or 'cooked' tea that was given to everyone else. Dry tea and sugar were also given to the attendants who cared for the sick and was justified on the basis that they worked very hard. When the guardians objected to this practice, claiming it was open to abuse, the medical officers responded with a strong letter emphasizing that the attendants needed more sustenance than the standard workhouse diet and outlining the possible consequences of a negative response from the board of guardians: 'If our ordering extras for those in attendance upon the sick be interfered with, it will be necessary in order to secure proper nursing to appoint at least ten additional paid nurses for our department.'[89]

Their appeal was rejected and the doctors were not able to enforce their demand for extra nurses. Edward Byrne wrote again in May 1879, stating the great risks to which these inmate attendants were exposed:

> I beg to say that I have had several instances of sick attendants contracting the disease in the smallpox hospital, three of which cases ended fatally; that two of the attendants in the fever hospital were buried on the 6th inst, having died from typhus fever contracted in the discharge of their duty and I have others at present incubating the disease.[90]

The board finally acquiesced and gave permission to supply an extra allowance of tea and sugar to the attendants. Within two weeks of his letter, Edward Byrne himself contracted enteric fever and was in a critical condition. The board received a letter from Joseph Byrne requesting leave of absence to care for his brother. Edward Byrne gradually improved and returned to work two months later. Other members of staff who interacted with infectious patients were not so fortunate. Revd Brandon, the Protestant chaplain, died of scarlatina in 1866 and the master of the workhouse, John Hornidge, died from typhus fever in 1871.[91] In 1882, the board decided to close all the fever sheds at Kilmainham and to transfer the fever patients to Cork Street Fever Hospital. After disinfection, the sheds were used as accommodation for infirm women.[92]

First clinical examinations

The board of guardians received a request from the Queen's University of Ireland in October 1869 seeking permission to examine students in the South Dublin Union for the diploma in medicine.[93] The board received a similar request in 1871 from James

Little, registrar of the College of Physicians, requesting permission for candidates for the licence to practise medicine to be examined in the workhouse infirmary. The board of guardians agreed to the requests 'subject only to the safeguards for the safety, comfort and regard of the feelings of the inmates of the workhouse infirmaries as our medical officers shall consider necessary in each case'.[94] These were the first clinical examinations to take place in the South Dublin Union. The registrar of Trinity College requested permission, in November 1890, to allow the surgeons Abraham Colles, Edward Halloran Bennett and Charles Bent Ball, to hold clinical examinations in the workhouse.[95]

The care of children

Joseph Byrne wrote a report in 1869 on the health of children, aged between 5 and 15 years, who had been admitted during the previous year. The total number of children admitted was 1,159, with a mortality of ten, which was less than one per cent, not withstanding the fact that there had been an epidemic of measles in the spring of that year and later one of whooping cough.[96] At this time infants were still being abandoned at or in the vicinity of the gate of the workhouse.[97] Deserted infants were also brought to the workhouse on a regular basis, most frequently by police officers.

As a result of the Irish Church Disestablishment Act 1869, it was no longer possible to register all abandoned infants as Protestants. From 1871 the religion of a deserted child was decided by the board of guardians. From then on, choosing a religion for an abandoned child led to frequent acrimonious debates at the meetings of the board of guardians. The Catholic chaplain was noted to have been 'undefatigable in assembling the Catholic guardians, in order to secure a majority whenever the religion of a child was to be decided by vote'.[98]

As the nineteenth century progressed, there was a growing realization that the workhouse was not a suitable environment for orphans and deserted children. Two philanthropic women, Ellen Woodlock and Sarah Atkinson, were absolutely convinced of this and in 1855 they established St Joseph's Industrial Institute in Richmond Road to take young teenage girls out of the South Dublin Union. Ellen Woodlock was the daughter of Martin Mahony, a woollen manufacturer in Blarney, Co. Cork, and a younger sister of Francis Sylvester Mahony, a writer who used the pseudonym 'Father Prout'. Sarah Atkinson was a well-known essayist who was born in Co. Roscommon. Woodlock and Atkinson planned to train the girls as domestic servants but this proved more difficult than they anticipated as the girls were already very institutionalized and as a result lacked both enthusiasm and initiative:

> [T]hey are so totally devoid of knowledge of the common things of life, that they
> make the effect at first of being completely deprived of ordinary intelligence. Most
> of them have never seen the interior of a dwelling-house, have never handled a

breakable article, or used a knife and fork; consequently they are so awkward, that they destroy a considerable amount of property ... one can imagine it would take a considerable time to train a cook who never saw a pot put on the fire, or beheld a whole joint of meat in its integrity.[99]

The staff at St Joseph's discovered that they had to begin by giving rudimentary lessons and then concentrate on each girl as an individual before any progress could be made. St Joseph's Institute became well respected as a model for the rescue of destitute girls but it had to close in the 1860s because of lack of funding. In 1872, Woodlock and Atkinson established a hospital for poor children, St Joseph's Infirmary for Children, at 9 Upper Buckingham Street. From 1876 it was run by the Irish Sisters of Charity and moved to a larger premises in Upper Temple Street in 1879 where it became known as Temple Street Hospital.[100]

Members of the Dublin Statistical Society, later renamed the Irish Statistical and Social Inquiry Society, were strong advocates of workhouse reform. The society took a particular interest in the plight of children and advocated a boarding-out system. A select committee of the house of commons was appointed in 1861 to inquire into the administration of the poor law in Ireland. It made a number of recommendations that were incorporated into the 1862 Poor Law Amendment Act. The act gave the board of guardians the legal authority of a parent in cases of orphaned or deserted children up to the age of 15 years. It also gave the board of guardians power to board these children, up to the age of 8, with families. The boarding-out programme for children was supervised by the guardians and it was classified as outdoor relief. Those willing to accept a child were paid £7 per year for a child aged under 1 year and £5 for an older child. Clothing was supplied for the child by the South Dublin Union and school fees were paid for older children. From time to time the children were brought before the guardians for inspection. This had the effect over time of shifting the care of these children into the community and out of the workhouse. The practice of boarding out became increasingly accepted as the best way of coping with deserted and orphaned children under 15 years.[101]

There were other developments in the second half of the nineteenth century that reduced the necessity to admit children requiring special care or supervision to the South Dublin Union. Several voluntary institutions were founded for the care of orphaned and deserted children and industrial schools were introduced to which children under 14 could be committed for a variety of reasons such as begging, being found guilty of minor offences and also for being without means of support.[102] The annual report of the poor law commissioners in 1864 suggested that those with intellectual disabilities should be supported by the poor law in special asylums. The first such institution, Stewart's Hospital in Dublin, was opened in 1869.

The board of guardians rented new buildings at Pelletstown on the Navan Road from the superioress of the Dominican Convent in Cabra in 1898. The buildings were used as a school for boys who were transferred from the workhouse. The experiment was a success and it became policy to keep children in accommodation outside the workhouse. The board of guardians bought the building and thirty-four attached acres from the nuns in 1900 with the intention of using it as a home for boys.

In 1872, the Local Government Board for Ireland was established. The board consisted of five members under the presidency of the chief secretary to the lord lieutenant. One member of the board had to be medically qualified. The board took over the functions of the poor law commissioners and remained the central authority for health services and local government until the 1920s.

Demand for salaried nurses

The increasing number of sick patients being admitted to the workhouse infirmary created a demand for better nursing and in particular for the employment of salaried nurses. The possession of a salary differentiated these nurses from pauper nurses. The adjective 'salaried' conveyed the idea of responsibility for carrying out the instructions of the doctors and for being kindly and attentive to the sick.[103] As the century progressed, it became increasingly apparent that nurses, like doctors, required systematic training, and nursing schools were created to meet this need. In 1890, a circular was sent by the Local Government Board to the boards of guardians 'urging the importance of trained and experienced nurses and pointing out that suffering is caused to the sick by the selection of incapable persons as nurses'.[104] The Local Government (Ireland) Act 1898 made it illegal to employ or use an untrained or uncertified person as a nurse.[105]

Supporting the destitute and sick poor

The recorder of Dublin, Sir Frederick Falkiner, speaking in 1881 observed, 'The current history of Dublin is a tale of two cities, a city of splendour and a city of squalor: diverse as the poles.'[106] During the nineteenth century Dublin had the highest mortality rate in the British Isles and one of the highest in Europe. William Wilde identified poverty, unemployment, overcrowding and unsanitary environments as the factors responsible for this. He demonstrated statistically, working on information from the 1841 and the 1851 censuses, that there was an unequivocal relationship between high mortality rates and bad housing. The average age of death in the better housing localities was 30–35 years while in the poorest areas the average age was 5–10 years. In most deprived areas over 60 per cent of children died before the age of 10.[107]

The South Dublin Union continued to play a significant role at times of social crisis in Dublin. There were very high levels of unemployment in the city in the late 1870s and considerable distress in many rural areas around the country. Many of those without work gravitated to Dublin where some of them helped to swell the numbers in the South Dublin Union. The Relief of Distress (Ireland) Act was passed in 1880 and this empowered unions to grant outdoor relief for a limited period to able-bodied men and their families. The relief was to be in the form of food and fuel and it was to be administered only by unions in the regions of greatest distress, which included the South Dublin Union.[108] The social historian Mary E. Daly has drawn attention to the increasingly significant role played by the South Dublin Union in the care of the sick poor towards the end of the nineteenth and beginning of the twentieth century. A study of the admissions to the workhouse in 1904 revealed that a total of 41.7 per cent of male admissions and 39 per cent of female admissions arrived with a medical recommendation. The diagnoses included injuries, rheumatism, debility and respiratory problems such as bronchitis, pneumonia and tuberculosis.[109] The South Dublin Union was serving a dual function as an infirmary for the sick poor and as a workhouse for the destitute. It would continue to fulfill both of these roles throughout the first 50 years of the twentieth century without adequate funding for either function.

7

The Mercy nuns and reform

The high grey walls of the workhouse shut out almost everything; they were a fortification against the life of the city, a barrier against time, which passed yet did not seem to pass. The visitors who came weekly were few; the inmates were many.[1]

There were complaints about the standard of care and nursing at the South Dublin Union in the latter years of the nineteenth century. It was alleged that the nurses were consuming 'medicinal comforts' prescribed for the sick and that property belonging to the institution was being stolen by members of the staff. The board of guardians was determined to raise standards by introducing appropriate reforms. Other workhouses, faced with similar challenges, had invited sisters belonging to religious orders to nurse their patients. It was fortunate for the South Dublin Union that the Mercy order had decided that the most appropriate way of celebrating its fiftieth anniversary was to devote itself 'to neglected patients of the South Dublin Workhouse Hospital'.[2] In 1880 a seven-member multidenominational committee, established by the guardians, visited workhouse hospitals around the country where religious sisters were employed as nurses.[3] The committee reported that all the workhouses where nuns had become involved as nurses had shown a dramatic improvement in standards.[4] A week later the board of guardians unanimously decided to appoint Catholic sisters to nurse Catholic inmates in the South Dublin Union Infirmary and to employ Protestant deaconesses as nurses on the Protestant wards.

The nuns and the South Dublin Union

Ten sisters of the order of the Sisters of Mercy were appointed as nurses at a salary of £30 per annum in November 1880. Two Protestant deaconesses were appointed from St Patrick's Nurses' Home in York Street,[5] which had been founded in 1876 by Amy Lee

Plunkett, wife of Archbishop Plunkett of Dublin. The institution trained general nurses to provide specialist home nursing for the poor.[6] Another deaconess from Dr Laseron's Evangelical Protestant Deaconesses Institution and Training Hospital in Tottenham Green, London, was appointed two weeks later.

The nuns took up duty on Monday 29 May 1881. Mother Walburga Grace and nine other Sisters of Mercy arrived at the South Dublin Union at 8:30 a.m. accompanied by Edward McCabe, the archbishop of Dublin. They were met by the chaplain, Revd John Carr, and by the master of the workhouse. The archbishop then presided over an inauguration ceremony that was of sufficient interest to be reported in the *London Tablet* on 4 June 1881. The writer described the occasion as:

> [A]n event that must forever be regarded as one of the most notable that have taken place in the life of that institution, and summer sun never shone on a more impressive spectacle than the function celebrated on Monday, by which those ladies were installed as nurses over some 900 of the poorest and most pitiable objects of human charity that one can look upon.[7]

The nuns face a challenge

The nuns, unlike the deaconesses, had no formal training in nursing, but they shared with them a determination to improve the sanitation and cleanliness of the wards and the nutrition and well-being of the patients. They were first accommodated in the female hospital, where the walls and floors were filthy and patients slept in verminous straw beds covered by sheets. The floor of the wards inclined towards a central channel running the length of the room to receive excreta. Two of the nuns became ill and had to be replaced. More suitable accommodation was found for the nuns in the three-storey Georgian building that still survives today and stands opposite the entrance to the Trinity Centre for Health Sciences.

During the first week in the workhouse, the nuns asked each other regularly, 'Do you think we will weather it?' However, they were determined to succeed, and their work soon began to yield results.[8] Wards and rafters were whitewashed, floorboards were scrubbed and strips of linoleum were laid in the centre of the wards. The nuns insisted on clean linen to cover the recently installed truckle beds and two nuns were placed in the kitchens to ensure that the food was properly prepared and safely delivered to the wards.

One of the Protestant deaconesses, Barbara Annan, was elected matron in February 1882.[9] She was replaced on the wards by another deaconess and two more deaconesses were appointed. In July 1887 the board of guardians decided to advertise for tenders to build a convent. The architect selected was William Mansfield Mitchell of 10 Merrion Street. Mitchell was a pupil of the distinguished Irish architects Sir Thomas Deane and Benjamin Woodward. He had rebuilt most of the buildings on

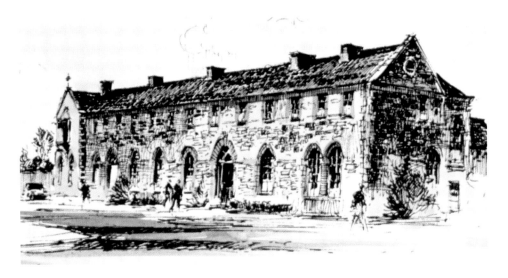

7.1   The hospital convent by Colin Gibson.

Grafton Street between Wicklow Street and Suffolk Street and among his other works was an extension to Mercer's Hospital in 1887. Initial progress on the construction of the convent was rapid and the nuns took up residence the following year. However, the building was not completed until 1902.

The nuns worked from 8 a.m. to 7 p.m., with short breaks from duty, seven days a week. They were relieved by teaching sisters and junior professed nuns when they wished to go on a short holiday or on retreat. Night duty was carried out by wardmasters and wardmistresses, who also saw to general supplies and to laundering. Writing in 1898, one of the visiting medical officers, Dr Samuel M. Thompson, commented on the significant improvements the nuns had achieved:

> The discipline and sanitary conditions, bedding and dietary have all been improved of late years, no epidemic has spread in the hospitals or house and by strict antiseptic measures and improved nursing etc. every operation performed of either major or minor character has been invariably successful.[10]

One of the nuns, Sr M. Rosalie, was a gifted gardener and she cultivated an area in the grounds of the hospital and converted it into a miniature botanic garden, with flowering trees, shrubs, flower beds and rockeries.[11]

Gradually the number of nuns increased and at the beginning of the twentieth century there were thirty-two nuns in the South Dublin Union. These nuns were known as 'The Invincibles' by their colleagues in other Dublin convents because of the difficult problems they had to face. Each nursing sister had between forty and forty-five patients under her care. The nuns were responsible for female and male

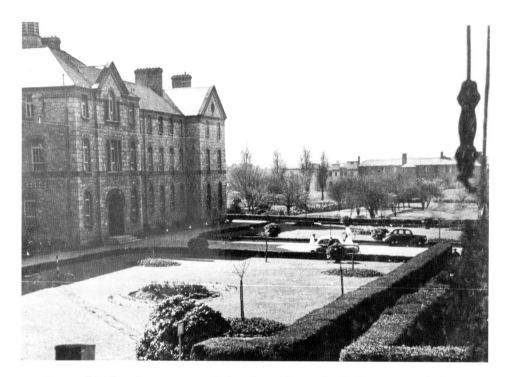

7.2   A nun walking from the convent towards the infirmary (Hospital 2–3). The convent was built opposite and parallel to the infirmary. In the distance, on the right, is the old Kilmainham Auxiliary Workhouse and, attached to it on the left is the Male Consumptive Hospital. These buildings were later refurbished to form the Rialto Chest Hospital and subsequently became Hospital 7. Private collection.

patients in Hospital 2–3, the isolation or tuberculosis hospital and the children's hospital. They were assisted in their work by nurses and by inmate attendants. The inmate attendants were 'selected by the matron for their good conduct while in the workhouse; some of them are widows of artisans, with one or more children in the workhouse schools'.[12] The appointment of inmate attendants had to be approved by the resident medical officer. They were not allowed to act as nurses and always had to be under the direct supervision of a trained nurse.[13]

For most of the nineteenth century wealthy patients were treated by physicians and surgeons in their own homes even if this involved surgery. With the introduction of antiseptic surgery and anaesthesia an increasing number of middle-class patients were being admitted to general hospitals for treatment. This created a demand for educated and 'genteel' nurses to work in these hospitals and nursing rapidly evolved into a respectable profession.[14] During the latter half of the nineteenth century, the Protestant-administered voluntary hospitals in Dublin began to develop small nursing schools and the Catholic Mater and St Vincent's Hospitals both established nursing

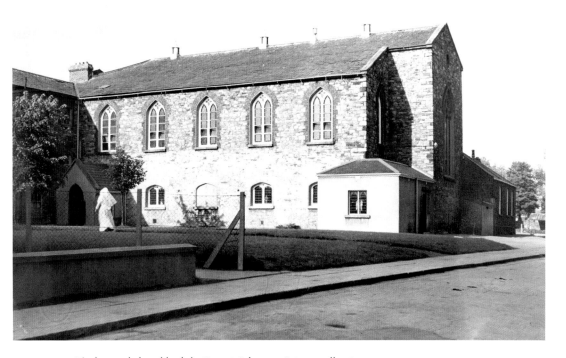

7.3   The hospital chapel built by Francis Johnston. Private collection.

schools in 1891. These nurses were trained primarily to staff the voluntary hospitals, but the nuns in the South Dublin Union managed to attract some of them to work with them in the workhouse infirmary.

Medical care

The 1911 census revealed that there were 3,539 inmates in the South Dublin Union and 2,184 or 62 per cent were listed with a specific illness. Of the latter group, 1,264 were in the hospital section. The principal conditions leading to admission were rheumatic (415), respiratory (390), frailty (334), skin disease (173), neurological (162) and heart disease (70). Trauma (67) including fractures (17), and hernia (39), were the most common surgical reasons for admission. There were 204 cases of tuberculosis in the South Dublin Union on the night of the census.[15]

Medical care was delivered in the workhouse by the resident medical officers and by the visiting medical officers. The visiting medical officers 'on account of their seniority and their longer and more varied experience' had overall responsibility for patient care and did daily ward rounds. The resident medical officers made the clinical decisions in the absence of the visiting medical officers and were obliged to see all the sick patients every night.[16]

There were two resident medical officers and one of them, Frank Dunne, in a letter to the board of guardians in 1903, described how their workload was divided:

> [T]he work of the two resident medical officers of this workhouse is divided so that Dr MacNamara has charge of the female departments and I have charge of the males.
>
> In the morning both of us attend to our own departments and the resident on duty for the day attends to any cases of emergency that may arise, and also examines all admissions up to 5 or 6 p.m. or until he is relieved by his colleague who comes on duty for the night.
>
> The resident on night duty carefully examines all admissions and any cases for the hospital are followed and visited and prescribed for ... and in addition all the wards of the hospitals are visited after 9 p.m. to see that everything is right for the night ... the workhouse opens at 6 a.m. in summer and 7 a.m. during winter months and I make it a practice to visit all the departments in my charge early in the morning and by so doing facilitating the work of the diet clerk, the stores, the apothecary and master's office, and what is more important still, I am able to ensure that any patient whose condition necessitates transfer to hospital may be seen and prescribed for by one of the visiting physicians before he leaves the workhouse.[17]

As in all hospitals of the period, therapeutic options were limited. Medicines such as mist cardiac, mist expectorant and sedative powders for patients who were noisy at night were kept in big Winchester bottles on the wards. The doctors could prescribe a range of creams and medications, some of which are still in use in medicine and homeopathy. These included aqua rosae, glycerine belladonna, glycerine boracis, phenacetin tablets, flower of sulphur, fer mustard leaves, tincture of senega, senna, gentian, cod liver oil, boric acid, liniment of turpentine, quinine sulphate, sodium salicylate, spirit of chloroform, ferrous iodide, tincture of opium, arsenic and cascara.[18] The Local Government Board made an attempt to enforce strict control over the types of medicine that might be prescribed for patients in the workhouse infirmary. However, the board of guardians defended the interests of the patients making it clear that they would 'continue to order for the sick poor what remedies their skilled officers prescribe for their patients and in the event of a surcharge for same being made upon the guardians, the guardians will appeal to the courts of justice of the country'.[19] The medical officers also took a principled stand:

> [T]he prescriptions for patients are dictated solely with proper regard to the due treatment of the sick placed in their charge and they cannot consent to be com-

pelled to prescribing remedies other than those, which in their opinion and professional judgement they decide to be necessary in each particular case.

We desire also to state that the workhouse hospital has developed into a very extensive curative institution and that its character as such can only be upheld by the use of all the means known to advanced science for the treatment and cure of disease.[20]

A major problem for both the medical and administrative staff was the adulteration of food and milk by suppliers. Dr Charles Cameron, the public analyst, analyzed milk from the South Dublin Union in 1871 and found that it contained '16 per cent of water above the natural proportion, while the proper weight of the fluid was cleverly made up by a liberal addition of salt'.[21] Water reduced the nutrient value of the milk and as the water was sourced from contaminated canals and rivers it increased the risk of transmitting dysentery, typhoid or cholera. The addition of salt could have serious consequences for infants in the workhouse.[22]

Commissioners for the *British Medical Journal*

Despite the best efforts of the nuns, nurses and doctors, they were just scratching the surface. The South Dublin Union needed a substantial investment and this was not forthcoming. The *British Medical Journal* sent a team of commissioners to study the administration of Irish workhouses in the mid 1890s. The report of the visit to the South Dublin Union, which was regarded by the authorities 'as somewhat of a model to other unions', was published in the *British Medical Journal* in 1896. It made very grim reading. It is clear from the report that the matron who took the commissioners around made no attempt to restrict them to the more presentable sections of the workhouse. They first visited the wards for the sick patients in the infirmary, which they found very overcrowded and with no day rooms. They observed that the patients were similar to the patients in any general hospital but that there were more cases of 'hopeless paralysis and senility'. There was a shortage of nuns or deaconesses, with often only one responsible for a ward of 45 to 50 beds. As a consequence, they found that there was far too much reliance placed on inmate carers or 'deputies' as they were called. Wardmasters and wardmistresses were still present on the wards but were subordinate to the nuns and deaconesses. At night there was only one nurse on the female side and one on the male side. 'By this arrangement', the inspectors observed, 'a large and important hospital is practically nursed by paupers at night.'

In another ward, known as the separation ward, the patients appeared to be looking after themselves or, at best, were in the charge of an inmate. They found the nursery for healthy infants under 2 years, which occupied two floors, untidy, dirty and showing want of supervision. There was an officer in charge of the nursery but they

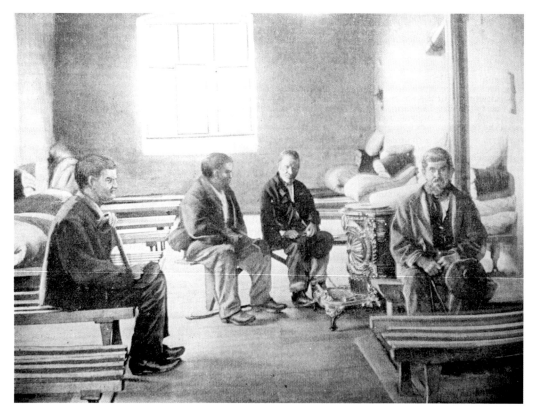

7.4   Harrow beds in an Irish workhouse. *British Medical Journal* (Sept. 1895).

observed that she was 'much handicapped in her work by the ignorant mothers, who are very difficult to manage'.

The aged and infirm were housed in blocks separated from the hospital buildings. The inspectors were impressed by the facilities for the women, describing them as:

> [O]ne of the best parts of the house; they are in small huts which run three sides round a garden where are seats, flowers, and grass, all of easy access from the wards. The wards themselves had a bright, home-like appearance, the cross-lights and the distance from the high buildings allowing of plenty of sunshine.[23]

The wards for the old men were not as good and were 'altogether destitute of the comfort that one looks for in old age'. The old men slept on 'harrow' beds which were widely used in Irish workhouses. About 2 feet 3 inches wide, each one consisted of five parallel wooden bars supported at the foot on an iron crossbar and two iron legs. The head rested on a continuous rail fixed on iron uprights about 6 inches from the wall. These old people were under the care of inmates and were locked into their wards at 7 p.m. with only commodes or pails to rely on for sanitary facilities.

The visitors also saw the 'lunacy' wards, which they found were very overcrowded and custodial in nature. The maternity section was near the main gate in a wing of the old Foundling Hospital and accommodated 40 beds in four wards. There were only 80 to 100 confinements each year. The visitors were surprised to learn that there were no sanitary appliances in this block, and the matron pointed out a privy 'at some little distance away, to which everything had to be carried'. However, a new sanitary system was being put in place in the South Dublin Union at the time, with new closets being added to the wards together with bathrooms with a hot and cold water supply. The wards were heated by steam pipes running round the skirting boards and by open fireplaces. The children's hospital made the most favourable impression on the visitors:

> The children's hospital is a bright and cheerful spot among these dreary surround-
> ings; the wards are large, walls painted in two colours, cots down the middle, and
> small bedsteads round the walls, with toys, pictures, and plants giving it a pleas-
> ant appearance. The boys' and girls' wards duplicate each other on the ground
> floor. There is also a good playground, but no dayroom to relieve the wards in
> bad weather. The children are treated here until the age of 14 or 15. The hospital is
> nursed by the nuns and the inmates.[24]

The commissioners concluded that the South Dublin Union had too many departments and that it was impossible to exercise efficient control over such a large and heterogeneous establishment. They commented on the need for more staff and the replacement of the inmate nurses or 'deputies' by trained nurses. They advocated 'asylum' training for the attendants in the lunacy wards and better assistants for the nursery. The commissioners emphasized the need for more resources and they pointed out:

> that after the first outlay, the work would be done with greater economy and effi-
> ciency, and the South Dublin Union would take the position that belongs to it of
> right – that of the pioneer in the matter of workhouse reform.[25]

The report of the commissioners led to an improvement in the standard of nursing care in the South Dublin Union and the Local Government Act 1898 prohibited the practice of assigning inmates to nursing duties.

Lady Jane Brabazon

Life was dismal for the large number of frail elderly women and men, many of them bed-ridden, who were housed in the overcrowded gloomy wards. There was little for them to do to break the monotony of their existence until their plight came to the attention of a young aristocrat, Lady Mary Jane Brabazon (later Lady Meath), who had a strong social conscience. She was born in March 1847, the daughter of Sir Thomas Maitland,

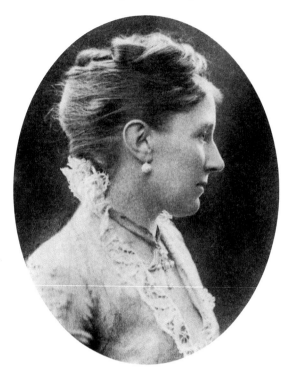

7.5 Mary Jane Brabazon, countess of Meath. Reproduced
from SICCDA, *Ladies of the Liberties* (Dublin, 2002).

11th earl of Lauderdale who, despite his wealth and social position, despised pretension and chose to live a simple life. His daughter inherited these characteristics and shunned a lifestyle of pleasure and privilege in favour of a life dedicated to the poor and disadvantaged in society.[26] She married Lord Reginald Brabazon, later the earl of Meath, in 1868. He shared her views and they collaborated on two books, *Social aims*, in 1895 and *Thoughts on imperial and social subjects*, in 1906. Lady Brabazon became the main driving force behind the Artisan's Dwelling Company, which by 1914 had built 3,084 new cottages in the Coombe area, housing 13,938 tenants. In 1886 she established trust funds for homeless and destitute children in Dublin and she laid out two playgrounds for children in the Liberties. She then turned her attention to improving the lives of the thousands of long-stay inmates in workhouses throughout the British Isles. In 1882 she wrote a paper entitled 'Need the infirmary paupers be unemployed?', which was read at a meeting in London of the Metropolitan Poor Law Guardians Association:

> I think I am accurate in stating that adequate work suitable to the capacities of the paupers is not provided. If so how is the dreary appearance of many of the wards to be accounted for, where such patients are found? Here sad clusters of men and women may be seen with hands lying idly before them, dreaming away precious weeks, months and years. Such an existence is not life ... to eat, to drink, to sleep

and dwell upon real or imaginary miseries, make up, it is feared, the sum total of many a sad existence.[27]

Introducing a new approach

Lady Brabazon began to introduce her ideas in Kensington Workhouse and in the South Dublin Union, where the long-stay patients were given some material to work on. In 1900 she established the Brabazon Employment Society to promote her idea of providing dependent residents of workhouses with what would now be termed diversional therapy. She arranged for volunteers to visit the South Dublin Union to teach the women sewing, knitting, crochet and lace making, and the men were taught carpentry and joinery. After a slow start the scheme was adopted by over 200 workhouses and other institutions housing frail and dependent residents throughout the British Isles. Every year she held an 'at home' in her residence in Kilruddery for officials working with the Local Government Board in Dublin and Wicklow so that she could discuss the current challenges facing workhouses and the progress of reform.

Support of the guardians for home rule

Throughout most of the nineteenth century there was a unionist majority on the board of guardians. However, at the end of the century this changed and the number of guardians with home rule sympathies increased significantly. Home rule supporters became the majority on the board of guardians following an election in 1899. At the first meeting of the new board in 1899 the following resolutions were passed:

1. That we the members of the board of guardians of the South Dublin Union, at this our first meeting desire to place on record our unalterable conviction that nothing short of legislative independence will ever satisfy the national aspirations of the Irish people.

2. It is our opinion that the claims of the Catholics of Ireland to equality in university education should be recognised, and that similar facilities should be afforded to them as those enjoyed by their Protestant fellow countrymen.[28]

They wished to see these aspirations achieved by political means rather than by violent revolution. The meetings of the board of guardians offered a wide political platform to the home rule supporters as the proceedings were reported in the national Irish and English newspapers and, on 4 September 1902, they were reported in the *New York Times* under the headline 'The "Proclamation" of Dublin':

> At a meeting of the South Dublin Union, says a telegram from Dublin to *The Times*, James Mullett moved a resolution protesting against the proclamation of Dublin City under the Crimes Act.

Mr Mullett said that the government was again repeating the events of twenty years ago, and was goading young men to crime by proclaiming places which, the officials admitted, were free of crime. He protested against the 'villainous conduct of the alien government ...'[29]

The proclamation under the Crimes Act of 1887 gave powers to the lord lieutenant to prohibit or suppress 'dangerous associations'.

Queen Victoria's visit to Dublin

Queen Victoria visited Ireland in 1900 at the end of the Second Boer War. Even though the war was very unpopular internationally, as many as 28,000 Irishmen fought in the British army against the Boers. The purpose of Queen Victoria's visit was to show her appreciation for this support and loyalty. However, 400 Irish nationalists fought with the Boers and both they and their supporters resented the royal visit.

A large children's party was planned to take place in the Phoenix Park as part of the queen's visit and this became the focus of nationalist protest. The party was condemned as British propaganda and it was claimed that the children were being used to portray Ireland as a loyal colony of the empire. The newspapers were inundated with letters either condemning or supporting the children's party. Some weeks before the queen's arrival the guardians of the South Dublin Union received a letter asking them to accept an offer of jam and toys, which could be given to the children to celebrate the first day of the queen's visit to Ireland. The guardians were also asked to allow the children of the workhouse to attend a garden party in the Phoenix Park on the fourth day of the queen's visit. There was a nationalist majority on the board of guardians and a heated debate took place on whether to accept or reject the offers. Eventually the guardians voted to reject the offer of jam and toys, but to allow the children to attend the party.

The adult inmates also had an opportunity to see the queen, as she and her entourage used the South Circular Road to travel to and from the vice-regal lodge in the Phoenix Park, where she stayed during her visit. It offered a more scenic route than travelling through the very populous Liberties.[30] On Friday 20 April at 4 o'clock in the afternoon, the queen set out from the vice-regal lodge to visit the Loreto convent in Rathfarnham and to call at the Meath Hospital on the way. The *Irish Times* reported that after crossing the Liffey by Island Bridge the royal carriage, escorted by six mounted policemen from the Dublin Metropolitan Police, headed for the South Circular Road:

The people at all points of the drive gave Her Majesty splendid ovations. The imposing institution kept by the Little Sisters of the Poor was passed, and at the turn of the road a large number of the inmates of the auxiliary of the South Dublin Union, who had assembled on the roadside in anticipation of the queen's coming, gave Her Majesty a delighted greeting, Rialto Bridge was now crossed, and the vicinity of Dolphin's Barn was traversed.[31]

After Queen Victoria's departure from Ireland a group of nationalist women formed the Ladies' Committee for the Patriotic Children's Treat, with the purpose of organizing a party in Phoenix Park for 'patriotic children'. There were eighty-five women on the committee and Maude Gonne played a prominent role. The 'Patriotic Children's Treat' took place on 1 July, but children from the schools and institutions that had accepted the invitation to go to the royal party three months earlier were banned from attending. The children in the South Dublin Union were among those excluded.[32]

Pressure for reform

At the beginning of the 1900s there was growing pressure for significant reform of the poor law and workhouse system. A vice-regal commission on poor law reform, which was established in 1903 and reported in 1906, recommended that a single workhouse should be retained in each county for the old and infirm and that these should be known as county alms houses. All the other workhouses should be closed. It stated that poverty in Ireland could only be dealt with adequately by the development of Irish resources: a very belated acceptance of Whately's proposals of 1838. The commission recommended that the various classes of inmates in the workhouses should be segregated into separate institutions and proposed the separation of the workhouse infirmaries from the poor law. In a radical move it proposed the creation of a state health service embracing the former workhouse infirmaries, county infirmaries and dispensaries, to be funded by the state, which would also pay the salaries of the medical staff. While the proposals were described by both the *British Medical Journal* and *The Lancet* as 'remarkable', in practice the report gathered dust and the workhouses remained in place.[33]

There were other acts unrelated to the poor law that were passed in the early years of the twentieth century which impacted on the role of the workhouses. These included the Old Age Pensions Act 1908, the Tuberculosis Prevention (Ireland) Act 1908, the National Insurance (Health) Act and the National Insurance (Unemployment) Act 1911, the Notification of Births (the Maternity and Child Welfare Schemes) Act 1915, the Public Health (Medical Treatment of Children) Act 1919 and the Blind Persons Act 1920.[34]

Voluntary hospitals under financial pressure

Access to the voluntary general hospitals became more difficult for poor people in the early years of the twentieth century. These voluntary hospitals relied on philanthropy to meet their costs as the patients were not charged for their care. The situation was exacerbated by the very significant growth in the population of the city in the late nineteenth and early twentieth century and the increasing numbers of people from other parts of Ireland seeking admission to the Dublin voluntary hospitals. The 1913 Dublin Lockout placed further pressure on acute facilities in the voluntary hospitals. From 28 August 1913 until 18 January 1914, over 20,000 workers were locked out of their workplaces in a dispute with their employers, which led to dreadful deprivation among the working class and the destitute.[35]

These pressures caused the voluntary hospitals to move from one financial crisis to the next and many of the hospitals began requesting fees from those who could pay. This brought in significant income and gave more stability to the management of the hospitals. The majority of the acute voluntary hospitals developed subscription fees which provided a steady income. Under these schemes subscribers contributed money to the hospital on a regular basis. The hospitals also took out substantial bank overdrafts. In December 1913, Mercer's Hospital carried an overdraft of over £4,000 and the Royal City of Dublin Hospital, Baggot Street, carried an overdraft of about £7,000.

The admission of fee-paying patients to the wards of the voluntary hospitals significantly reduced their capacity to cope with the very poor and destitute, and increasing numbers of poor patients who were acutely ill were admitted to the infirmary of the South Dublin Union. It was anticipated that there would also be a substantial increase in the number of social admissions as a result of hardship due to the Lockout, but to everyone's surprise this situation did not materialize. The main impact of the Lockout on the South Dublin Union resulted directly from the strikes, which made it difficult for the management to run the institution and to maintain vital supplies. The admission of increasing numbers of semi-private and private patients to the voluntary hospitals and the fall in admissions of the poor and destitute set the scene for friction between the government and the voluntary hospitals in the decades ahead.

Tuberculosis

Tuberculosis was a major cause of death in Ireland during the nineteenth century. It was responsible for half of all deaths between the ages of 15 and 35, and women were more likely to die than men.[36] Despite the fact that many of its victims were young, no special provisions were made for patients suffering from the disease. They were not welcome in the acute voluntary hospitals in Dublin as there was no known treatment for the disease and they tended to occupy beds for long periods. Many had no option but to seek admission to the infirmary of the South Dublin Union. Because of this, an expertise in caring for patients with tuberculosis gradually emerged in the institution. The pressure on existing wards made it necessary to build a hospital for tuberculosis patients near the Rialto entrance on the South Circular Road around 1870. In 1903, a Catholic church was built opposite the hospital to serve the patients. This replaced a smaller chapel that had been located in this area for around fifty years.

In the early years of the twentieth century, the campaign against tuberculosis was led by the Women's National Health Association of Ireland, under the auspices of the countess of Aberdeen, wife of the lord lieutenant. The association organized the Dublin Tuberculosis Exhibition as part of the International Exhibition in Ballsbridge in 1907. Frank Dunne, visiting medical officer to the South Dublin Union, gave a presentation on sanatoria and tuberculosis dispensaries at the exhibition. He underlined the importance of early diagnosis and stressed that, of over nine hundred cases of tuberculosis that were admitted to the South Dublin Union over a twelve-month period, less than 14 per cent pre-

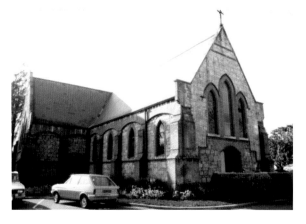

7.6   The Catholic church near the Rialto gate. Completed in 1903, it served the hospital and local community for over a hundred years. It was demolished in 2017 to make way for the construction of the new children's hospital. Private collection.

sented any prospect of cure. There was also a high mortality rate from tuberculosis among children. In the same period 152 children died in the South Dublin Union, 54 of them from tuberculosis.[37] The new tuberculosis hospital soon proved to be inadequate to cope with the demand on beds so Dunne persuaded the guardians to purchase two prefabricated ward units. At the National Exhibition in Ballsbridge, Dunne exhibited drawings and photographs of his female tubercular unit, which could accommodate sixty patients. There was a small laboratory adjacent to the unit. The male tubercular hospital housed seventy-two patients. Dunne, who was originally appointed to the South Dublin Union in 1902 as resident medical officer, travelled widely on the Continent to keep abreast of modern treatments for tuberculosis and was regarded as one of the leading experts on the treatment of the disease in Ireland. He used tuberculin, a therapy then in vogue in leading centres, to stimulate immunity against the disease. Dunne concluded his presentation at Ballsbridge with a tribute to the board of guardians:

> Before I close I should like to pay tribute to the board of guardians of the South Dublin Union who, as the premier union of Ireland, were the first poor law union to provide isolation hospital accommodation for their tubercular patients; and with the sanction and encouragement of the Local Government Board have provided a special tubercular diet and defrayed the entire cost of Professor Denys' tuberculin, which I have used for the past three years.[38]

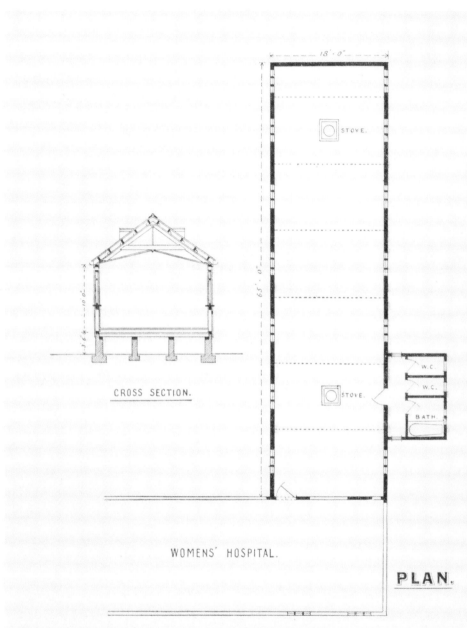

CROSS SECTION.

18'·0"

STOVE.

65'·0"

STOVE.

W.C.

W.C.

BATH

WOMENS' HOSPITAL.

PLAN.

Scale, 16 feet to 1 inch.

NEW WARD FOR WOMEN, IN WOMEN'S CONSUMPTION HOSPITAL,
SOUTH DUBLIN UNION.

Reproduced by kind permission of Messrs. Humphreys, Ltd.

7.7 The plan of a prefabricated ward for female patients with tuberculosis at the South Dublin Union. Reproduced from Countess of Aberdeen (ed.), *Ireland's crusade against tuberculosis* (Dublin, 1907).

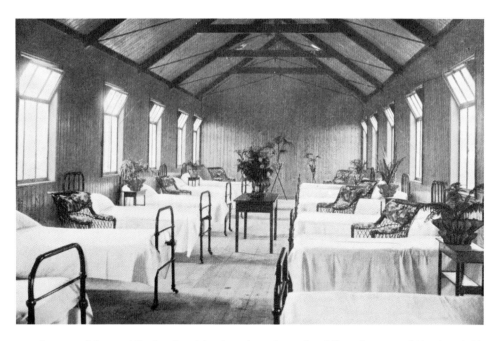

7.8   Interior of the ward for females with tuberculosis. Reproduced from Countess of Aberdeen (ed.), *Ireland's crusade against tuberculosis.*

The First World War

During the years of the First World War there was increasing pressure on the beds for tuberculosis patients and the guardians decided to open more accommodation for men in 1915.[39] The war also had other consequences for the tuberculosis service because a number of staff volunteered for active service. Dunne and a resident medical officer, Thomas Maguire, both obtained commissions in the Royal Army Medical Corps (RAMC) and they were granted leave of absence by the board of guardians in 1915. The first woman doctor to work in the South Dublin Union, Mary Welply, was appointed to cover Maguire's duties.[40] Several nurses were also given leave of absence to go to the front. Dunne served with the RAMC in Egypt. He found time to study Egyptian archaeology, and it became a life-long interest. He resumed his duties in the South Dublin Union after the war.

The board members of the South Dublin Union were sympathetic to the war effort and they allowed recruiting posters to be placed on the walls of the workhouse. They decided to take a more proactive role to boost recruitment in November 1915 when the master was instructed 'not to employ any man for temporary duty who is fit for military service'.[41] The board also passed a vote of sympathy to Mrs

Ada Redmond in March 1918 on the death in London of her husband, the home rule politician, John Redmond.[42] The meeting was then adjourned as a mark of respect to his memory.

Social distress

In a study of mortality rates in thirty cities worldwide published in 1906, Dublin had the highest mortality rate among the cities of western Europe. It recorded twice the death rate of London.[43] In the South Dublin Union there were 4,350 inmates in January 1908 and the institution was so full that it was necessary to place extra straw beds on the floor.[44] The unemployment rate was high and opportunities for work were limited. The number of people admitted because they had no abode rose from 11 per cent in 1875 to 16 per cent in 1904. Most of the rise was due to eviction and the work-house of the South Dublin Union was a refuge for people who would otherwise have ended up homeless on the side of the street:

> [A] substantial proportion used the workhouse for short-term relief when faced with illness, eviction or lack of accommodation. Women and children seem to have used the workhouse to tide them through a husband's absence seeking work, or a bout of domestic friction. Every register records the admission of several 'marriage cases'. The care which the workhouse provided may not have been popular, it was in most cases a last resort, but it must be seen as an integral part of the relief mechanisms available to the city's poor.[45]

The playwright and social reformer George Bernard Shaw was invited to deliver a lecture entitled 'The Poor Law and destitution in Ireland' on 3 October 1910 in the Antient Concert Rooms. As part of his preparation, he visited the South Dublin Union on the afternoon of the lecture. Later, in a hard-hitting talk that was reported in the *Irish Times* on the following day, he asked his audience what workhouses did in Ireland, and then answered his own question as follows:

> They took a number of people of all kinds, and threw them into a building, higgledy-piggledy. They took the most hardened scoundrels, and placed them side-by-side with comparatively innocent young men. They took a young woman whose only crime was to be poor [and placed her] in close association with other women whose company was extremely bad. He found, however, that in Dublin attempts were made at segregation and classification. They were very careful about skin diseases, but cared not in the slightest for soul diseases. The only con-clusion he could come to was that they believed people had skins, but did not believe that people had souls. The very worst skin disease was not so dangerous or contagious as a soul disease. ... Why should the epileptic and consumptive be put into the workhouses? They were not the proper places for such people,

who should be in hospitals, where proper nurses, and not pauper nurses, were employed to tend them. (Applause).⁴⁶

Shaw told his audience that children should not be placed in a workhouse under any circumstances:

> It was the fact of the child being there that helped to make the workhouses as horrible as they were. He did not want to appeal to their instincts of humanity, which might probably lead them wrong. He did not want to appeal to their sentimentality. He wanted to appeal to their economic sense, their sense of justice. Poverty was a crime – a crime not of the poor, but of the people who allowed them to be poor. Poverty was a crime of society – a preventable crime ... In going over the workhouse that day, the majority of the men he saw were respectable men – men who would take a job if they could get it.⁴⁷

Shaw went on to say that although he would not like to live in the South Dublin Union, it was a palace compared to the places in which thousands of people had to live in Dublin, and he placed the blame for this squarely on the shoulders of Irish society, which included his audience. The *Irish Times* described his lecture 'as a sermon on civic responsibility'.

The flotsam and jetsam of humanity

The workhouse had a forbidding appearance with high walls and barred windows and Dubliners referred to it as the 'Old Spike' because of its prison-like appearance. People arrived constantly, both day and night, seeking admission to the institution, and this began to cause problems for those living in its vicinity. The board received a letter in September 1908 from a Mr P. Kavanagh, forwarding a petition signed by ten residents of James's Street, asking the guardians to have the heavy knocker on the front gate removed and replaced by an electric bell 'as great noise is occasioned at night by persons continually knocking at the gate thereby making sleep impossible'.⁴⁸

Dillon Cosgrave, the Carmelite historian, described the workhouse as being 'like a haven where all the restless flotsam and jetsam of humanity is finally washed up'.⁴⁹ He wrote that the inmates wore prison-like clothes, a grey dress and shawl for the women and grey suits for the men. Although the majority of admissions were drawn from the poorer sections of the community there were inmates from all ranks of society, including army officers, priests, former matrons, professors, barristers and doctors. One, a medical doctor, who did not disclose his professional status, worked as a helper until he was finally located by his relatives, who took him home. The wife of Alex Fraser, master of the Union between 1882 and 1908, was surprised to come across her daughter receiving lessons in French from the cook in the kitchen of Garden Hill, the house of the master in the grounds of the South Dublin Union.

It turned out that the cook, Anne McCabe, had been educated in a convent in Paris. She married without her family's approval and when her husband died she was left destitute. McCabe was too proud to go back to her family so she sought refuge in the South Dublin Union. Although encouraged to leave the Union she stayed with the Fraser family until her death.

There was a social stigma attached to admission to the South Dublin Union, particularly among the so called 'respectable' poor. An elderly house painter who had seen better days begged for support from the Mansion House Relief Committee in 1906 so that he could avoid being admitted to the Union as a pauper. This, he said, would break the heart of his daughter, who was a nun in Castleisland convent.[50]

Parnell's sister dies in the Union

Emily Parnell, sister of Charles Stewart Parnell, was one of the most unexpected admissions to the workhouse infirmary. She arrived in Dublin from Wales on 13 May 1918 and spent a night in Maples Hotel, Kildare Street. She must have suddenly become ill or very confused in the hotel, as the next day she was seen by both Dr Healy, a dispensary doctor, who diagnosed senility and by Mr Blackburne, relieving officer for the South Dublin Union, who arranged her admission to the workhouse infirmary on grounds of destitution.[51] Her name was entered as Roberts, probably in error for Ricketts, which was her married name. She died five days later on 19 May and was buried in Rathdrum Cemetery. Her admission and death caused a sensation and were reported in the *New York Times*.

Plunkett's *Strumpet city*

The novelist James Plunkett described the great hardship and grinding poverty in Dublin during the years leading up to the First World War in his novel, *Strumpet city*. One of the characters, Miss Gilchrist, worked as servant and cook to the wealthy Bradshaw family for many years and she had a comfortable room in the house. She had a mild stroke and when she failed to make progress Mr Bradshaw arranged her admission to the South Dublin Union. There she lived a lonely existence:

> The high grey walls of the workhouse shut out almost everything; they were a fortification against the life of the city, a barrier against time, which passed yet did not seem to pass. The visitors who came weekly were few; the inmates were many. Carts passed in and out on stated days with a jingling of harness and a creaking of shafts and a stumbling of hooves on the uneven cobbles, but these meant little to the old women who hobbled about the grounds in shapeless grey dresses, and nothing at all to those lying in the close-packed wards, their eyes fixed on the high ceilings for hours of silence. Here, too, Death came

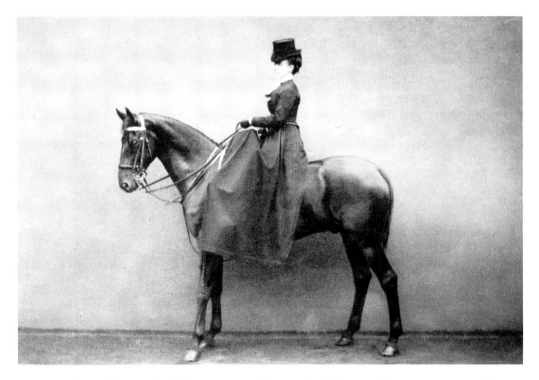

7.9   Emily Parnell, sister of Charles Stewart Parnell. Reproduced from E. Dickinson, *A patriot's mistake: being personal recollections of the Parnell family* (Dublin, 1905).

most frequently and with no noise at all. From where, Miss Gilchrist sometimes wondered; through the great arched gateway whether closed or open, up from the deep earth or down from the insubstantial sky? Three times it had come for her in the space of almost three years: once in daylight, when from beyond the screens about her bed the voices of the others and the clatter of crockery told her it was tea-time; once in the small hours when the candle in the hand of the sister lit the priest's bending face; once when a giantlike thumb stretched down to anoint her from a limitless absence of either light or darkness.[52]

Miss Gilchrist was very distressed by the prospect of being buried in a pauper's grave and she asked Father O'Connor, a friend of her former employers, to appeal to the Bradshaws to claim her body and arrange her funeral. Mrs Bradshaw, who felt guilty over the way they had deserted Miss Gilchrist, gladly acceded to the request when it was put to her by Father O'Connor. She said she would also like to visit Miss Gilchrist, but Father O'Connor thought it would be too much for a woman of her class and sensitivities:

Father O'Connor insisted that it was out of the question. He told her again about the kind of place it was, about the inmates, their coarseness, the overpowering combination of age and ignorance and illness. Mrs Bradshaw would find it too distressing.[53]

Mrs Bradshaw took the priest's advice and did not visit her former housekeeper.

Amalgamation of the North Dublin Union and the South Dublin Union

During the early years of the twentieth century there were several proposals to amalgamate the workhouses and administrative areas of the North Dublin Union and the South Dublin Union. In January 1901 the South Dublin Union rejected an approach from the North Dublin Union to consider amalgamation. In their letter of response, the guardians of the South Dublin Union stated that 'it would not be to the advantage of this union to become amalgamated with the North Dublin Union, and we respectfully decline the conference proposed on that subject'.[54] Matters did not end there, and in 1908 a vice-regal commission recommended the amalgamation of the Dublin unions.[55] Some years later, Dublin Corporation and the Local Government Board also urged some form of amalgamation.[56] The primary motivation behind the move was a desire to reduce the substantial costs associated with running both unions. In 1916, the boards of the two unions were considering attempts to rationalize the working policies of two auxiliary workhouses used for children, one in Cabra, which was linked to the North Dublin Union and one in Pelletstown, which was linked to the South Dublin Union. These discussions led again to consideration of the advantages of an amalgamation of the two unions.[57]

In 1918, military events brought an unexpected new urgency to the issue. On 3 July the board of guardians of the South Dublin Union was informed by the Local Government Board that they had received a communication stating that the military authorities intended to take over the North Dublin Union's workhouse to provide winter quarters for the troops.[58] Plans for the amalgamation now proceeded rapidly, and after intensive negotiations it was agreed to unite 'in their entireties' the two unions. The boards of guardians were amalgamated and they became the Dublin Union.[59] The first inmates from the North Dublin Union were transferred to the South Dublin Union in July 1918. Over the following two months 931 inmates from the North Dublin Union were transferred. There were already 3,208 inmates in the South Dublin Union before the transfers took place.

The new joint board met for the first time on 2 October 1918. Economic hardship and dire poverty were still forcing many, including widows and orphans, to seek admission to the Dublin Union and, because of this, the new board decided to double outdoor relief. It made good economic sense as it cost £31 per annum to support an individual in the workhouse, whereas outdoor relief cost £6.10 per annum.[60] Care in the community was greatly increased by the commencement of home nursing by the Sisters of Mercy in eight dispensary districts in May 1919. This was a significant and pioneering development. Eight sisters were appointed to undertake this role and a ninth to oversee the work.

Despite the increasing medical workload in the hospitals of the Dublin Union, the medical cover had not changed significantly since the mid nineteenth century. There were four visiting medical officers on the staff in 1919 – William C. Cremin, Frank Dunne, Patrick D. Sullivan and Lewis Farrell – and they each had a substantial workload. Sullivan attended 435 patients, Farrell 373, Dunne 325 and Cremin 210. The Local Government Board sanctioned the appointment of a fifth visiting medical officer, Thomas Maguire, in September 1919. The guardians decided in 1919 that the two resident medical officer posts should have a tenure of three years.[61] A further significant development occurred in 1920 when two rooms, a pantry and store on the ground floor of Hospital 2–3, were altered to establish the first X-ray department.[62]

The foundation of the Legion of Mary

A group of young men from the St Vincent de Paul Society began to visit the male wards of the South Dublin Union during 1918. They belonged to the St Patrick's conference of the society and they met in Myra House in the parish of St Nicholas of Myra, Francis Street. The hospital visitations were suggested and encouraged by the president of the conference, a young civil servant named Frank Duff, because he realized that many of the patients in workhouse hospitals received few visitors. The visitors were also welcomed by the Sisters of Mercy. Membership of the St Vincent de Paul Society was confined to men at that time, but women were frequently at Myra House because of their involvement in establishing a branch of the Pioneer Total Abstinence Association. A council was established to run the Pioneer Association in 1918, and this brought members of the St Vincent de Paul Society

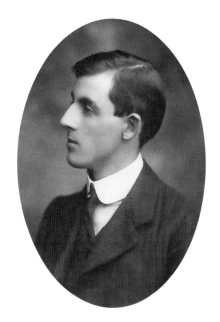

7.10   Frank Duff c.1912. Photograph courtesy of the Legion of Mary.

into regular contact with the women from the Total Abstinence Association. Monthly meetings were held at which it became the practice for groups involved in various charitable endeavours to report on their work.

A report on a visitation to the Dublin Union was presented to a meeting by one of the visitors, Matt Murray, in the summer of 1921. According to Frank Duff, founder of the Legion of Mary, this report was the 'spark' that led to the establishment of the new movement.[63] A few of the women present were moved by the description of the work in the Dublin Union and asked Frank Duff if it would be possible for women to visit the female wards. He was encouraging, so they invited similarly motivated women to join them and they agreed to meet on the following Wednesday evening at Myra House. This meeting on the 7 September 1921 is recognized as the foundation meeting of the Legion of Mary.[64]

Elizabeth Kirwan, an office cleaner from New Zealand, was appointed president of the group which was known initially as the Association of Our Lady of Mercy. Four years later the name was changed to the Legion of Mary.[65] Membership was confined to women at first, with Frank Duff attending in an advisory capacity, and with Fr Michael Toher as spiritual director. Men were admitted as members in 1927. The first work the new group undertook was visiting the cancer wards of the Dublin Union. A system was devised to give structure and stability to the visitations. There

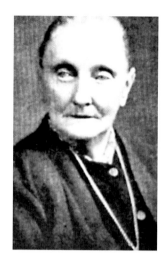

7.11   Elizabeth Kirwan, first president of the Legion of Mary. Photograph courtesy of the Legion of Mary.

was to be a regular weekly visit to the Dublin Union and two people would go together to the wards selected for visitation. Each visitor concentrated on different inmates but they both became known on the ward so that if one of the visitors was unavoidably prevented from visiting, the other would be familiar to everyone and so disappointment would be avoided. This practice of visitation in pairs became one of the hallmarks of the Legion of Mary.[66] There was a weekly meeting of the group to plan the visits and ensure regularity. Although their primary motivation was to bring spiritual solace, the visitors also performed many practical tasks for the patients such as writing letters for them and seeking out relatives or friends and encouraging them to visit.[67]

From these modest beginnings in the Dublin Union, the Legion of Mary developed into a worldwide organization with 3 million active members, including a quarter of a million members under the age of 18.[68]

The great influenza pandemic

The influenza pandemic of 1918–19 has been described as 'the deadliest plague in history' infecting an estimated 20 per cent or more of the world's population and resulting in 50 million deaths.[69] The origin of the 1918 influenza virus is still uncertain but recent research suggests that the virus may have originated in North American domestic and wild birds.[70]

The pandemic arrived in the British Isles in May 1918 and lasted for twelve months. It came in three waves, with the first abating in July, the second running from mid October to December and the third from mid January 1919 to mid March.[71] Most deaths occurred during the second wave. Older, frail individuals and those with dampened immune defence systems were seriously at risk, but the epidemic was very different to previous or subsequent epidemics of influenza as it was extremely aggressive and appeared to target young adults.[72] Healthy people going about their normal daily routine might suddenly feel unwell and be dead by nightfall. It is estimated that about 800,000 cases of influenza occurred in Ireland, infecting about one-fifth of the population.[73] While 20,057 people were certified as having died from influenza, this is considered to be a conservative estimate as many doctors were under so much pressure that they were unable to keep abreast of the paperwork.[74] The playwright Seán O'Casey remembered the stacks of coffins outside the premises of Dublin undertakers, 'towering barricades of them already sold, yet many more were needed for those who died'.[75]

Mortality from the flu was higher in Dublin than in the rest of Ireland during all three waves of the epidemic. People living in the slums and tenements of inner-city Dublin were particularly at risk and this placed great pressure on the Dublin Union. On an evening in February 1919, the caretaker in Corporation Buildings broke into a room occupied by a family named Phelan, who had not been seen for several days. He was shocked by what he found:

> Inside the dilapidated room, he found four bodies in a single bed. Twenty-seven-year-old Frances Phelan, a domestic servant, was already dead, the autopsy later revealing that a bout of influenza had been quickly followed by pneumonia, leaving her lungs in an 'advanced stage of congestion'. Lying beside her were her husband Peter and their only child Nicholas, a baby of fourteen months, still with his comforter in his mouth. Draped across the foot of the bed lay Peter's sister. The latter three were unconscious but alive.[76]

The caretaker arranged for the three who were still alive to be taken to the infirmary of the Dublin Union but all three died within hours of admission.

People living in large institutions were particularly vulnerable. Under normal circumstances, the death rate in winter in the Dublin Union ranged from fifteen to twenty people each week. Every year the death rate rose during the winter because of the spread of infectious disease. However, during the great flu of 1918, the death rate rose dramatically, and at the peak of the epidemic fifty patients died in one week. During the epidemic the nuns did double duty and nuns from the Mercy headquarters were sent to support them. Many of those who died were young and the agitation arising from the fear of infection became so great that the master of the Union had to call in the police to quell a disturbance. The medical and nursing staff struggled to cope with the large numbers of critically ill patients. Other staff and volunteer inmates did heroic work, knowing that their own lives were at risk. Many of them became ill and the words 'sick and unable for duty' appear repeatedly in the minute books of the Dublin Union throughout the epidemic.

The visiting medical officer, Dr William Cremin, played a leading role in dealing with the crisis from the beginning. On 6 November 1918, he recommended that infirm male patients and those with ulcers should be transferred to the Garden Infirmary, making four wards available in Hospital 2–3 for the admission of patients with influenza. He also requested four nursing sisters to take charge of the four wards. During the week of his request, 172 patients were admitted suffering from influenza, of whom 49 died. A man was specially employed to speed up the removal 'in proper time' of the bodies of those who died during the night.[77] Just over a week later, Cremin found it 'necessary to take over the apartments in Hospital 11 (subsequently Hospital 7) occupied by the assistant medical officer and nurse. This will increase our accommodation by 24 beds.'[78]

The situation was similar in the Dublin voluntary hospitals. The throughput of sick and dying patients was very high, 'yet only half of the usual compliment of staff was available to care for them'.[79] The dispensary doctors were overwhelmed and exhausted and it is not surprising that many of them developed the flu. Donough MacNamara, who was the house physician in the Mater Hospital, wrote a graphic account of the experiences of a young Irish doctor caring for patients with the flu in Dublin. His experience would have been replicated in hospitals all over Dublin, including the infirmary of the Dublin Union:

> The symptoms were the usual ones associated with any fever. The onset was rapid with raised temperature (though this was often moderate, and a poor guide to the real condition of the patient), fast pulse, headache, great weakness and pains all over the body. But the one thing that was almost constant in all the patients I examined and they must have run well into four figures, was the finding of moist rales at the lung bases, usually with but little cough to account for them. The cough, alas, often came later, and with it a coalescing of all the little spots in the lung into patches of consolidation, which spread until almost the whole lung was one solid mass …
>
> I have examined a freshly admitted case at 4 p.m. and examined another patient in the same bed three hours later, the first patient having died and been removed to the mortuary, only to make room for the second in that short space of time.[80]

The chaplain of the Dublin Union, Revd Richard Dillon, faced an almost superhuman task in his efforts to administer spiritual care to the sick and dying and other priests were brought in to assist him.[81]

Although so many people died and everyone lived in fear at the time, the flu of 1918–19 was rarely mentioned subsequently in newspapers, books or the media.

This has been attributed to a form of collective amnesia.[82] Several factors have been postulated to explain this amnesia, including the time of the pandemic's emergence at the end of a horrific war and its comparatively short period of impact compared to other pandemics. Interest in the 1918 flu rose during the closing years of the twentieth century, with the emergence of new threats such as HIV/AIDS, SARS, avian flu and ebola.

8

The South Dublin Union and the 1916 Rebellion

But in the wards it was a dreadful sight, the killed brought in and the wounded lying close up to the poor old paupers, who were of course shrieking with fear. I have never seen a more horrible sight and I have seen some.[1]

At the turn of the twentieth century, the South Dublin Union was like a small town. It contained a maze of streets and lanes between tall grey buildings, but there were also some open spaces and fields within the high perimeter walls. The staff and inmates all knew their place in the strictly regimental, generally peaceful and protected environment. The whole institution was 'somewhat reminiscent of a great monastery'.[2] Alexander Fraser was the master of the Union at this time. He lived with his wife, Agnes, and their eight children in Garden Hill, a spacious Victorian house situated at the Rialto end of the South Dublin Union, with a long avenue leading to it from Mount Brown:

> Garden Hill combined these urban surroundings and the terrors of the workhouse – the drunks, the toughs playing cards hidden in the cabbage field, the lunatics – with the setting of a country house. There was a paddock, a stable yard, a field for cricket and hockey, hammocks under cedar trees, and an escape across fields to an orchard where apples could be bought for a penny. Certain trespassing in the Union was allowable, to visit the night watchman's hut and brew cocoa or to go to the convent, but the children only saw the kitchen on a Christmas tour, when they helped to stir vats of fruity rice pudding, and admired huge barmbracks.[3]

Fraser had joined the staff of the South Dublin Union Workhouse as the master's clerk in 1876 and had been appointed master in 1882.[4] He spent his life trying to improve conditions in the workhouse in spite of the opposition of a 'bullying hierarchy'. He was a popular master, and when he married in 1885 the officers of the

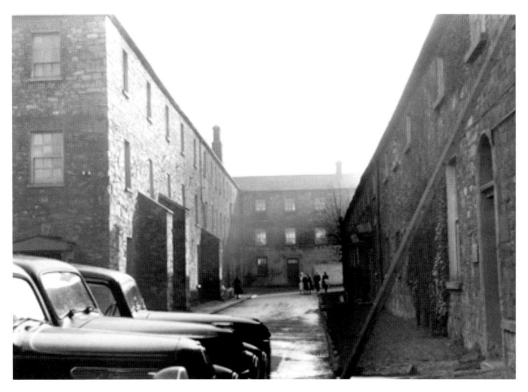

8.1 One of the narrow streets in the South Dublin Union, formed by buildings from the Foundling Hospital period. Hospital 1 (old numbering) is on the left and No. 2 Auxiliary Ward (the long, low stone building, which now forms part of the Trinity Centre for Health Sciences) is on the right, with part of the female Roman Catholic Hospital facing. BMH/IE/MA/P/42/22. Courtesy of the Military Archives, Ireland.

8.2 Garden Hill in 2017. Photograph: Anthony Edwards.

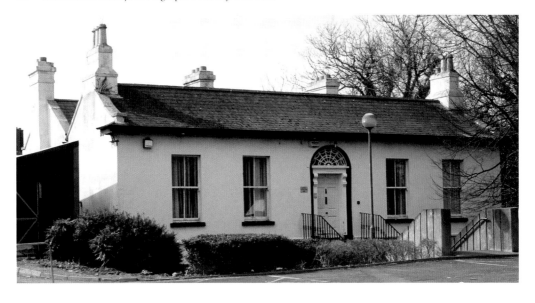

Union presented him with an illuminated scroll. Fraser had grown up on a number of country estates where his father had served as estate agent. He enjoyed riding fast horses and shooting and he kept a grey named Shamrock in a paddock at Garden Hill. In 1908, he broke his knee in an accident and died from pneumonia a short time later at the age of 57.[5] Edward Doyle succeeded him as master.

Several of the more senior staff lived with their families in the grounds of the South Dublin Union. Jim Branigan, better known as 'Lugs' Branigan, who achieved fame as a garda on account of his pragmatic approach to street violence in Dublin, was born in 1910 in the South Dublin Union. His father, John Branigan, was a wardmaster and he, his wife and four children lived in a house just inside the front gate and to the right. The house was demolished during the expansion of the Trinity Centre for

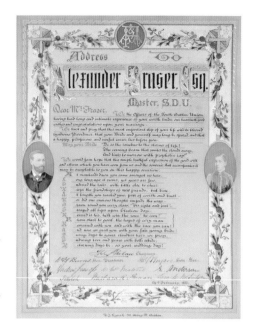

8.3   Illuminated scroll presented to Alexander Fraser by the officers of the South Dublin Union on the occasion of his marriage to his wife Agnes. Courtesy of Ian Fraser Clark.

Health Sciences at the end of the twentieth century. The Branigans, in common with the families of other officers, had inmates as servants. In the Branigan household, these were a cook and two male house servants.

The children who lived in the grounds of the South Dublin Union rarely moved outside it other than to go to school. By and large they found their playmates among the other children who also lived in the Union. Jim Branigan recalled this period later in his life:

> [A] lot of officials and their families lived in officers' quarters ... Also residing in the Union was the master of the institution and his wife, who was the matron; Mr and Mrs Edward Doyle and their family, the assistant matron Miss Mannion and the assistant master Mr Hennessey, his wife and family. All the children were within a few years in age of one another. It was easy for the young people to keep in the institution as there were miles of roads, a ball alley and several fields. The boys were always cycle-racing along the road as there was little or no traffic.[6]

As a child he was to witness the beginning of the most tumultuous event in the Union's history on Easter Monday, 24 April 1916. At around noon on that day, there

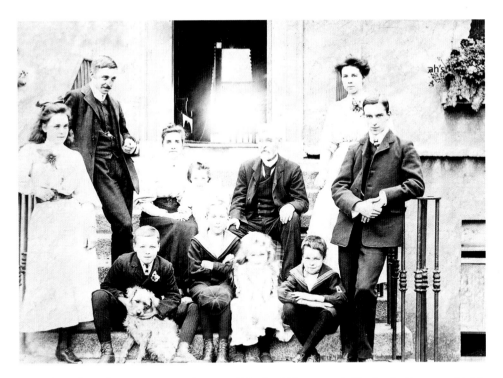

8.4   Alexander and Agnes Fraser on the steps of Garden Hill, surrounded by family. Courtesy of Adele Crowder and Ian Fraser Clark.

was a knock on the Branigans' door and Jim's mother answered it. 'Ah Willie, come on in,' Jim heard his mother say. It was William (W.T.) Cosgrave, who had grown up on James's Street, across the road from the Branigans, and who was well known to the family. There was a young man with him, whom Cosgrave introduced. 'This is Éamonn,' he said, 'he is in command here.'[7] The young man was Éamonn Ceannt, commandant of the 4th Battalion of the Irish Volunteers.

The Easter Rebellion

On Easter Monday, the South Dublin Union was occupied by the 4th Battalion of the Irish Volunteers under the command of Ceannt and Vice Commandant Cathal Brugha. The battalion had assembled earlier in the morning in Emerald Square, a small square of workmen's cottages, off Cork Street in Dolphin's Barn. Of a nominal strength of 700, only 130 men had assembled.[8] 'Today you're going into action!' Ceannt told his men, 'An Irish Republic has been declared and we are marching on the South Dublin Union.' They also planned to place outposts at Watkins' Brewery in Ardee Street under the command of Captain Con Colbert, at Jameson's distillery in Marrowbone Lane under Captain Séamus Murphy and at Roe's Malt House

179

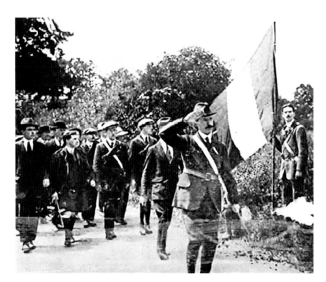

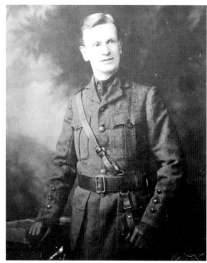

Left 8.5   Commandant Éamonn Ceannt leading the 4th Battalion in a march past the flag. Courtesy of the Irish Volunteers Commemorative Organisation.

Right 8.6   Captain Séamus Murphy, commanding officer of the Marrowbone Lane garrison. Courtesy of Nessa Rowan.

in Mount Brown under Captain Thomas McCarthy. The purpose of these outposts was to support the Union garrison, and of these outposts, Jameson's proved the most strategic. Its role was to protect the southern wall of the South Dublin Union and to block troops who might attempt to march along Cork Street, which could be seen from the end of Marrowbone Lane. At 11:30 a.m. the battalion left Emerald Square to occupy all these positions. Ceannt led a party of forty-two men along the canal bank to the Rialto bridge and they entered the Union by the back gate. They cut the telephone wires and took possession of the keys, to the great surprise of the porter, who thought they were merely on weekend manoeuvres. Meanwhile, Cosgrave guided another party, under the command of Brugha, along side streets to the main gate of the South Dublin Union, which they entered. The remaining Volunteers occupied the designated outposts without incident.

The South Dublin Union was chosen for occupation by the leaders of the 1916 Rising because of its strategic position, being close to the Richmond and Islandbridge barracks and to Kingsbridge railway station.[9] It was also a short distance from the Royal Hospital Kilmainham, the British military headquarters in Ireland. However, the decision to place a garrison in the South Dublin Union, which housed over 3,000 sick and destitute inmates, when, it is argued, other locations would have served the purpose, remains controversial.[10]

The leaders of the volunteer forces in the South Dublin Union

Éamonn Ceannt was born in Ballymoe, Co. Galway, in 1881. The family moved around the country before eventually settling in Dublin. As a young man he joined the Gaelic League and learned to play the uilleann pipes, becoming very proficient. It was through the Gaelic League that he met his wife, Áine Brennan, whom he married in 1905. Aine was the daughter of a wardmistress in the South Dublin Union and she lived with her mother in one of the houses on its grounds.[11] After a number of changes of accommodation, the Ceannts settled at 2 Dolphin's Terrace, now 283 South Circular Road, a short distance from the South Dublin Union. Ceannt was a member of the small group of men within the Irish Republican Brotherhood who began formulating plans for the Rising as early as 1914, and he was also one of the seven signatories of the Proclamation of the Irish Republic.[12]

Cathal Brugha was born in Dublin in 1874 and attended secondary school in Belvedere College. He had to leave school early because his father's antiques business failed. In his spare time he became an enthusiastic supporter of the Gaelic League and travelled around the country promoting the Irish language. He was a senior figure in both the Irish Volunteers and the Irish Republican Brotherhood. In 1914 he led a party of Volunteers to receive the delivery of arms that Erskine Childers had smuggled into Howth aboard his yacht, the *Asgard*.

W.T. Cosgrave was a lieutenant with B Company, 4th Battalion under Cathal Brugha. His father, Thomas Cosgrave, was a publican and grocer at 174 James's Street, which was opposite the main entrance of the South Dublin Union and was where W.T. Cosgrave was born in 1880. Thomas Cosgrave was a guardian of the South

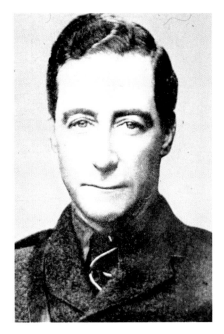

8.7   Vice Commandant Cathal Brugha. Courtesy of Cathal MacSwiney Brugha.

8.8   Lieutenant William T. Cosgrave. Reproduced from Francis Vane, *Agin the governments* (London, 1929).

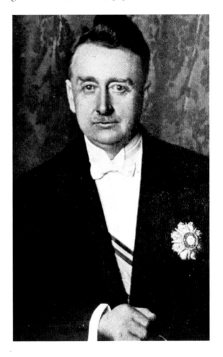

Dublin Union until his death in 1888. W.T. Cosgrave was active in Sinn Féin and was elected to Dublin Corporation in 1909. He became chairman of the corporation's finance committee in 1916.[13] He played an active role as a reforming politician, one of the factors that helped to have his death sentence commuted after the collapse of the rebellion. His brother, Philip, was one of the Volunteers who occupied Jameson's distillery in Marrowbone Lane and their step-brother, Frank Burke, fought in the South Dublin Union.

Deployment of Volunteers

There was considerable activity within the South Dublin Union as the Volunteers began to take up their positions. Ceannt would have had some familiarity with the institution as his wife Áine had friends there. After the rebellion, a seemingly innocent visit by Éamonn and Áine to one of these friends in the Union was seen in a different light, as the assistant matron, Anne Mannion later recalled:

> I remember that Miss White, who resided next door to me, told me that about a week prior to Easter Sunday 1916, Eamonn Ceannt and his wife paid her a visit to collect a toy gramophone for their little son who was ill. During the visit Eamonn Ceannt said that he would like to see the grounds, and Mr Dooley, a wardmaster, took him through the Garden Infirmary. Ceannt simply walked around, and examined the views that could be obtained from the windows.[14]

Immediately after the occupation, the Volunteers concentrated on erecting defences. The main gate was blocked and the passages were barricaded. The large minute books of the board of guardians and other substantial ledgers were stacked around windows as part of the defences. Ceannt had anticipated before the rebellion that he would have an adequate number of Volunteers to defend the complex. However, due to the low muster, he never had more than sixty-five men to deploy throughout the grounds. On Ceannt's instructions, George Irvine and twelve Volunteers occupied a long shed near the Rialto entrance, with sides and a roof of thin corrugated iron, which housed six dormitories for male patients with mental illness. The patients were placed together by their wardmaster in the last of the six dormitories. The Volunteers used mattresses to give some protection at the windows. Ceannt sent an officer and five men to cover the canal wall and another five Volunteers were sent to guard the eastern wall. He placed twelve men in McCaffrey's fields, which backed on to the north-western wall of the Union, on elevated ground overlooking Kilmainham and he also placed men in the boardroom above the arched entrance to the South Dublin Union.

One of the main objectives of the Volunteers in the South Dublin Union was to prevent soldiers from entering the city through Mount Brown and James's Street. The Union was flanked on its western side by a series of open spaces, which included McCaffrey's estate (or fields), the orchard fields and the master's fields, stretching

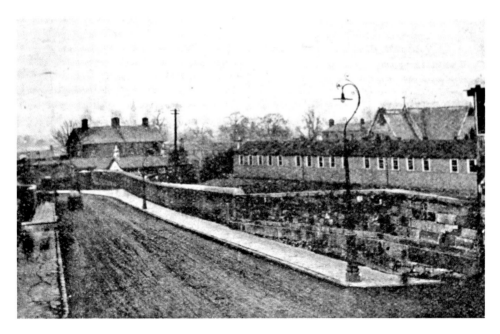

8.9   The 'lunatic' wards that were occupied by George Irvine and a detachment of Irish Volunteers. *Catholic Bulletin*, June 1918.

from James's Street south to the canal; these formed a small farm for the Union.[15] The fields bisected the institution with the main dense group of buildings to the north-east of the open space and the Kilmainham auxiliary workhouse and sheds to the south-west, at the Rialto gate. Soldiers advancing along Mount Brown would have to pass McCaffrey's fields. These fields were bounded by the Union wall and by Brook-field Road and are now largely covered by the houses of Ceannt Fort. Ceannt, Brugha and their quartermaster, Peadar Doyle, identified the buildings suitable for defence purposes with the aid of an Ordnance Survey map of the Union and then posted men in each of them. Eight Volunteers were placed in Hospital 2–3.[16] This was a large build-ing in the centre of the complex that became known as Hospital 3 after the buildings were renumbered in the middle of the twentieth century. Six men were positioned on the top floor and two on the ground floor.[17] Ceannt also placed men in the female Catholic hospital, from which the patients had been vacated.

Overleaf 8.10   Section of map of the South Dublin Union made by the architect J.J. Inglis in 1911 showing the western end of the complex. Hospital 2–3 and the convent can be seen on the right, and the Catholic church (1903), the male and female 'lunatic' wards and the male and female 'consumptive' wards can be seen on the left or Kilmainham section. Irvine and his men occupied the male lunatic ward. Reproduced by permission of St James's Hospital.

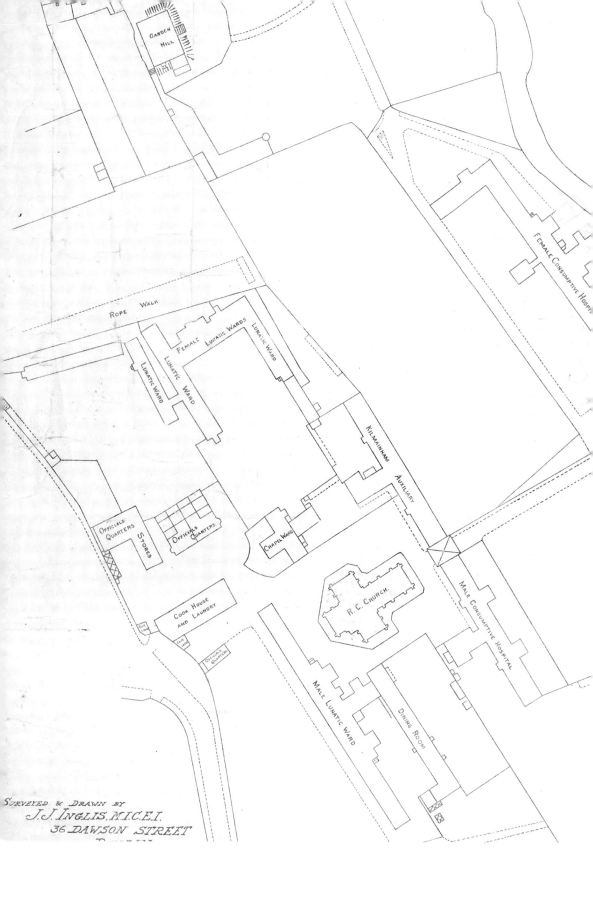

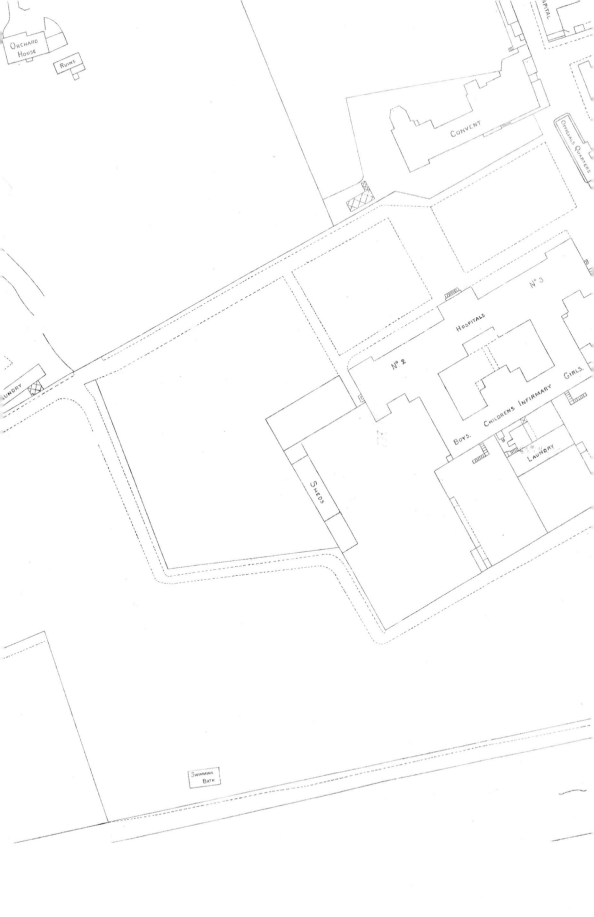

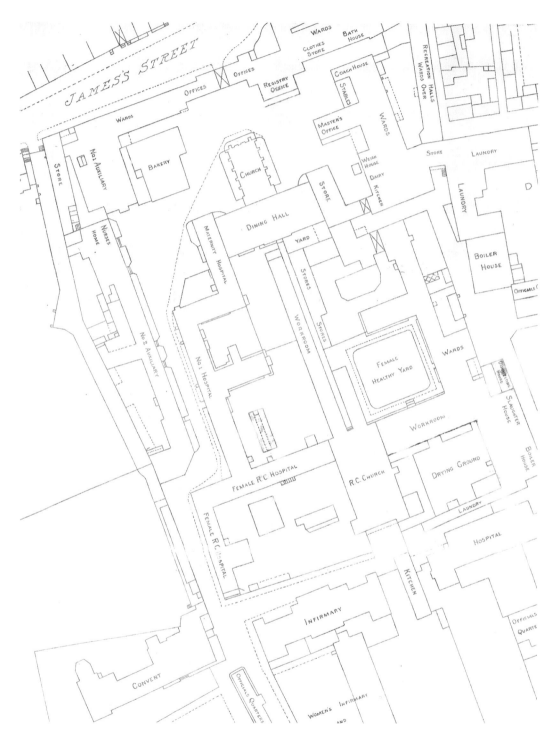

8.11 Section of map of the South Dublin Union made by the architect J.J. Inglis in 1911 showing the eastern end of the complex. The most intense fighting of Easter Week took place around the nurses' home, which can be seen on the upper left-hand side of the map. Reproduced by permission of St James's Hospital.

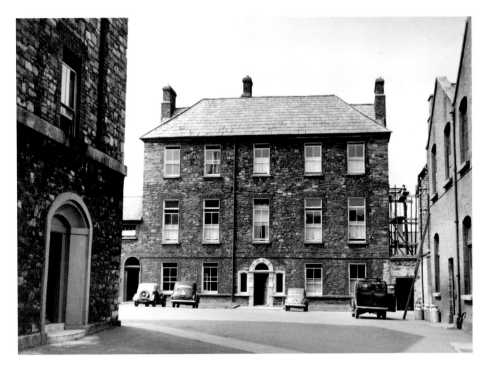

8.12 The night nurses' home, with the dining hall on the left and the bakery on the right. BMH/IE/ MA/42/3. Courtesy of the Military Archives, Ireland.

Nurses' home becomes headquarters

Large red flags were placed on the hospital buildings not occupied by the Volunteers, and staff members were given the option of leaving, but many chose to stay to look after their patients. On the advice of W.T. Cosgrave, Ceannt made the night nurses' home his headquarters.[18] This was a solid three-storey house with commanding views over Mount Brown, Brookfield Road and the Rialto gate. The building housed fifty-eight nurses and two superintendent nurses. It was situated on the west side of the courtyard immediately inside the front gates and at a right angle to James's Street, from which it was separated by the No. 1 Auxiliary Ward. The house has been conserved and now forms part of the Trinity Centre for Health Sciences. The night nurses were asleep when Ceannt requisitioned the building, and the Volunteers had to wake them and move them to another location.[19] When the resident medical officer, George McNamara, saw all the preparations, he realized that the Volunteers were getting ready for an armed conflict. He became very agitated and demanded that the Volunteers should immediately remove the barricades. When they refused he grabbed a telephone but dropped it when he found himself at the point of a bayonet. After the nurses' home had been secured, most of the windows were smashed, barricades were erected and marksmen were placed at the back windows overlooking Mount Brown.[20] Ceannt also positioned men in the boardroom and offices on the first floor, over the entrance to the Union on James's Street.

The battalion quartermaster, Peadar Doyle, was instructed to order a number of able-bodied Union inmates to take boxes of ammunition into the night nurses' home. Doyle felt uneasy about this and opted instead to agree a price for the job with the men, who accomplished the task with considerable enthusiasm. Ceannt then gave William Murphy, the storekeeper of the Union, an order for provisions. During the following week, Murphy showed great courage delivering supplies to the hospitals throughout the institution wearing a white coat and holding a white flag attached to the handle of a broom.

Doyle was sent to the convent, which occupied a central position in the grounds. He knocked on the door, which was answered by a nun who inquired, 'Have you come to read the gas meters?'[21] As they prepared their positions, members of the 4th Battalion could hear the strains of a military band coming from Richmond Barracks, which was situated a short distance away on Emmet Road in Inchicore.

Royal Irish Regiment

The 3rd Battalion (Special Reserve) of the Royal Irish Regiment was quartered in Richmond Barracks. The battalion was formed in 1914 and supplied men to other battalions of the Royal Irish Regiment then on active service on the Western Front and in Macedonia. There were just over four hundred soldiers in the barracks, most of them young Irish men, some with no combat experience and others who had just returned from active service in France. The Royal Irish Regiment, which was first raised in 1684, was one of eight Irish regiments recruited and garrisoned in Ireland. It was commanded by Lieutenant Colonel Lawrence Owens. For some time before the Easter Rising, a picket of a hundred officers and men was kept in readiness to proceed at a moment's notice wherever required. At about noon on Easter Monday, Owens received a telephone message from Dublin Castle ordering all troops in barracks to go at once, fully armed, to the castle. Major Philip Holmes, the officer commanding the picket, was ordered to proceed immediately to the Castle. Holmes was originally from Cork and was one of thirty-two RIC district inspectors who were seconded to the army in 1914.[22] The route would take the picket through Mount Brown and past the South Dublin Union, where members of the 4th Battalion were lying in wait.[23]

First soldiers attacked

The column of soldiers approached Mount Brown shortly after midday. Holmes noticed some of Ceannt's men in McCaffrey's fields and halted the column near Brookfield Road. A sergeant and five troops were sent forward as a probe but the

Volunteers did not fire on them. Holmes then sent a party of twenty men forward under the command of Lieutenant George Malone. The Volunteers waited until the soldiers came quite close and then opened fire. Three soldiers fell on the road and the rest sought cover by breaking into the houses and buildings facing the Union. Three soldiers ran through a door of a tanyard that had been forced open but a fourth soldier was shot and killed before he could follow them. Malone was badly injured in the hip as he tried to drag the dead soldier into the tanyard. Once sheltered, the soldiers began to return fire. Volunteer John Owens, aged 24, was killed in this exchange. Meanwhile, Lieutenant Colonel Lawrence Owens arrived with another 200 soldiers and decided to launch an attack on the South Dublin Union.

Owens, who was born in Dublin in 1860, was a very experienced officer, who had fought in the Second Boer War. He sent a party with a Lewis machine gun to the Royal Hospital Kilmainham, which overlooked the South Dublin Union. Snipers were positioned in the upper windows of the Royal Hospital. Some soldiers were sent up the avenue that linked the road to the master's house. These soldiers kept up a continuous barrage of fire for over two hours, targeting the Volunteers in McCaffrey's fields.[24] Owens also sent two companies along Brookfield Road towards the Grand Canal to prepare for an attack on the Union from the Rialto end, under the command of Major E.F. Milner, Captain Alfred Warmington and Lieutenant Alan Ramsay. Both Ramsay and Warmington were Irish. Alan Ramsay was 26 and a son of Daniel Ramsay of Ballsbridge, Dublin. His family was involved in horticulture and had a nursery.[25] Alfred Warmington was born in Queen's County (Laois). In 1885, when he was about 15, his family moved to Naas, where his father was appointed manager of the Munster

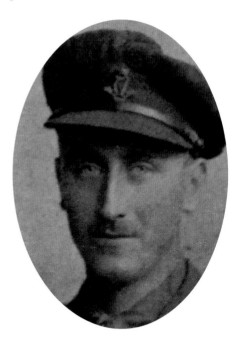

8.13   Lieutenant Alan Ramsay. Reproduced with permission of the South Dublin Libraries/ Our Heroes.

8.14   Captain Alfred Warmington. Reproduced with permission of the South Dublin Libraries/Our Heroes.

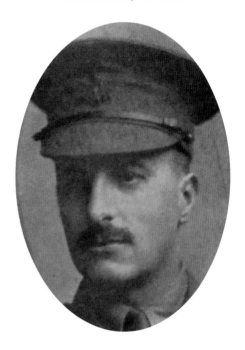

and Leinster Bank. Like Owens, Warmington had also fought in the Second Boer War, and had subsequently returned to Ireland, where he worked with the Great Southern and Western Railway Company. He joined the Royal Irish Regiment on the outbreak of the First World War and fought in Flanders.[26]

Assault on the Union

The assault began just before one o'clock. The Volunteers in McCaffrey's fields were the first to feel the ferocity of the full attack. They came under a hail of continuous rifle fire and began to retreat, leaving behind two wounded Volunteers and the body of John Owens. As they crawled across the fields to gain the shelter of the work-house buildings, the Lewis gun on the roof of the Royal Hospital opened fire on them. A small group of Volunteers remained in the field and took positions closer to the nurses' home. A second volunteer, Richard O'Reilly, aged 16, was mortally wounded.[27] At the same time as the fighting began at McCaffrey's fields, Ramsay led an assault on the Rialto gate at the rear of the hospital. Warmington followed him with a second group of soldiers. They could not get through the main gate, which was locked, but the soldiers were able to break open an adjacent smaller door. Ramsay charged through the door and was shot in the head by the waiting Volunteers.[28] The Volunteers allowed a stretcher party to remove the officer to the nearby female epileptic hospital, where he died. Warmington, no doubt incensed by the death of his colleague, attempted to lead a party of soldiers further into the Union but before he could make any progress he too was shot dead. His body was placed on a bed next to Ramsay.[29]

The Volunteers, led by George Irvine, found that their building at the Rialto entrance offered little protection.[30] Bullets cut through the thin walls of the shed, ricocheting and striking the iron bedsteads. They pierced the wooden partitions, which divided the building into six individual dormitories, as if they were tissue paper. Fortunately, none of the inmates who had been moved to the dormitory furthest from the fighting, was injured, but a bullet did pierce the wardmaster's coat.[31] In the fighting 17-year-old John Traynor, one of the Volunteers, was fatally wounded and another, Patrick Morrissey, was badly wounded in the leg. The Volunteers tried to retreat a short distance to the male tuberculosis hospital but the gunfire was so intense that they had to abandon the attempt and return to the shed. As the fighting continued, the rifles of the Volunteers became so hot that they had to take turns firing to give the guns a chance to cool. When the soldiers realized this was happening they launched an assault on the shed and broke into it using a heavy lawnmower as a battering ram. The Volunteers inside surrendered. Morrissey, the wounded volunteer, was brought by the soldiers to a ward, from which he escaped in a milk cart a few days later.[32]

Master's house surrounded

James Cribbin, who was a district clerk in the South Dublin Union, was in administrative charge of the institution on Easter Monday. In an interview he gave to the *Kildare Observer* on 25 May 1916 he said:

> Our position once the fight commenced was perilous in the extreme. I myself had several very narrow escapes, a soldier on one occasion being shot dead within a yard or two of me by a Sinn Féin bullet, fired from the boardroom ... We were obliged to open a temporary burial ground to provide for those killed, and in all we buried 14 or 16 bodies of soldiers and Sinn Féiners, and some of our own officers and inmates.[33]

Garden Hill, the residence of the master, Edward Doyle, had extensive gardens, which stretched down on one side to the epileptic department near the Rialto gate. On Easter Monday he and his wife and older children were enjoying the races at Fairyhouse and had left the three youngest children at home. These children were terrified when their home was surrounded by soldiers who believed that the rebels had occupied the house. The children watched the soldiers from one of the windows as they crawled over the lawns. The soldiers then opened fire on the house, shattering the window of the dining room. As there was no return of fire, the soldiers gained access to the house and found the children, whom they evacuated to friends later that evening.[34]

Volunteers retreat

As the assault continued, another group of soldiers made their way along the canal bank in an attempt to gain entry to the South Dublin Union through a door in the southern wall, close to the doctors' residence, where Mercer's Institute for Successful Ageing now stands. These soldiers came under heavy fire from the Volunteers in Jameson's distillery in Marrowbone Lane and from six men that Ceannt had sent to defend the canal wall. Eventually the soldiers managed to break down the door and gain entrance to the grounds. A military party of fifteen men occupied the front rooms of Rialto Buildings, which stood on the south bank of the canal, a position that completely dominated the open grounds of the South Dublin Union inside the canal wall. Long range fire from the Royal Hospital Kilmainham continued to sweep across the fields.[35] The defenders tried to retreat under heavy gunfire and, while attempting to cross a field to Hospital 2–3, two of them, 18-year-old Brendan Donelan and 42-year-old James Quinn, were killed and another sustained serious injuries.[36]

In the early afternoon fifty British soldiers entered through the gate in the canal wall and they began an assault on Hospital 2–3. Although they came under furious

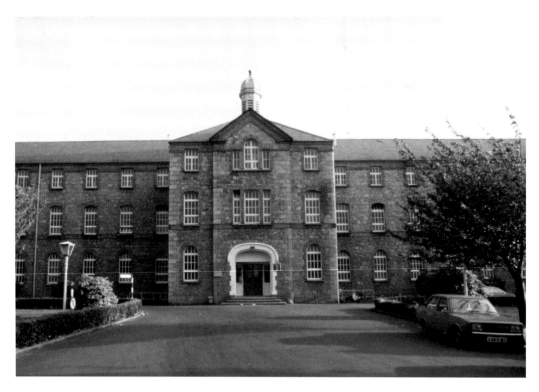

8.15   Hospital 2–3. Private collection.

fire from the upper windows of the hospital they succeeded in reaching the hospital walls and broke into the ground floor. Two Volunteers, Dan McCarthy and James Kenny, posted earlier by Ceannt in an empty ward on the ground floor, were taken by surprise when they heard soldiers in the corridor. They opened the ward door and fired on the soldiers, who promptly retreated. The Volunteers then decided to retreat, and the soldiers pursued them along the corridors of the hospital. The two Volunteers stopped at the end of each corridor to fire back at the advancing soldiers. They then tried to escape from the building by jumping through a ground-floor window. As they dashed across the grounds, McCarthy was wounded by a bullet and fell. Kenny continued to run and when he turned a corner by the Protestant infirmary he came across Ceannt, who was tending to a badly wounded Volunteer. Ceannt entered the infirmary and informed the staff of the plight of the wounded man and immediately a nurse and two inmates were sent with a stretcher to collect him. Ceannt and Kenny were about to dash across some open space when a nun opened a gate for them, allowing them access to the female Roman Catholic hospital. They then made their way back to the headquarters in the nurses' home under a barrage of covering fire from the Volunteers.[37]

The shooting of Nurse Kehoe

Having secured access to Hospital 2–3, the soldiers now concentrated on capturing the Volunteers who were on the top floor. There was an exchange of heavy gunfire, followed by a lull at about 1:30 p.m. One of the nurses, Margaret Kehoe, expressed relief that the fighting had stopped, but she had hardly spoken when rifle fire recommenced on the floor beneath. Nurse Kehoe ran down the stairs with the intent of checking on some patients.[38] However, two soldiers had taken up positions in a corridor on the ground floor and when Nurse Kehoe appeared they opened fire, believing she was a rebel, killing her instantly.[39] Speaking of Nurse Kehoe's death, James Cribbin said:

> Few losses any of us sustained were more poignantly regretted than that of Miss Keogh. She had been nursing there for nearly 20 years, and a more popular, conscientious or capable officer we never had … A pathetic incident in connection with her death was the terrible sorrow of her attendant, a man named George Browne, about 50 years of age. When she was shot he went about restlessly in the building mourning her death, and wishing, too, that he were dead. Poor fellow, his wish was satisfied, for the very next day he fell with a bullet through his heart as he went to look out through a window.[40]

Margaret Kehoe was from Leighlinbridge, Co. Carlow, and was a daughter of the coroner for the county. She was aged 49 at the time of her death.

Meanwhile, the seriously wounded volunteer, Dan McCarthy, was brought into Hospital 2–3. He was bleeding profusely from an abdominal wound and he was admitted to one of the wards, where he lay with his revolver under his pillow. Shortly after his arrival British soldiers entered the ward and made straight to his bed. Some of the soldiers threatened to kill him with their bayonets but an officer intervened. One of the patients in the ward then called out to the officer that McCarthy had a gun under his pillow. The officer took possession of the revolver and McCarthy was promptly moved to another ward, where he was kept under close guard.[41] A large party of soldiers continued to search through Hospital 2–3 for rebels.[42] Many of the patients were hysterical and over the din of screaming and shooting, the staff shouted appeals to both sides to stop the madness.[43]

After a further encounter on the top floor of Hospital 2–3, six Volunteers were captured. The soldiers then forced access to the female Catholic hospital, and after an exchange of fire the seven Volunteers occupying the building retreated through the wards, chased by the soldiers. The Volunteers managed to escape from the building and made their way to the nurses' home. The troops now wished to push on and attack the buildings at the front and capture the rebel headquarters in the nurses' home. Their advance was thwarted by their lack of knowledge of the maze of lanes and streets, and the Volunteers pinned them down, firing on them from vantage points in the surrounding buildings.

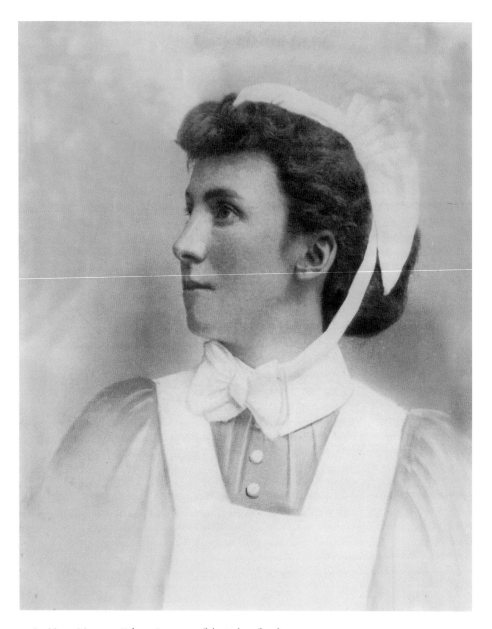

8.16   Nurse Margaret Kehoe. Courtesy of the Kehoe family.

During the fighting the military searched houses on the South Circular Road overlooking the Union, and when each search was completed a soldier was posted in each
house. One house owner confronted a soldier, 'Look here boy,' he said, 'that is a hospital. Be careful,' and the young man replied, 'Don't I know it well. Didn't I often go
there to visit my grandmother.'[44]

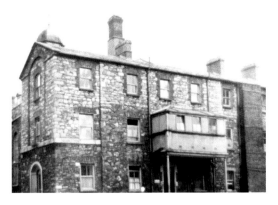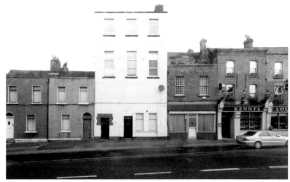

Left 8.17   The maternity building from which British snipers fired on the night nurses' home, which stood opposite and at a short distance. Private collection.

Right 8.18   Crimea House (centre). Rosanna Heffernan was killed by a bullet that entered through a window on the first floor. The birthplace of William T. Cosgrave is the red-brick house on the right with 'Kennys' over the door. Photograph: Anthony Edwards.

By late afternoon the firing began to die down and the soldiers maintained their positions for the night. They had met with stiff resistance from the Volunteers during the day and the regiment had not been able to advance towards Dublin Castle. However, with nightfall, eighty-six soldiers of the regiment did manage to reach Dublin Castle.[45]

Fighting on Tuesday

From daybreak on Tuesday, intense fighting recommenced, with machine guns in the Royal Hospital Kilmainham spraying the Union buildings with bullets. Soldiers gained access to the dining hall of the old Foundling Hospital and, taking up positions at the windows, they began to fire on volunteer positions in the offices fronting James's Street. A British sniper, positioned in a building that housed the maternity wards, opposite the nurses' home, killed 19-year-old Frank Burke, stepbrother of W.T. Cosgrave, who was on the top floor of the nurses' home. Cosgrave had persuaded Burke to become involved in the National Volunteers movement and the death of his stepbrother affected him deeply for the rest of his life, as he blamed himself for involving Burke in the rebellion.[46] In the intense crossfire it was inevitable that there would be civilian casualties. William Halliday, on holiday from Belfast, was shot on the South Circular Road and Mrs Rosanna Heffernan, who lived in a large house known as Crimea House in James's Street, was killed by a stray military bullet. Crimea House stood opposite the Union, and it was given its name because shirts had been produced there for the soldiers who were sent to fight at Balaclava in the 1850s.[47]

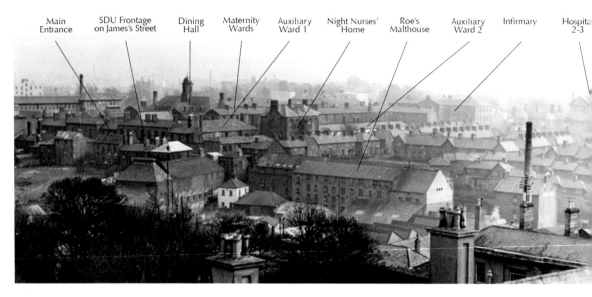

Main Entrance   SDU Frontage on James's Street   Dining Hall   Maternity Wards   Auxiliary Ward 1   Night Nurses' Home   Roe's Malthouse   Auxiliary Ward 2   Infirmary   Hospital 2-3

8.19   The South Dublin Union as seen from the Royal Hospital Kilmainham. BMH/IE/MA/P/42/4. Courtesy of the Military Archives, Ireland.

The soldiers now controlled most of the South Dublin Union, apart from the Volunteers' headquarters and the offices and boardroom that fronted James's Street. Lieutenant Colonel Owens intended to continue and complete the assault on the remaining positions held by the Volunteers. Much to his amazement, he received orders to take his soldiers out of the grounds and to withdraw to Kingsbridge station, which he did under protest.[48] His superiors had decided that Dublin Castle was secure and that it was not necessary to continue the assault. However, British forces continued to pin down the Volunteers in the nurses' home with machine-gun and sniper fire.

The Volunteers erected a five-foot-high strong barricade across the hallway of the nurses' home, facing the front door. The stairs behind the barricade turned at right angles onto a landing that ran parallel to both the front of the house and to the barricade in the hall. They erected a second barricade, a foot in height, on this landing. This allowed them to lie on the landing and fire into the hallway over the main barricade. The purpose of these barricades was to have successive lines of defence if the soldiers succeeded in getting through the front door. Such a breach was unlikely to happen, as Volunteers covered the front door from the upper windows. The one attempt to take the house from the front during the week was successfully rebuffed.

On Tuesday morning the assistant matron, Anne Mannion, returned from Belfast, where she had been for the Easter weekend. She had great difficulty in gaining access

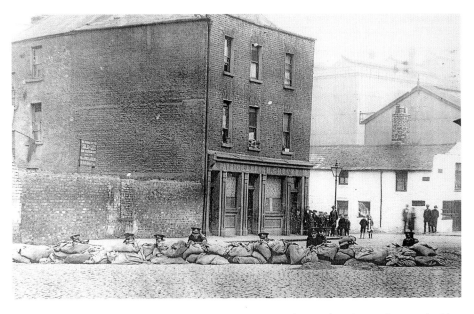

8.20   British soldiers near James's Street. From S. O'Broin, *Inchicore Kilmainham and District* (Dublin, 1999).

8.21   Hallway of the night nurses' home showing the arched doorway that Volunteers barricaded. Reproduced from Cliff Housley, *The Sherwood Foresters in the Easter Rising, Dublin 1916* (Dublin, 2015).

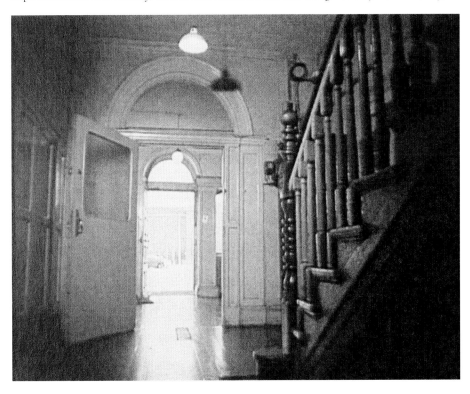

to the Union because of the barricade at the entrance on James's Street and the constant gunfire. She succeeded eventually and immediately set about delivering food and supplies under a Red Cross flag. The staff continued to work throughout the week, caring for the frail and sick. Later on Tuesday the bodies of five Volunteers, which had been removed to the small laundry shed at Rialto, together with the bodies of Nurse Kehoe, Mr Halliday and inmates of the Union who had either been killed in the action or had died of natural causes, were buried temporarily in a plot in the master's fields.[49]

Battle for the Union

Thursday saw the most intense fighting of the week. The early part of the day was quiet and staff took the opportunity to begin moving patients from the immediate area around Ceannt's headquarters. One of the Volunteers, Michael Lynch, found time to visit his aunt who was a wardmistress.[50] Patrick Smyth, a wardmaster, went to the bakehouse for bread. He had to step over a dead soldier to enter and was immediately halted by another soldier, holding a rifle. The soldier was 'shaking all over' and it took a while for Smyth to convince him that he was not one of the Volunteers. Meanwhile the Volunteers in the boardroom broke through the walls of the offices fronting James's Street into the adjacent No. 1 Auxiliary Ward so that they could move freely between the boardroom and the nurses' home.[51]

On Thursday afternoon, two battalions of Sherwood Foresters left Ballsbridge showgrounds with instructions to march to the Royal Hospital Kilmainham. They made their way along the South Circular Road without incident until they arrived at Rialto, where they came under heavy fire from the Volunteers in Jameson's distillery, who were under the command of Séamus Murphy. Panic ensued and their horses began to stampede. The soldiers were unable to cross the exposed Rialto bridge and their commanding officer, Colonel W.C. Oates, ordered the column to halt and sent an appeal to Portobello Barracks for assistance. Sir Francis Vane, a major in the Royal Munster Fusiliers, was in charge of the defence of the barracks at Portobello and was about to go out on a patrol with a party of fifty experienced men and five officers.[52] He set off 'at the double' with his men for the South Dublin Union. Vane, described by Desmond Ryan as 'an unusually capable commander', was invited by Oates to take command of the attack on the rebel positions.[53] Vane and his men entered the Union grounds and, meeting up with a company of Sherwood Foresters, Vane assumed overall command.[54] He began his assault on the rebel positions at 4 p.m.[55] The soldiers advanced 'by sectional rushes, in files and open formation, pouring a curtain of fire or unceasing stream of bullets into all objects in the line of advance. As each line of some fifty men approached, another line was seen advancing close behind them from Rialto, and it soon became evident that the nurses' home was their main objective.'[56]

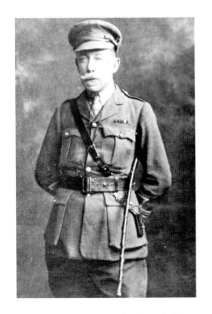

8.22 Sir Francis Vane. Reproduced from *Agin the governments* by Francis Vane (London, 1929).

8.23 Captain Michael Martyn. Reproduced from 'The Robin Hoods': the 1/7th, 2/7th and 3/7th Battns, Sherwood Foresters, 1914–1918 (Nottingham, 1921).

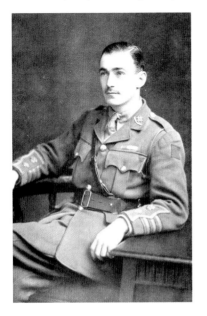

Meanwhile, a convoy of eight wagons of supplies travelling from Kingsbridge station to Portobello Barracks was halted by the action. The convoy was guarded by two officers and fifty men under the command of Lieutenant Monk Gibbon, who would later become a distinguished Irish writer. In his autobiography, *Inglorious soldier*, Gibbon describes the scene:

I remain to help Vane. He is very cool and has been walking about under fire carrying just his little cane. The Union is being attacked across a field. The little party I have brought with me are to support. We lie on the grass at the rear. Other troops are advancing by short runs in front, a party of about twenty. They signal us up and we dash up and lie down on the grass in an orchard about twenty yards behind them, getting what cover we can. There is little or none, and the rebels are pouring a steady fire from the windows of the Union ...[57]

Assault on the nurses' home

Vane described the action on Thursday afternoon in a letter to his wife written a few days later:

Well I have been in some fights but never in such an odd one as this for we commenced by open fighting in fields and so far as right flank was concerned fought up to literally 3 feet of the enemy. But everything was bizarre on that day for we advanced through a convent where the nuns were all praying and expecting to be shot poor creatures, then through wards of imbeciles who were all shrieking – and through one of poor old women, until we zapped our way right to the wall of the house occupied by the enemy.[58]

As the fighting continued Captain Michael Martyn noticed No. 2 Auxiliary Ward, a long low two-storey building to the left of the nurses' home and connected to it.[59] Martyn led the way across to the building, which was originally a manufactory for the Foundling Hospital, but which in 1916 was being used as wards for older people. He proceeded through the ground

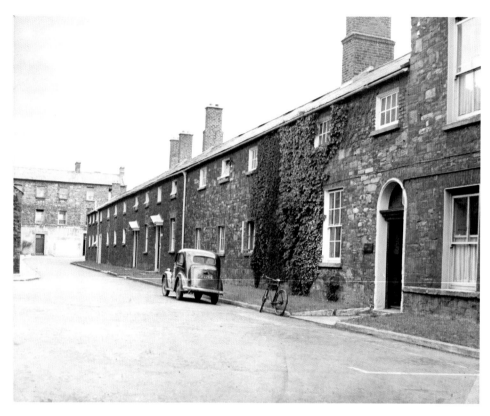

8.24   The long, low building (No. 2 Auxiliary Ward) attached to the night nurses' home. Private collection.

floor ward until he came to the side wall of the nurses' home. The soldiers broke a hole in the wall and then crawled through it. They found themselves in a room that opened into the lobby, or front hallway, of the nurses' home. Two privates, George Barrett and Arthur Warner, rushed into the lobby followed by Martyn and Corporal Walker. The two privates were shot and killed as they ran towards the barricade.[60] However Martyn and Walker managed to crawl to the barricade. They were followed by Captain John Oates, son of the commanding officer. Oates later recalled what he saw in the lobby:

> I shall never forget that scene. I was looking into a lobby. To my right was the main door of the nurses' home, which had been blocked up with all sorts of rubbish. To my left was a wide doorway or archway – a kind of ornamental affair dividing the lobby. This had been barricaded with the most extraordinary conglomeration of everything you could possibly think of – sandbags, stones, rocks, furniture, mattresses. Opposite me was a door. It was open and I could see that it led into some kind of offices with a big barred window at the far end.

'Mickey' Martyn and Sergeant Walker were stretched flat on the floor just under the barricade with the Sinn Féin rifles sticking out of the barricade just over their heads. The rebels, apparently, were unable to depress them to the right angle. I saw Walker take a pin out of a bomb and try to throw it over from where he lay. Unfortunately there were only a few inches of space between the top of the barricade and the ornamental arch and it was not an easy thing to do. Instead of going over, the bomb hit the top of the barricade and fell back into the room. I thought 'My God – that's the end of them!' and I'm ashamed to say, I ducked back. Then I heard a tremendous explosion.[61]

Martyn and Walker were not killed, as the former had grabbed the hand grenade and thrown it over the barricade where it exploded on the far side. Martyn was awarded the Military Cross for this act of bravery.[62]

'The British are in'

When the soldiers broke into the front hallway of the house, Ceannt realized that the situation was desperate. He led the Volunteers out of the nurses' home and into a room on the top floor of No. 1 Auxiliary Ward, which stood just north of their head-quarters. There they were joined by the Volunteers from the boardroom. Believing that the soldiers would take the nurses' home, the Volunteers decided that they would not surrender and that they would fight to the finish in the boardroom and adjacent offices. Cosgrave argued that the military had not in fact taken the nurses' home and urged Ceannt to return.[63] Meanwhile Brugha, who was on the second floor of the nurses' home, heard shouts of 'the British are in!' Believing that the soldiers had penetrated the building, he slowly made his way down the stairs, gun at the ready. It was at this moment that Martyn threw the grenade. Brugha took the full force of the blast as he came down the stairs, and he was severely injured. John Joyce, who had been firing from the top floor of the house, was the last man to come down the stairs and he found the seriously injured Brugha lying on the ground. Despite his injuries he was pointing his 'Peter the Painter' pistol at the barricade, intending to defend the position on his own. Joyce made his way out of the house to the room where the remaining men of the battalion had assembled, and he informed them of Brugha's serious condition.[64] Ceannt left immediately, taking Peadar Doolan, the battalion's first-aid officer, and Cosgrave with him. As they approached the back of the house they heard Brugha singing 'God save Ireland'. Brugha had propped himself against a wall and was firing at the barricade intermittently to stop the soldiers from crossing over it. Brugha's courage inspired the Volunteers to take up positions again in the nurses' home and they sent a deafening barrage of gunfire across the barricades.

As one of the Volunteers, James Foran, was making his way back to the boardroom, he saw about thirty soldiers behind the bakehouse. Foran ran back to warn the Volunteers and the soldiers started an intensive assault on the house. Some of the soldiers heard voices coming from a ground-floor room of No. 1 Auxiliary Ward. One of the men climbed up to a barred window about 8 feet above the ground level and dropped a hand grenade inside. The room was used for storing clothes but some inmates had gathered there believing it was safe. The grenade killed one man and injured several others.[65] The Volunteers in the nurses' home were now surrounded, but just when things looked very bleak, the assault suddenly stopped. The British were fired on from behind by their own men, and thinking that they were surrounded by Volunteers, they withdrew.[66]

Meanwhile, in the nurses' home, the soldiers had withdrawn, apart from Captain John Oates, who remained in a room off the hallway. There were two boxes near him containing forty-eight bombs. He began to throw a bomb into the lobby every two or three minutes:

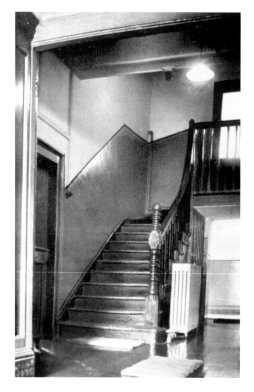

8.25   The stairs and return where Cathal Brugha was severely injured. Reproduced from S. Ua Ceallaigh, *Cathal Brugha* (Dublin, 1942).

> I felt sorry for the old people behind me in the Ward – the noise must have been horrible – but I never heard a sound from them. Every now and then these chaps kept firing into the lobby and then I'd give them another one. I'd got through one box and was half-way through the other, beginning to wonder what I was going to do next, when Martyn returned. He said, 'It's all right now – brigade and the transports have got through – we've managed to keep these chaps so busy that they haven't had time to give trouble. Orders now are to withdraw.'[67]

The soldiers withdrew from the buildings surrounding the nurses' home at 8:30 p.m. The battle had lasted nearly five hours.[68]

Surrender on Sunday

There was no fighting on Saturday and the Volunteers did not become aware of the general surrender ordered by Patrick Pearse on Saturday until the following morning, when Thomas McDonagh arrived from Jacob's Biscuit factory to inform

Ceannt, who then briefed his men of the decision of headquarters. The men were reluctant to surrender, but they had no other realistic option. The garrison then paraded in the courtyard before marching out through the main gate.[69]

The surrender was witnessed by 12-year-old Cissie Keenan, who lived in the square on Bow Lane. In 1994, when she was 91-years-old, she recalled the events of Easter Week 1916. When the fighting stopped towards the end of the week she was allowed on the lane. One of her friends, Paddy Byrne, ran over to her and said, 'Let's go up to the Union, Ceannt is surrendering.' She remembered clearly:

> There wasn't a soul on the road. You could see all the way down James's Street as far as the post office.
>
> The only action on the road was a British officer, a soldier, maybe a sergeant, in front carrying a white flag and a Church Street [Capuchin Franciscan] priest. They walked slowly up the road until they reached the main gate of the Union with its heavy wooden doors and enormous arch.
>
> They knocked on the gate and it was some minutes before the gate was opened. I think they had to remove some barricades. The three went in.

8.26   A guard-duty roster found in the night nurses' home by the matron, Anne Mannion, following the surrender. BMH, WS297, by Anne Mannion. Courtesy of the Military Archives, Ireland.

After twenty minutes someone shouted that Ceannt and his men were marching out. She then heard another say, 'Take a good look at him for it is the last time you are likely to see him.' Throughout her long life the sight of Ceannt exhausted and limping at the head of his men lived vividly in her memory.[70]

Following the surrender, a Red Cross ambulance took the wounded men out of the South Dublin Union. Cathal Brugha and Dan McCarthy were taken in the same ambulance to an improvised hospital in Dublin Castle. The British soldiers expected a much larger force to emerge and were astonished that such a small garrison could have held the South Dublin Union. Vane had estimated that there were two hundred men fighting against his force in the region of the nurses' home on the Thursday.[71] In a letter to his wife on 2 May he wrote, 'I am sorry for our poor fellows who were killed. They fought splendidly. So did the enemy.[72]

The assistant matron, Anne Mannion, recalled that after the Volunteers had vacated the South Dublin Union, the gates were thrown open and crowds went through the nurses' home looking for mementos.[73]

The Union takes account

The day after the surrender, the guardians formed a committee for the purpose of feeding the poor living in the immediate areas around the South Dublin Union. It was Tuesday, 2 May, before John Condon, the clerk of the Union, was able to re-enter his office for the first time since the Rising had begun. He was shocked by what he saw. He told a meeting of the board of guardians on 10 May that 'the office was in a deplorable state. The windows were riddled with bullet holes, all the presses and cabinets were broken open, and their contents scattered broad cast over the whole place ...' He attempted to restore some order with the help of two of his office staff and they started by 'taking the minute books from the windows where they were used as barricades, and bore evidence of their use as such, many of them being pierced with bullet holes'.[74]

The master, Edward Doyle, gave his report on the events of the rebellion to the same meeting. He summarized the conflict and described the Volunteers as 'the invaders'. He then went on to praise the staff and to describe measures he took to ensure the welfare of the inmates under his care:

> He cannot too strongly praise the courage and devotion to duty of the great majority of the workhouse staff, ministers, priests, nuns, storekeeper and his assistant, wardmasters, wardmistresses, nurses etc., they all behaved splendidly under very trying circumstances also some of the inmates.
>
> Whilst it is invidious to mention names he cannot refrain from mentioning the master baker and his two assistants Kynes and Kelly, who attended here daily and with the assistance of inmates, kept the bakery running with the result that we had plenty of bread not alone for our own requirements but were able to give to the poor and others who were unable to procure bread elsewhere for love or money. On Tuesday, he had the dead bodies of the Volunteers collected and brought to a temporary morgue near the back gate, where all save one have since been identified.[75]

The master informed the meeting that George McNamara, the resident medical officer, who had been on continuous duty throughout the week of the rebellion, had been arrested by the military on Saturday, 29 April, and was still being detained. McNamara resumed his duties on 18 May. At a meeting of the board on the 17 May the guardians expressed their sympathy on the death of Nurse Kehoe.[76] One of the nuns, Sr M. Austin Frost, who worked in the cancer ward of the South Dublin Union, received leg injuries from a bullet wound which left her with a permanent disability. Several members of staff were subsequently awarded bonuses because they had 'during the recent disturbance carried out their own duties and any other duties allocated to them with fearlessness and self-sacrifice'.[77] Revd Richard Dillon was the Catholic chaplain to the South Dublin Union during the fighting of 1916.

He spent the week in the Union and it was said of him that 'his spiritual duty was his only consideration, and with the utmost impartiality he assisted the wounded and dying among the combatants'.[78]

Fate of the leaders of the Volunteer forces in the South Dublin Union

Éamonn Ceannt was tried before a military court on 3 and 4 May. He was found guilty 'of taking part in an armed rebellion and in the waging of war against his Majesty, the King'. He was executed by firing squad on 8 May in Kilmainham Jail.[79] Con Colbert, who fought in Jameson's distillery was found guilty on the same charge and was also executed early on the morning of 8 May. Ceannt and Colbert were the only two leaders from the 4th Battalion to face death by firing squad.

W.T. Cosgrave was sentenced to death but was reprieved and sentenced to penal servitude for life. He was sent to Portland Prison in Dorset and later moved to Lewes Jail in Sussex, where many of the rebels were held.[80] He was released from prison in June 1917. Cosgrave went on to play a leading role in Irish politics and was elected president of the executive council of the Irish Free State in 1922. He held the post for a decade and played a key role in establishing Irish democracy.

Cathal Brugha eventually recovered. The serious nature of his injuries probably saved him from execution, as he was not expected to survive. His heroic stand soon became part of the folklore of the rebellion, and it is commemorated in the rebel song 'The foggy dew': 'O had they died by Pearse's side, or fought with Cathal Brugha'.

2016 commemoration

St James's Hospital and Trinity College Dublin held a joint commemoration for the centenary of the Easter Rising on the weekend beginning Friday 6 May 2016. It was organized in collaboration with the 4th Battalion Dublin Brigade 1916 Relatives' Group and the Rialto-Kilmainham 1916 Commemoration Committee. The weekend began with a two-day symposium on the Easter Rising in the Trinity Centre for Health Sciences, which was opened by the late Liam Cosgrave, former taoiseach and son of W.T. Cosgrave. On Saturday, a ward in the hospital was named in honour of Nurse Margaret Kehoe; the lord mayor of Dublin, Críona Ní Dhálaigh, opened an exhibition of photographs relating to the Rising and an evening of readings and music took place in the Trinity Centre for Health Sciences. On Sunday 8 May, a plaque was unveiled in the central square of St James's Hospital by David Ceannt, grand-nephew of Éamonn Ceannt, and by Cathal MacSwiney Brugha, grandson of Cathal Brugha. The weekend of commemoration concluded with a recital from the locally based St James's Brass and Reed Band, which was established in 1800 and has played at many events of national significance since then.

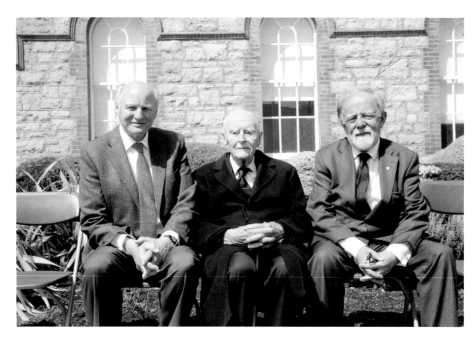

8.27   At the Easter Rising commemoration at St James's Hospital on 8 May 2016: David Ceannt (left), grand-nephew of Éamonn Ceannt; the late Liam Cosgrave (centre), former taoiseach and son of William T. Cosgrave; and Cathal MacSwiney Brugha (right), grandson of Cathal Brugha. Photograph: Mark Maxwell.

8.28   Easter Rising commemoration on 8 May 2016 in the central square of the hospital. Photograph: Mark Maxwell.

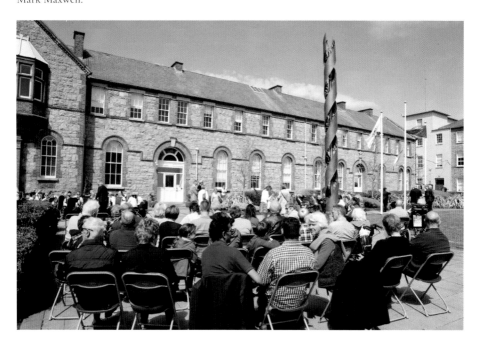

9

War and politics

This anachronistic symbol of an alien government.[1]

At first the rebellion of Easter Week was perceived to be a failure, but the execution of fifteen leaders over ten days caused great reaction throughout Ireland and a demand for independence. Most members of the board of guardians, in common with the majority of the people of Dublin, did not support the 1916 rebellion. However, after the executions, support on the board for the nationalist cause grew rapidly. This change was signalled in a very dramatic way by the co-option of Áine Ceannt, widow of Éamonn Ceannt, onto the board of guardians in March 1918 and her election as deputy vice chairman a few months later.[2]

The general election of December 1918 gave Sinn Féin a decisive mandate to create an independent Irish parliament in Dublin. Dáil Éireann met for the first time on 21 January 1919 and established a provisional government. The programme adopted by the First Dáil included the following declaration:

> The Irish republic fully realises the necessity of abolishing the present odious, degrading, and foreign poor law system, substituting therefore a sympathetic native scheme for the care of the nation's aged and infirm, who shall no longer be regarded as a burden but rather entitled to the nation's gratitude and consideration.[3]

Nationalist control of the Dublin Union

In local elections held in January and June 1920, supporters of Sinn Féin were elected onto several local county councils and boards of guardians. A sufficient number of nationalists were elected onto the board of guardians of the Dublin Union to give them a majority. Margaret Pearse, mother of Patrick and Willie Pearse, was among those elected onto the board and Áine Ceannt was returned. A guardian with republican sympathies, Michael Ó Fogludha, was elected as chairman at a meeting on 23 June 1920.

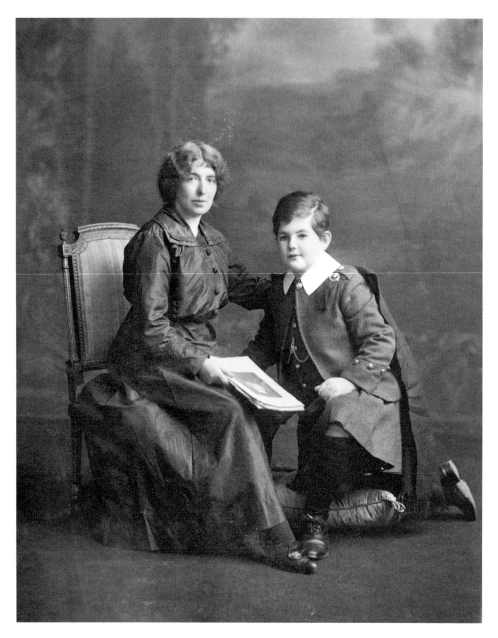

9.1   Áine Ceannt and her son Ronan. Image courtesy of the National Library of Ireland.

The British forces now regarded the Dublin Union as an institution under republican control and a potential refuge for rebels. The Union was surrounded by military on 1 January 1921 and a detailed search of the wards and of several departments was carried out. The only thing that the search yielded was a packet of sporting cartridges on top of a cupboard in the master's office.[4] The residence of the master was also subjected to military raids. Edward Doyle, who was the master at the time, had already been through the traumatic events of 1916. He was known to be a Parnellite and members of the Doyle family recalled years later that they were subjected to constant harassment by the Black and Tans. One of Doyle's daughters, Pauline, recalled seeing an older brother:

> being held by a Tan at the point of a bayonet while his comrade questioned her parents whom they had interrupted at a meal.
>
> The commanding officer suddenly broke off his questioning, gazing at a picture on the dining room wall, of a major in the British Army. He asked who it was and my father replied that it was my mother's brother. The search was immediately called off and we were left in peace after that. It transpired that the C.O. had been in school with my uncle.[5]

On 2 February 1921, the board of the Dublin Union received a circular demanding full allegiance to Dáil Éireann and its agencies. The guardians were instructed to cease all communications with the British Local Government Board and to communicate only with the Local Government Department of Dáil Éireann. The board complied with these requests.[6]

Uncertain times

The unsettled nature of the times made it difficult to ensure cash flow and income, and there was also a significant demand for outdoor relief. As a consequence, the board was well over £35,000 in debt to its bank in early February 1921. The bank refused to honour any further cheques until something was done to reduce the large overdraft. The guardians were put in a very serious position as the contractors threatened to cease supplies if their accounts were not paid. The supply of flour was the first to be affected, but the contractors also threatened to stop the supply of other essential commodities, such as milk and meat. The guardians realized that unless the situation changed, they would be unable to keep the institution open, as there were 3,858 inmates to be fed, of whom 1,700 were sick and receiving hospital treatment, and there were a further 8,000 people dependent on outdoor relief.[7] A number of astute deals by the master with suppliers, and eventual lodgements from Dublin Corporation and Dublin County Council, eased the situation, although the bank continued to refuse to increase the overdraft and also refused to honour certain payments.

Political allegiance

Despite these financial problems, the political allegiance of the guardians never wavered. At their meeting of 18 May 1921, they passed a motion of sympathy to the relatives of Revd James O'Callaghan, who was shot during a military raid on a house in Cork where he was a visitor, and to the relatives of Daniel O'Brien, a member of the IRA who was executed in Cork for being in possession of a revolver.[8] Michael Ó Fogludha was re-elected chairman of the board of guardians in June 1921. The proposer and seconder both spoke in Irish and Ó Fogludha's response was also in Irish. Later in the year, in the hope of improving the financial situation, the board of guardians agreed to the appointment of a commissioner by the Local Government Board of Dáil Éireann with a remit to reform the administration of the Union. Séamus Murphy, who had commanded the Volunteers in Jameson's distillery during the Easter Rising, was appointed as commissioner and he was given plenary powers by the board of guardians.[9]

The workhouse system was regarded by nationalists as an integral part of the British legacy in Ireland. During the War of Independence, several workhouses were closed and this had a direct impact on the Dublin Union, as many displaced inmates from the country workhouses made their way to the city and sought admission to the Dublin Union. The increase in numbers was a source of great annoyance to the guardians, as it was an extra cost for which they were not compensated. Another source of grievance was the non-payment by the British military for the occupation of the North Dublin Union. The military owed a sum of nearly £7,500 for goods purchased from the North Dublin Union and £18,000 in rent for the three-year occupancy.[10] After the Anglo-Irish Treaty in 1921, which established the Free State, the military authorities suggested that the guardians' claim 'was one for financial adjustment between the Imperial and Free State governments'.[11]

Refugees from Belfast's sectarian conflict

Between 1920 and 1922, sectarian conflict raged in Belfast, beginning in July 1920 with riots in the shipyards. Loyalists marched on the shipyards and forced over 2,000 Catholics and socialist Protestants out of their jobs. This led to rioting in residential areas, resulting in the deaths of twenty people. The rioting was followed by recurrent violence, particularly in the first half of 1922, which included the burning of Catholic-owned houses and the eviction of large numbers of Catholic tenants.[12] Catholics fled Belfast in large numbers, seeking refuge in Glasgow and Dublin. By June 1922, about 1,500 refugees were being lodged in Dublin, in mostly unsuitable accommodation. The provisional government re-housed 500 refugees at Marlborough Hall, a teacher-training college in Glasnevin. On 9 June, W.T. Cosgrave, then minister for local government, appealed to the master of the Union to provide accommodation for refugees. Cosgrave asked that the refugees not be listed as destitute inmates, but be recorded under a separate system.[13] The refugees included men, women and children, and 393 had been admitted to the workhouse of the Dublin Union by 21 June 1922.

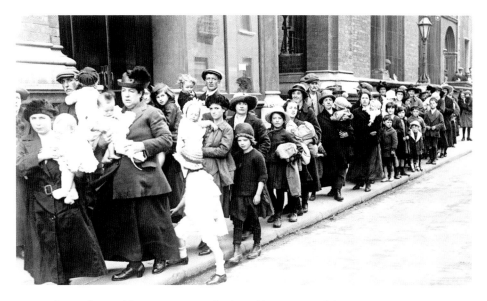

9.2   Refugees from Belfast queuing outside the Kildare Street Club (now Alliance Française) in Kildare Street at the end of May 1922. Photograph: Getty Images.

9.3   A refugee child with her doll, outside the Kildare Street Club at the end of May 1922. Photograph: Getty Images.

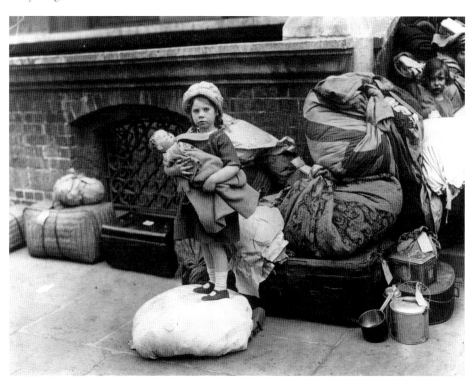

The Dublin Union and the Irish Civil War

A substantial number of republicans opposed the Anglo-Irish Treaty and rejected the authority of the new Irish Free State. The majority of the nationalists on the board of guardians supported those who opposed the treaty. At the annual general meeting of the board of guardians on 14 June 1922, Michael Ó Fogludha was again elected as chairman, Mary J. McKean was elected as vice chairman and Margaret Pearse as deputy vice chairman. The election of McKean and Pearse reflected the strong representation of women on the board of guardians.

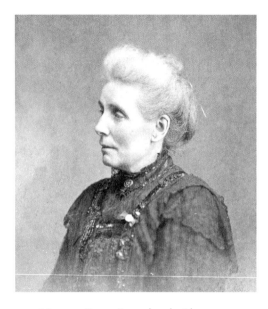

9.4 Margaret Pearse. Reproduced with permission of the Pearse Museum/OPW.

Civil war erupted on 28 June 1922 when Free State soldiers attacked the Four Courts, which was held by anti-treaty forces. The conflict took place very near the Dublin Union and the board of guardians met on 3 July 1922 to set in place measures to relieve the distress of the local population. The clerk read the minutes of 3 May 1916, which showed the steps taken by the board of guardians to help the local population during the 1916 Rising. They then passed a resolution empowering the relieving officers and the officers of St Vincent de Paul to grant provisional relief to deserving cases of distress by providing credit notes with traders or by the distribution of money.[14] Food was distributed to those in need as well as bedding and surgical dressings. Trains were not running and as a consequence milk was in short supply. Fifty-five people were admitted to the Dublin Union either for their own protection or because they had been made homeless by the military operations.[15]

The guardians made no secret of their support for the anti-treaty forces in the Civil War. Government soldiers attacked hotels in O'Connell Street that were being used as the headquarters of the Dublin Brigade of the Irish Republican Army. Cathal Brugha, who had fought with such tenacity in the South Dublin Union and who was now a leading member of the anti-treaty forces, was shot dead when he refused to surrender. At a meeting of the board of guardians on 12 July the following resolution was passed unanimously:

> That we, the Dublin board of guardians tender our sincere sympathy to Mrs Cathal Brugha and family on the death of her husband who during his life and unto death had laboured for the cause of Ireland, and who did so much for the revival of the

Irish language and the upholding of the republic which he was instrumental in establishing.[16]

On 2 August, a vote of sympathy proposed by Margaret Pearse on the death of Harry Boland, another prominent republican, was passed unanimously.[17] She was a strong supporter of Éamon de Valera and the anti-treaty cause, and she claimed that her sons would never have accepted the Treaty.[18]

Opposition to summary executions

The members of the Third Dáil met for the first session on 5 September 1922. The meeting was overshadowed by the growing success of the guerrilla warfare being waged throughout the country. There were doubts about the effectiveness of the army and fears that the pro-treaty government forces might be defeated. It was in these circumstances that the public safety bill was introduced in the Dáil on 27 September. The bill empowered the army to establish military courts that could impose the death sentence for a number of offences, including the possession of arms or aiding attacks on government forces. The board of guardians expressed strong opposition to this policy. The first executions – of four men who were apprehended carrying arms – took place on 17 November, and a further three anti-treaty IRA men were shot two days later. The arrest of the author Erskine Childers for carrying a gun at his cousin's house in Co. Wicklow, and his execution on 24 November 1922, was quickly condemned by the board, which passed the following resolution unanimously: 'That our board offers its sympathy and condolence to the friends and relatives of all those who on either side and non-combatants, have lost relatives in this deplorable conflict.'[19] The board then went on to pass a second motion, condemning the execution of Erskine Childers and the other republican prisoners.[20] On the 6 December 1922, in a motion proposed by Margaret Pearse, the guardians expressed their horror and indignation at the execution of more republican prisoners of war, and they tendered their sympathy to the relatives of three men.[21]

As the violence escalated, on 7 December, the day the Free State government was officially established, a pro-treaty Dáil deputy, Sean Hales, was shot dead in a Dublin street. The Free State ministers met immediately and decided that four republican prisoners, who had surrendered in the Four Courts, would be executed in reprisal. The summary executions of untried and unconvicted men produced a shocked reaction in Ireland and abroad. The board of guardians met on 13 December. It was a short meeting at which only three motions were proposed and they were all passed unanimously. They first deplored the shooting of Sean Hales and tendered the sympathy of the board to his relatives.[22] The second stated their abhorrence of the raiding and burning of the houses of pro-treaty TDs. The third, proposed by Margaret Pearse, condemned the executions of the four republican prisoners and, as a protest against the 'illegal executions', the board meeting was adjourned.[23]

End of the Civil War

The Irish Republican Army was defeated by the government forces and the hostilities ended in May 1923. Some members of the board of guardians now began to use their positions on the board to campaign for the release of republican prisoners. In July, a motion seconded by Margaret Pearse demanded better conditions for female prisoners being held in the buildings of the North Dublin Union.[24] In October the board of guardians received a deputation, led by Hannah Sheehy-Skeffington, in relation to the republican prisoners on hunger strike in a number of jails. Following the discussions, the board passed the following resolution: 'That we are of the opinion that the prisoners now on hunger strike should be unconditionally released and that we ask this in the name of humanity and peace.'[25] Copies of the resolution were sent to General Risteárd Mulcahy, President W.T. Cosgrave, Kevin O'Higgins, Lord Glenavy, chairman of the senate, and to the governor general. This was to be the last political act of the guardians, as within three weeks the government would dismiss the board.

Dismissal of the board of guardians

An inspector, James MacLysaght, was appointed by Séamus Burke, the minister for local government, to investigate the affairs of the Dublin Union. In the years after 1916 there had been regular allegations of poor management, maladministration and lax accounting.[26] MacLysaght presented his report in November 1923 and it contained several significant criticisms of the administration of the Dublin Union. The minister acted at once by sending a copy of the report, together with a letter, informing the guardians that he was dissolving the board 'in the interest of effective and economical public administration', and enclosing an order appointing Séamus Murphy, in his position as commissioner, to take over the functions of the board of guardians.[27] The guardians were angered by their summary dismissal and they passed the following motion:

> That this board, after close on 3½ years diligent work on behalf of the rate payers and the poor, strongly protests against being dissolved at such short notice as even not to allow of its dealing with today's agenda or without being given an opportunity of discussing the inspector's report.[28]

Murphy was born in 1887 in Terenure, Dublin. He attended Synge Street School and left at the age of 15 to take up a position with Hely's stationery shop in Dame Street. During the Easter Rising he had been captain of the garrison that occupied Jameson's distillery, whose purpose was to attack British military attempting to enter the southern grounds of the South Dublin Union. After the Rising he was imprisoned in Knutsford in Cheshire and in Frongoch in Wales. He was released from prison in December 1916 and spent some time in Galway, where he edited a newspaper and was undercover for the IRB. After the Civil War he returned to Dublin, where he joined the civil service in the Department of Local Government. Now, seven years after the Rising, he was in administrative charge of the Dublin Union. Within a short period, two other commissioners, Dr William C. Dwyer and Jane Power, were appointed. One of the suggestions MacLysaght had made in his report was that 'the hospital should be separated from the body of the house and be under distinct control'.[29] He also advocated the discharge home of patients who had recovered from an acute illness rather than the existing practice of transferring them to other parts of the institution, where they would stay for long periods. Murphy issued instructions to the master and medical staff banning the transfer of successfully treated patients from the acute wards to other parts of the Union. A further attempt to reform the admission system was made in 1924, when the commissioners decided that all children being admitted should have a doctor's note of referral.[30]

Acute hospital proposal

Murphy proved himself to be a very able commissioner. He was the first to propose the development of a well-equipped acute hospital on the site. He outlined his ideas in a letter to Frank Dunne, honorary secretary of the medical staff of the Dublin Union. Murphy envisaged structural alterations to Hospitals 2–3 to make them more suitable for admitting seriously ill patients. He proposed the training of probationer nurses, the building of a nurses' home for the student nurses, the development of X-ray and bacteriological departments and the establishment of facilities for lectures and examinations. He aimed to effect immediate change and, even though his proposals 'might embody a highly equipped hospital', he believed this could be accomplished by a carefully instituted 'step by step' plan.[31]

We shall never know if Murphy's enthusiasm for these changes would have made them possible, as he ceased to be a commissioner early in 1924 and was replaced by James MacLysaght. Murphy's plans, which involved moving inmates between different buildings so that facilities for acute patients could be rationalized, was seen as a threat to the segregation of inmates on religious grounds and caused alarm in the Church of Ireland. The commissioners received a letter from the Church of Ireland archbishop of Armagh, Charles Frederick D'Arcy, stating:

> that Mr E.M. Bateman, Church of Ireland chaplain, Dublin Union, informs him that there is in contemplation a very drastic re-organisation of the hospital's arrangements, which will change altogether the present arrangement whereby Protestant patients are kept together. Asking the commissioners to receive him together with certain of his city clergy in order that he may learn from the commissioners exactly what the proposals are.[32]

The objections were successful and Murphy's plans to develop an acute hospital were not progressed. Dublin City Corporation was dissolved in 1924. In the same year,

Murphy was appointed as chairman of three commissioners who took over the functions of the corporation. He held this post until 1930, and during his tenure he accomplished major reforms.

Rural and urban poverty

From the early 1920s, the Irish government undertook the daunting task of tackling rural and urban poverty in the newly independent state. The Civic Survey (1925) noted that 39 per cent of Dublin's population were paupers; there were 5,338 inmates in the Dublin Union and there were 121,135 paupers on outdoor relief of some kind, out of an estimated total population of 327,000.[33] The government took over the administration of the Irish poor law in 1920 and the boards of guardians were replaced around the country by county boards of assistance. These changes were initiated under informal 'county schemes', but later became law under the Local Government (Temporary Provisions) Act 1923. This act reduced the number of workhouses in the country but kept one central workhouse for each county. The changes in local government administration, introduced in 1923, left the poor law administration in the Dublin Union area almost unaltered.[34] Under the Ministers and Secretaries Act 1924, the Department of Local Government and Public Health, with its own minister, became the statutory central authority for the Irish poor law services that previously had been under the control of the Local Government Board.[35] This situation continued until a separate Department of Health was established in 1946.

Despite the best intentions of the commissioners of the Dublin Union to bring about change, they were overwhelmed by the sheer volume of people seeking both indoor and outdoor relief and by the lack of financial investment. The Dublin Union continued to function largely as it had done in the previous century. It fulfilled the functions of a county home, but also continued to provide hospital services for the poor of Dublin.[36] Writing in 1927, the Carmelite historian Dillon Cosgrave described how those admitted to the Dublin Union were distributed among the different sections of the workhouse:

> The inmates are divided roughly into three classes, the allocation to a particular class being based on the health or rather the degree of ill health, of the individual. In the first class called 'The Healthy Yards' the able-bodied, healthy inmates reside. The term 'able-bodied healthy' is a misnomer when applied to these poor people. They show very often from their appearance that lack of nourishment and comfort during their lives has rendered them infirm and prematurely old. Amongst this class the frequent outbreaks of influenza find a heavy toll of victims.
>
> The next class is called 'The Garden Infirmary'. Here the sick among the inmates serve, so to speak, a time of probation before they enter what are known as the Regular Hospitals. The Regular Hospitals are the third class. For neatness and

efficiency they compare favourably with any of the city hospitals. A visit to this division of the Union would serve to dispel the constant prejudice of the poor that degradation or shame is attached to the acceptance of the city's charity. Besides these main divisions, there are smaller ones called 'Isolated Wards'; two for consumptives, one for epileptics and those suffering from kindred diseases, and two for the mentally deficient. In these divisions there is altogether an average population of nearly four thousand.[37]

In the 1920s, an attempt was made to improve the image of the Dublin Union by introducing the name 'St Kevin's Institution'. The name was chosen because St Kevin was a patron of the archdiocese of Dublin. Although this name was used in official correspondence and documents, the general public continued to refer to the institution as 'the Union' or 'the Union Hospital'. Further confusion was introduced in the mid 1930s when the title 'St Kevin's Hospital (Dublin Union)' appeared on official notepaper. The institution was entered under this name in the *Irish medical and hospitals directory*, which was first published in 1937, and it was described as a general rate-aided hospital.[38] This remained the name used to describe the institution in the directory over the following decade until it was changed to 'St Kevin's Hospital' in the late 1940s. Yet, over the whole of the same period, the hospital was described in legal and government documents as the hospital of the Dublin Union.

The last master

The last master of the Dublin Union, Edward Doyle, resigned in 1929 in somewhat contentious circumstances. The auditor of the annual accounts of the Dublin Union had criticized the standard of the account-keeping in a number of audits. He was particularly critical of the failure to collect rents for grazing lands belonging to the Union. Both Doyle and the clerk, John Condon, were questioned about the matter at a meeting of the Dublin Union commissioners. The clerk blamed the master and argued that he did not have sufficient staff to deal with the issues raised in the audit, whereas the master placed the blame on the clerk for overlooking the matter. Both made strong arguments in their own defence. Doyle argued that recommendations from previous auditors' reports had been 'honestly and well carried out', and that since his appointment:

> he had successfully conducted the institution to the general satisfaction of the ruling authorities, and with sympathy and kindness to those under his charge. That period embraced the Great War, the 1916 Rising, 'the pogroms in the North of Ireland, which entailed the reception into the workhouse and catering for a large number of refugees' and also the 'exceptional distress period'.[39]

However, all pleas and arguments were to no avail. It would appear that the outcome of the inquiry had already been decided, as a letter to the commissioners from the secretary to the Free State's Department of Local Government and Public Health expressed the dissatisfaction of the minister, and went on to state that:

> little or no improvement can be effected without a thorough reorganisation of the entire staff. The minister is of the opinion that in view of the nature of this report and those of former audits, both the clerk and master should be called upon to tender their resignations with a view to effecting the necessary reorganisation.[40]

The master and the clerk were accordingly asked to submit their resignations and they complied. Doyle was asked to stay in his post until the proposed new arrangements were in place. Within a week, the commissioners forwarded their views on the reorganization of the administrative structures to the minister of local government and public health. They recommended the appointment of a resident medical superintendent (RMS), who would have overall responsibility for the supervision of the Union, and a chief clerk. The commissioners considered that an RMS was necessary because:

> the Dublin Workhouse Institution was developed on lines on which eighty per cent at least of the institution must come directly under medical supervision and that any lay person appointed no matter how active, would be stunted if he had not got some particular qualifications.[41]

Ten days later the commissioners wrote a further letter to the secretary of the Department of Local Government and Public Health, enclosing a twenty-four page memorandum regarding the staffing of the 'Dublin Workhouse and Dublin Union'.

Resident medical superintendent

Although proposed as a key reform, several of the duties of the RMS as outlined in the memorandum still reflected the ethos of the workhouse, beginning with the title of the post, 'resident medical superintendent of the workhouse'. The institution was referred to as the workhouse throughout the document, which contained a detailed list of the duties of the post, thirty-five in all. The RMS had to ensure that every poor person admitted was to be 'searched, cleansed and clothed; to be medically examined; and to be placed in the ward appropriate to the class to which he appears to belong …'[42] He had to 'provide for and enforce the employment of adult male inmates in such duties as they may be capable of performing and to allow none who are capable of employment to be idle'.[43] He also had duties of care for 'sick inmates' and was responsible for the supervision of the medical officers, including the visiting medical officers. Furthermore, he was required:

> to keep the hospital departments of the workhouse available for affording clinical instruction to students of medicine and surgery and instruction to probationary

nurses in accordance with rules to be prescribed by the board with the approval of the minister.[44]

The memorandum also outlined the duties of other senior staff and, as in the case of the RMS, these posts had a strong 'workhouse flavour'.

William C. Dwyer was appointed RMS in 1930 by the Local Appointments Commission. Born in Merrion, Co. Dublin in 1891, Dwyer had an unusual career. He was on the clerical staff of the South Dublin Union for thirteen years and while in this post he studied medicine, graduating in 1921. He served as a commissioner to the Dublin Union from 1923 to 1930, when he was appointed to the post of RMS. Dwyer also served as a commissioner for Dublin Corporation and played a large part in developing new housing schemes so that people could be relocated from the appalling slums in central Dublin. The RMS lived in the former master's house, Garden Hill, thus underlining the link with the previous administrative system. Dwyer resigned in 1943 because of ill health. The position was filled by Rose McLaverty in an acting capacity. She joined the staff of the Dublin Union as a resident medical officer in 1930. She worked in a variety of positions in the Dublin Union and in St Kevin's and resigned in 1946 for health reasons.

At this time there were two resident medical officers and the posts were much sought after. A candidate usually needed political support on the Dublin Board of Assistance if he or she was to be successful. The salary was £250 a year and included accommodation in a fine red-brick house that had a lawn, a tennis court and a garage. Resident medical officers were also assigned a maid to look after them.[45] An appointment was held for two years and responsibilities included the day-to-day care of patients and the administration of anaesthetics to patients undergoing surgery. Staffing on the wards was still very dependent on inmate labour and the resident medical officers were frequently asked by the nuns to prescribe 'mist. stim.' (a small whiskey) for the male workers.

Physicians and surgeons between the world wars

Despite the reforms of the early twentieth century, the number of consultant staff had remained unchanged since the South Dublin Union era. There were two surgeons, William C. Cremin and Patrick D. Sullivan, and two physicians, James J. Flood and Lewis J. Farrell. Cremin was born in Effin, Charleville, Co. Cork and he matriculated from Mungret College, Limerick in 1897.[46] He studied medicine in the Royal College of Surgeons in Ireland (RCSI), qualifying in 1903. He was awarded a diploma in public health (DPH) in 1905 and in the following year he became a fellow of the RCSI. He served as medical superintendent for Pembroke Urban District Council, which consisted of a large area stretching from Donnybrook to Ringsend, before his appointment to the staff of the South Dublin Union. Sullivan was a native of Limerick and studied medicine in the RCSI, graduating in 1905. Following postgraduate training in anatomy and surgery, he was appointed surgeon to St Kevin's Hospital and held the position until his death in 1940.[47]

James Flood was born in Dublin and educated at the Christian Brothers' School, North Richmond Street and at Castleknock College. He served initially at the North Dublin Union but following the merger of the unions he was appointed as a visiting physician to the Dublin Union, where he worked until his sudden death in 1937.[48] Flood was very interested in art and played an active part in the cultural life of Dublin. Lewis J. Farrell studied medicine in the RCSI and was appointed physician to the South Dublin Union hospital in 1911. He took a keen interest in sport and as a young man he was one of the early players for Bohemian Football Club, serving as goalkeeper for the team.[49] He was on the staff of the hospital until 1938, when he died, aged 64.

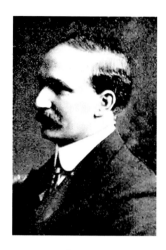

9.5   Dr William C. Cremin. Reproduced from the *Mungret Annual* (1948).

T.C.J. (Bob) O'Connell was appointed surgeon in 1941 to succeed Sullivan. O'Connell graduated from University College Dublin in 1930. He travelled to Berlin in 1933 to work in the clinic of the leading chest surgeon of the period, Ferdinand Sauerbruch, and he worked subsequently in the Brompton Hospital in London. O'Connell was responsible for providing a general surgery service to the hospital and he also established a special thoracic unit. At about the same time he began to develop a practice at St Vincent's Hospital. He eventually found that he could not cope with the burgeoning workload in both hospitals. This led to his resignation and departure from St Kevin's Hospital in 1945.[50]

William O. (Billy) Cremin, son of William C. Cremin, was appointed physician to St Kevin's in December 1939. He graduated from University College Dublin in 1933 and was awarded an MD three years later. He worked in the Mater Hospital, Dublin, and the Brompton Hospital, London. Father and son were both on the staff until the death of William C. Cremin in 1948 and they had a very lucrative practice in their residence at 120 St Stephen's Green West.[51] W.C. Cremin had a major collection of art and antiques, which included works by Brueghel, Canaletto and Rembrandt and many other famous painters. His son, Billy, a reserved and private man who never married, went on a cruise for three weeks every year and read medical books during the cruise. He also spent some time in London each year at a medical conference. He spent most of his day seeing patients in the hospital and at his residence, and went on house calls in the evening in a chauffeur-driven car.

Despite the improvements in healthcare, there had been no major capital investment in the institution and neither was there an appreciable change in the manner in which the institution functioned. Inmates still occupied grim old buildings that were in bad repair and many of the hospital's patients were housed in similar buildings. The onset of the Second World War would delay for another decade any attempts to make significant changes to the fabric of the hospital.

The Dublin Board of Assistance

The three commissioners continued to administer the institution until 1931, when the Local Government (Dublin) Amendment Act 1931 replaced them with the Dublin Board of Assistance. The Dublin Board of Assistance administered the poor law in the Dublin city area together with the part of Dublin county that was formerly a part of the Celbridge Union, around Rathcoole and Lucan. This body was composed of nominees of Dublin Corporation and Dublin County Council, which both supplied, through the rates, the funds required to support the institution. These administrative changes had little impact on day-to-day life within the Dublin Union, which still retained most of the characteristics of the Union workhouse. In the rest of the country, with the exception of the Cork Union, separate provision was made for patients incapacitated by chronic illness, for the elderly and for acute care. All of these categories were still to be found in the Dublin Union/St Kevin's Institution.

Accommodation for patients

There were six male hospitals, four female hospitals and the Rialto Hospital in St Kevin's (Dublin Union) in 1935. The male patients were housed in hospitals 1 and 2–3 (old numbering), in the male skin and epileptic hospital, which also accommodated cases of venereal disease, and in the Protestant hospital (now Hospital 2). The latter had its own matron and staff. Hospitals 2–3 were contained in one large granite building, which, while intended to accommodate only acute medical and surgical cases when it was erected in 1876, in fact housed a large number of chronically ill patients and only the top floor was reserved for surgical cases. There was a small two-roomed pathology laboratory on the ground floor of the acute hospital, which was run by two members of staff: a temporary pathologist, Michael F. Dodd, who was a commandant in the Army Medical Service, and his technician, John Duffy. The hospital was also equipped with an operating theatre. Hospital 1 was devoted mainly to chronic patients, as was the skin and epileptic hospital. The male Protestant hospital was also mainly for chronic patients.

The four female hospitals included the main female hospital, which housed both acute and chronic patients and had an operating theatre; the skin and epileptic hospital, which contained mostly chronic patients; the female Protestant hospital, which housed primarily chronic patients; and the maternity hospital. The maternity hospital had historically been quite busy but by 1935 most of its activities had been transferred to an auxiliary workhouse at Pelletstown.

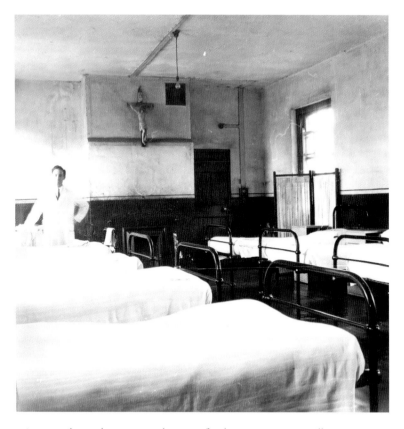

9.6   A ward attendant stops work to pose for the camera. Private collection.

The Rialto Hospital had 175 (female and male) beds for patients with pulmonary tuberculosis. This hospital was jointly managed by the Dublin Board of Assistance, because it was in the Union grounds, and by the public health authorities of Dublin city and county, because management of tuberculosis was perceived as a public health rather than a poor law concern. In addition to the above mentioned hospitals, St Kevin's provided separate accommodation for the old and infirm, both male and female, for sick children, and for the 'able-bodied destitute'.[52] A new four-storey building, Hospital 6, was constructed for male inmates at the front of the institution in 1934. It was a long narrow building with steel-framed windows and it was christened the 'Queen Mary' by Dubliners because it resembled the contemporary Cunard liner of that name.

Development of a radiology department

In January 1930, there were 4,366 residents in the Dublin Union/St Kevin's Institution and 1,230 of these were described as 'hospital cases'.[53] Despite the aspirations of the commissioners in their early reports, the hospital did not yet have a proper pathology

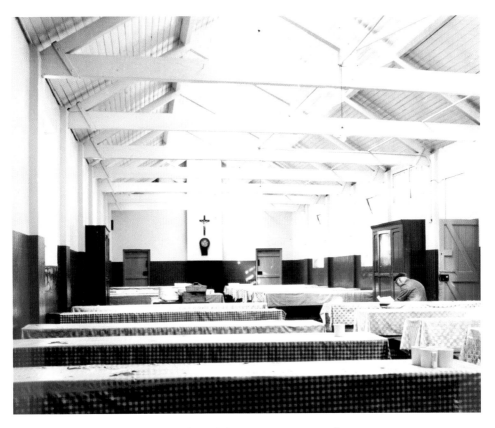

9.7   A man reading in a dining room for ambulant inmates. Private collection.

or X-ray department, but it was about to acquire both. One of the visiting surgeons, William C. Cremin, wrote to the commissioners in April 1930 asking them to purchase the X-ray and deep X-ray therapy apparatus formerly used by the radiologist Maurice Hayes. Hayes had a private radiological practice in 35 Upper Fitzwilliam Street where he had an extensive range of equipment. Following the acquisition of the apparatus, it was placed in a vacant building adjacent to Hospitals 2–3.[54]

An X-ray department was opened in 1931 and a year later William P. Murphy was appointed as part-time radiologist.[55] Murphy had graduated from University College Dublin in 1927 and decided to specialize in radiology early in his career. He did postgraduate work in Cambridge and in St Bartholomew's Hospital, London, before returning to Ireland where he was the first radiologist to be appointed as a permanent member of the hospital staff. He was supported by one part-time radiographer. He was also radiologist to Temple Street Children's Hospital. He was only 36 when he died of pneumonia in 1936. His obituary in the *British Medical Journal* stated that, following his appointment to St Kevin's Hospital, 'he did much work in founding and building up the department of radiology, which as a result of Murphy's work, is now one of the best in the city'.[56] He was succeeded by Richard A. Reynolds, who served as part-time temporary radiologist for twelve years before his appointment to the permanent post at the age of 55. He was also radiologist to Temple Street Children's Hospital and to Our Lady of Lourdes Hospital in Dún Laoghaire, which specialized in treating patients with spinal tuberculosis (the latter is now the National Rehabilitation Hospital). Reynolds carried out the first mass radiographic surveys in Ireland. His studies concentrated on institutions in Dublin and Cork and he found that 17 per cent of the children had active primary tuberculosis.[57]

A sheet of blotting paper

St Kevin's also provided accommodation for 'casuals', destitute men and women who were provided with sleeping accommodation but who had to leave during the day. Families evicted from their homes were also given shelter. The 'casuals' section continued to exist until major reforms were introduced in the middle of the twentieth century. The institution held very negative connotations for the local inhabitants who still called it 'the Union', and many people dreaded the possibility of ever being admitted there. Local children also feared 'the Union', a fear often instilled in them by the older generation, as the Dublin historian Eamonn MacThomais, who grew up in the neighbourhood, recalled:

> One morning as I passed the Union gates and turned into Pigtown, I noticed that women were sitting outside their whitewashed cottages, one woman asked me 'did you pass the Union gate by yourself?'. 'I did', I replied. 'Well you will want to watch out', says she, 'that they don't pull you in and give you the blue pill'. The children in school had the same story and a story about the dead nun who came through the side wall at twelve o'clock at night … The story of the dead nun and the blue pill, the children in school, and the old women in Pigtown, all had a terrible impression upon my childish mind … I ran like the hammers-of-hell past the Union gate. One day I heard the gate cringe as if to open: I got such a fright that I dropped my school bag and I did not wait to pick it up; but a man picked it up and came flying after me. 'My goodness the devil must be chasing you', he said. 'No mister', says I, 'it's the blue pill and the dead nun'. The man laughed and got on his bike and rode away.
>
> Another morning an unusual thing happened. As I was getting into my gallop to come past the Union gate I had to stop suddenly to allow a horse and car to come out of the big brown gate; it was a funny looking car, a black square box. I was later to know that it was the charity hearse. When the horse and car pulled out, I stopped and peeped into the Union gate. There was a big clock hanging on the wall with a brass frying pan, I thought, swinging back and forth. To the right of the clock was an office with a glass partition and looking out through the glass partition was a nice friendly-looking man with silver hair, he smiled at me and I smiled back. 'Come in' says he. I approached the gate cautiously and the man came

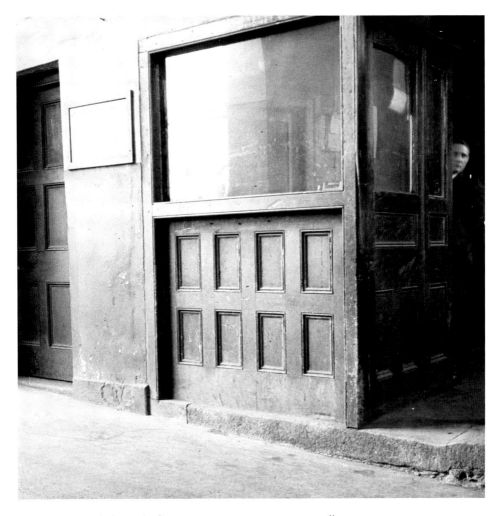

9.8   The porter's lodge at the front gate on James's Street. Private collection.

out the door. 'Are you going to school? Would you like a piece of blotting paper?'
And out of a big white pad was pulled a sheet of snow-white blotting paper. He
handed it to me and it felt warm and soft and nice.[58]

A poet's recollection of the Union

Thomas Kinsella, who is recognized as one of Ireland's great urban poets, was born
in 1928 and was familiar with the Union and the myriads of streets and lanes which
surrounded it when he was a child. His father was born in Bow Lane and his mother
in Basin Street. Kinsella recalled his childhood visits to this area and he remembered

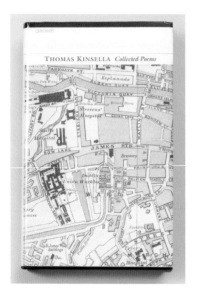

9.9 *Collected Poems* by Thomas Kinsella (2001). Reproduced with permission of the publisher.

a native Irish speaker named Dick King, who lived in one of the lanes and who worked on the Great Southern Railway. The young Kinsella became very attached to King, who subsequently died in the Dublin Union.[59]

Years later Kinsella wrote a poem in King's memory, which included these stanzas:

> Clearly now I remember rain on the cobbles,
> Ripples in the iron trough, and the horses' dipped
> Faces under the Fountain in James's Street,
> When I sheltered my nine years against your buttons
> And your own dread years were to come:
>
> And your voice, in a pause of softness, named the dead,
> Hushed as though the city had died by fire,
> Bemused, discovering ... discovering
> A gate to enter temperate ghosthood by;
> And I squeezed your fingers till you found again
> My hand hidden in yours.
>
> I squeeze your fingers:
>
> Dick King was an upright man.
> Sixty years he trod
> The dull stations underfoot.
> Fifteen he lies with God.
>
> By the salt seaboard he grew up
> But left its rock and rain
> To bring a dying language east
> And dwell in Basin Lane ...
>
> And season in, season out,
> He made his wintry bed.
> He took the path to the turnstile
> Morning and night till he was dead.
>
> He clasped his hands in a Union ward
> To hear St James's bell.
> I searched his eyes though I was young,
> The last to wish him well.[60]

10

A hospital for the sick poor

We feel the time has come – if it be not overdue – to tackle this problem in a big way and with the vision it requires; and that if it be done, lasting benefit will result to the State, the local authority and the poor.[1]

Abject poverty was still common in Dublin in the 1940s. Tuberculosis, diphtheria, typhoid, respiratory disease, arthritis and gastrointestinal infections were rampant. The life expectancy for a male infant born in the city was ten years less than that for a male infant born in Connacht, and there was a seven-year gap for female infants.[2] The paediatrician, author and social campaigner Robert Collis described the city's broad streets and affluent squares as its 'outer garment', but if you lifted the hem, he wrote, 'you will find suppurating ulcers covered by stinking rags, for Dublin has the foulest slums of any town in Europe'.[3] In 1938, there were 6,307 tenement houses in the city occupied by 111,950 persons and many of the houses were in a dangerous condition.

The Irish Hospitals' Sweepstake

The acute hospital services in Dublin were provided by voluntary hospitals that had been founded by philanthropic individuals or bodies. These hospitals were not under a statutory obligation to accept all the sick poor of Dublin in need of hospital care, and they admitted large numbers of patients from around the country. In contrast, the Dublin Board of Assistance had an obligation to provide hospital accommodation for all those in the city who needed it. After the First World War, funding became a major concern for the voluntary hospitals; with the advent of expensive new technologies, the cost of running acute hospitals was rising, inflation had reduced the value of endowment funds and charitable donations had fallen significantly. The hospitals were forced to fall back on their own resources and began to charge patients who had sufficient means for their treatment.[4] As a consequence,

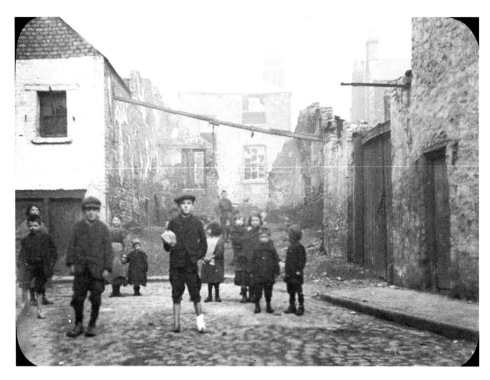

10.1   Children playing in Magennis Court, off Townsend Street, in 1913. Photograph: W.J. Joyce. Courtesy of Dublin City Library and Archive.

the proportion of patients being treated without charge in the voluntary hospitals had fallen to 40 per cent by 1935.[5]

The financial problems of the voluntary hospitals were eased considerably after 1930 with the creation of a lottery known as the Irish Hospitals' Sweepstake.[6] Hospitals that benefitted from this were required to allocate at least 25 per cent of their beds to non-paying patients, but there was no statutory requirement to maintain these free beds once the grant was awarded. Initially, only voluntary hospitals could benefit from the sweepstake, but from 1933, public hospitals could also seek support from it.[7]

Plans for a municipal hospital

Members of the Dublin Board of Assistance were highly critical of the voluntary hospital system and were eager to develop their own hospital to treat the poor. They submitted plans to the minister for local government and public health in 1933 for the development of a big new hospital of 600 beds in the grounds of the Dublin Union, adjacent to the existing acute facilities. This new municipal hospital would have its

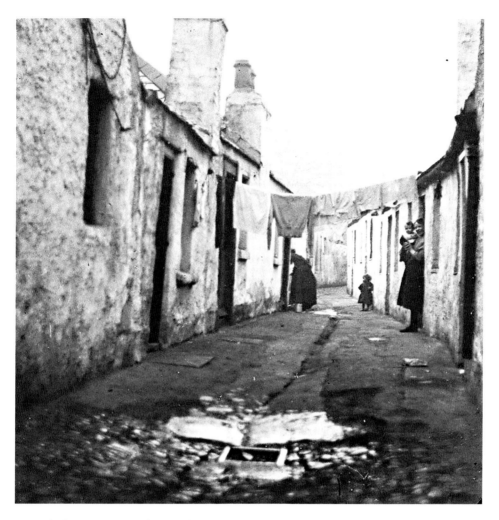

10.2   Plunkett's Cottages, off Sandwith Street, in 1913. Photograph: W.J. Joyce. Courtesy of Dublin City Library and Archive.

own separate entrance from Mount Brown or from the South Circular Road. The acute facilities would be called St Kevin's Hospital, after the patron of the archdiocese of Dublin, to distinguish it from the residential component for inmates, which would become known as the 'homes section' of the Dublin Union.[8] The minister submitted the proposal for the new hospital to the Hospitals Commission, which was established by Sean T. O'Kelly, minister for local government and public health, in 1933. Its role was to survey hospital facilities throughout the country and to advise the minister for local government and public health on the distribution of funding from the Hospitals' Sweepstake.[9] The Board of Assistance did not get a prompt response and, in February 1936, the following resolution was passed:

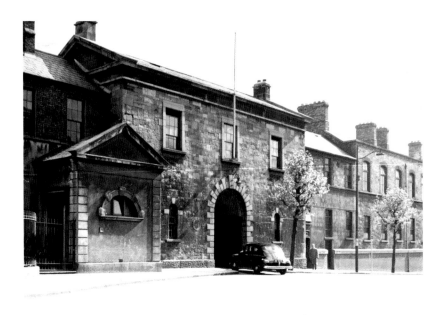

10.3   Entrance to the Dublin Union from James's Street c.1950. Private collection.

As the provision of a municipal hospital is admitted by all sections of the committee to be an urgent necessity, we further wish to draw the attention of the minister for local government and public health and the Hospitals Commission, to the delay in attending to the proposals of the board, submitted over two and a half years ago.[10]

The emergence of a strong lobby for a municipal hospital in Dublin caused great anxiety to the medical establishment associated with the voluntary hospitals. A joint meeting of members of the sections of medicine, surgery and pathology of the Royal Academy of Medicine in Ireland was held in May 1935 to discuss the state of the voluntary hospitals and to emphasize the importance of the research and teaching functions of these institutions. They met 'not alone with the object of clarifying our own opinions, but also with a view to helping, if they will be good enough to consider it a help, the members of the Hospitals Commission in the solution of their formidable and difficult problems'.[11]

The Hospitals Commission

In 1936, the Hospitals Commission published its first general report, which was very critical of the Dublin hospitals. According to the report, there were too many small hospitals, many of them using antiquated facilities. There was little cooperation between

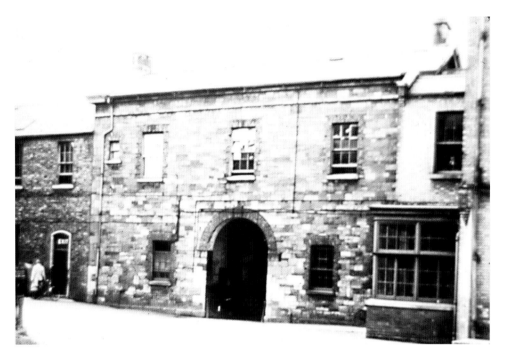

10.4   Entrance to the Dublin Union as seen from the inside c.1950. Private collection.

10.5   The eastern frontage of the Dublin Union on James's Street c.1950. Private collection.

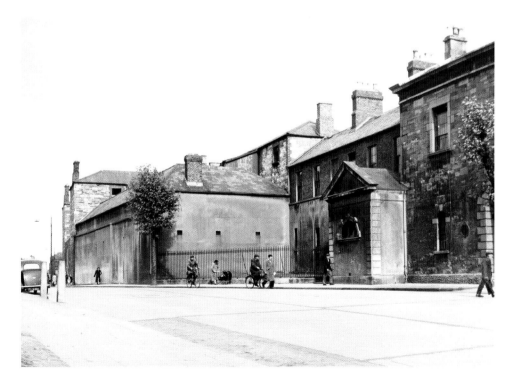

consultant specialists, and teaching was dropping behind international standards.[12] The report explored the advantages of a federation or amalgamation of hospitals and recommended that there should be two general hospitals in north Dublin and two in south Dublin. On the north side, the Mater and the Richmond Hospitals were identified for development. On the south side, the report recommended the construction of two large hospitals; one would consist of an amalgamation of Sir Patrick Dun's, Mercer's, the Royal City of Dublin (Baggot Street) and the Meath Hospitals, and the other would be a considerably enlarged St Vincent's Hospital on a new site. St Vincent's Hospital was situated at that time on St Stephen's Green in the city centre.

Should the voluntary hospitals be unable to respond to the challenge of providing the necessary accommodation for the poor, the commission suggested that St Kevin's Hospital should be developed as the chief hospital and clinical teaching centre in Dublin. This was a clear shot across the bows of the voluntary hospitals. The commissioners estimated that there were approximately 500 acute medical and surgical beds in St Kevin's Hospital. They expressed the view that 'this figure may be regarded as equivalent to the number of rejections through lack of accommodation by the voluntary hospitals'. As a consequence, they concluded that an assessment of the bed requirements of Dublin city would be incomplete if it did not take into account the 500 beds at St Kevin's Hospital.[13]

Strong opposition from the voluntary hospitals

Clinicians in the voluntary hospitals were generally pleased with the report as it had not advocated the development of a municipal hospital as a first option. A general meeting of the Royal Academy of Medicine in Ireland was held on 1 May 1936 to discuss future hospital policy for Dublin. The purpose of this meeting appears to have been to bury any further consideration of a municipal hospital. Henry Moore, professor of medicine at University College Dublin, was the main speaker and he did not beat about the bush: 'the present hospital managed by the Dublin Board of Assistance (St Kevin's) is not a teaching hospital and, in my view, never will be, however large it may become'.[14] Moore argued that the municipal hospital would not attract first-class consultants and would not be able to afford the range of specialists needed, and he rejected the idea of salaried medical staff. Consultants in the voluntary hospitals did not receive salaries and their incomes were dependent largely on private practice; working in a voluntary hospital made a consultant and his work known to family doctors, who would then refer private patients to him. Another speaker, J. Robert Rowlette, professor of materia medica at Trinity College Dublin, also condemned the use of salaries to support hospital consultants: 'the appointment to a paid post and the provision of a livelihood for life in public service not infrequently leads to a conservatism of outlook which is impossible to a man whose reputation and livelihood depend on his possessing a progressive mind'.[15] There were other prestigious speakers, including Thomas G. Moorhead, Regius professor of medicine at Trinity College; the pioneering neurosurgeon Adams A. McConnell; and the surgeon and historian William Doolin. All the speakers, apart from one, roundly condemned the concept of a municipal teaching hospital. The only speaker to disagree with his colleagues was William C. Dwyer, the RMS of St Kevin's and, although he was not vigorous in his support of a municipal hospital, he sought to convince his eminent colleagues that a doctor who accepted a salary did not 'become a mere vegetable, devoid of interest in his work or in humanity'. He argued with 'much force' that for the poor person, who cannot pay fees, the salaried doctor might be more acceptable than the doctor who depends for his livelihood only on those patients who can pay fees. The meeting concluded by passing the following resolution:

> That the future development of the Dublin hospital system being a matter of deep concern to the Royal Academy of Medicine in Ireland, the academy agrees with the opinion expressed in the Hospitals Commission's report that in view of all the circumstances the commission favours the development of the principal Dublin voluntary hospitals as against the creation of a Dublin municipal hospital, and feels certain that those Hospitals will be ready to enter into agreements, satisfactory to the minister, to ensure that the public interest would be safeguarded, particularly as regards the ready admission of poor patients.[16]

Acute cases in St Kevin's

The Hospitals Commission wished to establish the contribution of St Kevin's Hospital to the overall care of acutely ill patients in the Dublin area. This proved a difficult task. Officials of the commission, in collaboration with officers of the institution, could only achieve what was described as a 'more or less arbitrary classification' of the 1,582 patients considered hospital cases. The commissioners decided to rely on the impressions of the RMS, William Dwyer, 'who has had a considerable and lengthy experience of the South Dublin Union', to determine how many of the 1,582 beds could be designated as acute.[17] The RMS was of the opinion that there were, on average, about 300 acute cases in the hospital at any one time. All of these patients were cared for by twenty-four nurses and twenty-six nuns.[18] In 1936, the Hospitals Commission approved a grant of £166 towards adapting existing accommodation to support the development of a pathology department at St Kevin's Hospital because of the major medical and surgical work being carried out there.[19]

The best and most logical solution

In its second general report, the Hospitals Commission estimated that the Dublin Board of Assistance would need at least another 1,200 acute beds in order to meet the needs of the sick poor.[20] The solution which the commissioners proposed was the reorganization of the voluntary hospitals together with an expansion of their capacity. The commissioners reached this conclusion despite stating in the body of their report that the development of St Kevin's Hospital (Dublin Union) into a municipal teaching hospital offered the best and most logical solution. They considered that the development of St Kevin's might act against the interests of the voluntary hospitals, so ultimately they did not support it. In effect, the commissioners yielded to the vested interests of the voluntary hospitals and their powerful consultants. The commissioners argued that the close relationship of the Dublin medical schools with the voluntary hospitals would nullify any attempt to develop St Kevin's as a municipal teaching hospital.[21]

In its third general report, the Hospitals Commission recommended that St Kevin's Hospital should concentrate on:

> the provision of suitable hospital facilities for the long-term medical and surgical cases who cannot be admitted to the general hospitals. A hospital for this purpose should have at its disposal the services of permanent and consultative medical staff, somewhat equivalent to those functioning in a general hospital. It is probable that the nursing staff would not be as numerous as in a general hospital, in view of the smaller turnover of patients, but the demands of training and skill on the nursing staff would not be less.[22]

The commissioners made a modest sum available to refurbish the acute wards in St Kevin's. The medical staff estimated that the refurbishment would provide facilities for 180 male and 180 female acute patients. Although ultimately the recommendations of the minister and the commissioners favoured the voluntary hospitals, the seeds of the concept of developing St Kevin's into a major municipal hospital serving the poor had been sown.[23]

The creation of a bed bureau

At this time it was very difficult for family doctors to source hospital beds for their poor patients. They often had to ring one hospital after another in search of a bed. The commission responded to this situation by deciding to establish a centralized bed bureau, which would identify hospital beds for non-paying patients. The voluntary hospitals strongly resisted the formation of a bed bureau, as they perceived it as yet another attempt by the government to interfere in the internal workings of the hospitals and as a consequence weaken their independence. James Hurson, secretary of the Department of Local Government and Public Health, began negotiations with representatives of the voluntary hospitals in 1936 to try and establish a mutually acceptable scheme. The negotiations dragged on and appeared to be going nowhere until Hurson threatened to proceed with the commission's alternative proposal to establish a municipal hospital. The Dublin Hospitals' Bureau eventually began its work in 1941.[24] It was operated by the Hospitals Commission and had an advisory committee composed of one representative from each of the hospitals participating in the scheme. The bureau, which provided a twenty-four hour service, found beds only for patients who were eligible for admission to public beds. These included local authority patients and national health insurance patients as well as patients who could not contribute anything towards their mainte-nance. Private and semi-private patients were referred directly to a voluntary hospital. St Kevin's Hospital took part in the bed bureau from the beginning, and it accepted 127 patients from the bureau in the first twelve months of its operation. This compared favourably with Mercer's Hospital, which admitted 124 patients and the Meath Hospi-tal, which admitted 143. Dr Steevens' Hospital and St Vincent's Hospital admitted 337 and 457 patients, respectively.[25]

The Dublin Hospitals' Bureau gave the Hospitals Commission very valuable information about the admission policies of the Dublin hospitals. It soon became clear that the voluntary hospitals were generally reluctant to admit patients over the age of 60 who were suffering from medical or surgical conditions such as strokes and fractures. For instance, in 1949, over 489 applications were made by the bed bureau on behalf of patients over the age of 60; of these only 213 were admitted to the voluntary hospitals and St Kevin's Hospital on its own accepted 207. This happened despite the fact that it was the practice of the bureau to seek admission of patients to the voluntary hospitals before approaching St Kevin's. In order to encourage the voluntary hospitals to take more older patients, a scheme was intro-duced to speed up the transfer of patients considered chronic from the voluntary hospitals to the homes section of St Kevin's Hospital.[26]

The Second World War

The Second World War placed further pressure on the Dublin Board of Assistance. There were 2,835 patients and welfare cases in St Kevin's in 1939, reflecting the degree of poverty in the city. Air-raid precautions became a priority and the bedridden and infirm were moved to wards on the lower floors. An air-raid shelter was constructed in the cellars of the Foundling Hospital by reinforcing the arches with concrete walls. The cellars could accommodate 600 people. The homes section of St Kevin's still continued to function in many ways as a workhouse, nearly twenty years after independence. There was still an area for male and female 'casuals' to sleep in overnight, the Foundling Hos-pital buildings were still being used to house a large number of people, children were still living in the institution and infants were being nursed there. Robert Collis paid an unannounced visit to the homes section of St Kevin's during Christmas 1939 and sub-sequently shared his experiences in a wide-ranging paper, 'An examination of Dublin's public-health services', which he read to a meeting of the Irish Labour Party:

> If you go to the Dublin Union, you will find the old people, the mothers and fathers of Dublin, who have been put away, forgotten, abandoned. No, the Union is not an

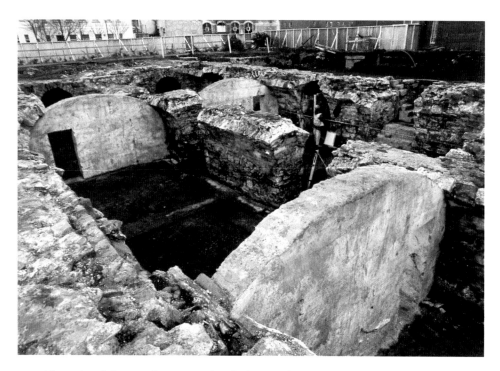

10.7   The vaults of the Foundling Hospital with their reinforced concrete walls. The vaults have been preserved under the Trinity Centre for Health Sciences. They were exposed during the construction of the second phase of the Trinity Centre in 1999. Courtesy of Professor Seán Duffy, Trinity College Dublin.

unkind place. The people who run it are human, and show the love of God in their faces. The inmates smiled on me when I visited it the other day and wished me a Happy Christmas, but I went away very ashamed, for I had never visited it before. I did not know that over one hundred women slept in an attic, built, I judge, two hundred years ago. I did not know that old men with epilepsy, and skin diseases, are left to die in a building no prison department in the world could pass.[27]

Suspension of Dublin Board of Assistance

During the Second World War, the Dublin Board of Assistance wrote to the minister for local government and public health informing him of a shortage of coal, 'without which the heating, cooking and other services in the board's hospitals and institutions cannot be maintained'.[28] The board began to experiment with the use of turf. Despite repeated unsuccessful appeals to the government for aid, the board was castigated in a public broadcast in 1941 by the minister for supplies for its failure to provide coal for the destitute poor.

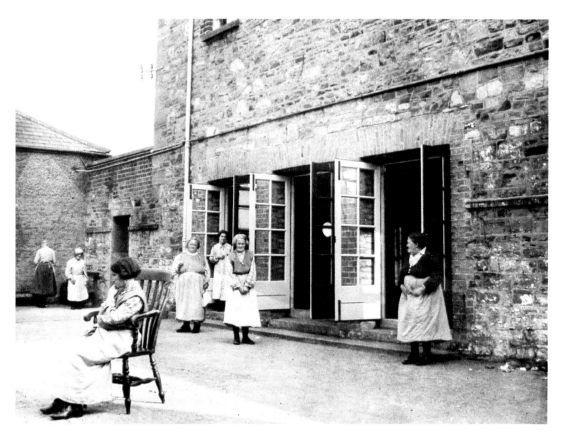

10.8   Women in institutional clothing, outside a day room in the Dublin Union/St Kevin's Institution. Private collection.

The unfavourable publicity gave the minister for local government and public health, Sean MacEntee, the opportunity to suspend the Dublin Board of Assistance in April 1942, following a sworn inquiry into maladministration. Three commissioners were appointed directly by the minister to take over the duties of the Dublin Board of Assistance, which had responsibility for St Kevin's, as well as the wider responsibility for distributing welfare relief throughout the union.[29] The three commissioners appointed were Séamus Murphy, Mary J. McKean and Edward M. Murrray. Séamus Murphy, who was appointed chairman, was an inspector from the Department of Local Government and Public Health. He had wide experience of local government and institutional reform and had already served as chairman of the Dublin Union commissioners who were appointed in 1923. Mary McKean, who had been elected to the board of guardians in 1922, was an experienced voluntary worker in childcare and had taken an active part in the administration of the Dublin Infant Aid Society. Edward M. Murray was an accountant with the Electricity Supply Board (ESB) at the time of his appointment and

had a background in the management of
stores and supplies.

The brief of the commissioners
included an inquiry into the administration of the affairs of the Dublin Board of
Assistance. The commissioners focused
their attention on St Kevin's Hospital, beginning with an investigation
into the staffing and the main departments and sections in the institution.
At this time, between the hospital and
the homes section of St Kevin's and the
Rialto Hospital, there were 106 nurses,
25 of whom were nuns; 39 wardmasters;
38 wardmistresses; and 36 tradesmen.

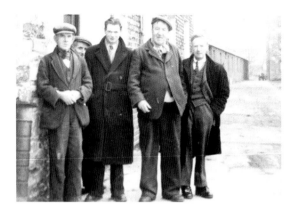

10.9   A group of male inmates. Private collection.

There were tradesmen's shops, a farm, a nurses' home, bath houses, workrooms,
kitchens, a laundry, a bakery, a butcher's shop and a forge situated within the walls
of the institution. In a preliminary memorandum, the commissioners also described
the various groups of patients and inmates and their locations, as follows:[30]

Location	Number of patients
Acute hospitals	294
Female Catholic Hospital	416
Maternity Hospital	36
Rialto Hospital	155
Female Skin & Epileptic	85
Male Infirmary	222
Male Healthy Department	47
Children's Infirmary	64
Hospital 1	135
Protestant Hospital	120
Old Women's Infirmary	102
Male Skin & Epileptic	56
Old Men's Infirmary	168
Female Healthy Department	97

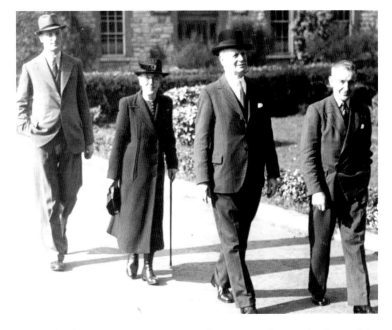

10.10 The three commissioners appointed in 1942 to take over the duties of the
Dublin Board of Assistance (left to right): Edward M. Murray, Mary J. McKean
and Séamus Murphy (chairman), accompanied by the medical superintendent,
Dr W.C. O'Dwyer. Courtesy of Teresa Murray.

The commissioners held meetings with the RMS and the visiting medical staff and
prioritized a number of actions: to appoint a house surgeon and house physician,
to install a new kitchen, to finalize the handover of the Rialto Hospital to Dublin
Corporation and to press for the appointment of a pathologist. The control of
visitors to the wards and of traffic through the hospital was also discussed in the
commissioners' report:

> When we took up duty the institution was practically a public thoroughfare.
> There was no restriction on visitors and the place was used freely by the public
> as a short cut between James's Street and Rialto. The medical officers had com-
> plained of the number of visitors in the wards. The general traffic has been
> stopped ... the admission of visitors is restricted to visiting days (Thursday and
> Sunday), to seriously ill or 'dead' passes and to organizations like St Vincent de
> Paul and Legion of Mary.[31]

The commissioners were critical of the work ethic within the hospital and as a result
of their findings three wardmasters were 'punished' and one 'nun nurse' resigned.

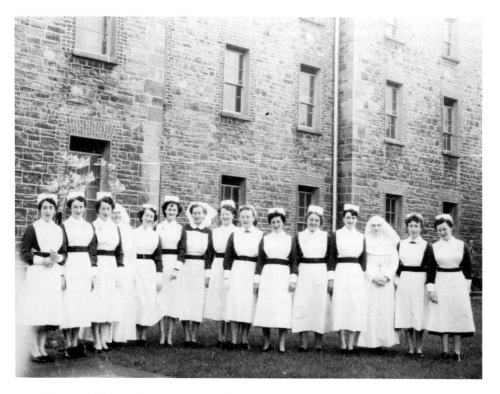

10.11　The nurses' choir in the 1940s. Private collection.

Development of the acute facilities

Significant progress was made in improving the standard of acute medical and surgical care at St Kevin's in the mid 1940s. One of the first developments was the construction of a pathology laboratory. A full-time pathologist had not yet been appointed and the specimens were being sent to the pathology department of the medical school in Trinity College. Another sign of the developing services was the appointment in 1942 of the first junior staff, a house surgeon and a house physician, at a salary of £50 per annum. The number of nursing positions increased in 1941 when the hospital was still under the administration of the Dublin Board of Assistance. At this time opportunities for employment were scarce and political interference in nursing appointments was rampant. In 1941, there were 318 applications for twenty-five positions. An interviewing committee of senior medical and nursing staff selected the twenty-five nurses on merit, eight of whom were chosen because they had special skills for particular areas such as the operating theatre. The politicians on the Board of Assistance were furious that the selection committee had chosen the nurses for appointment and demanded that they should see all the

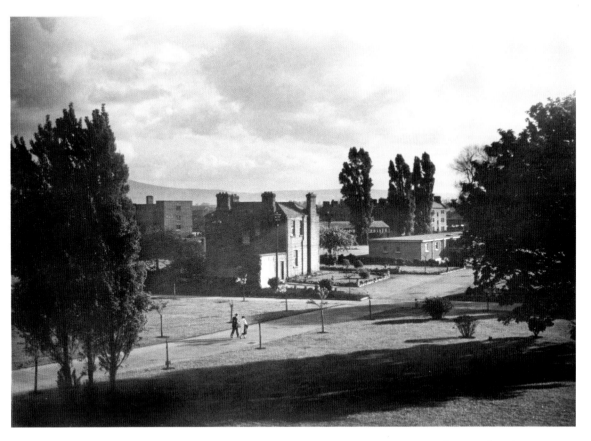

10.12   Two doctors walking in the grounds c.1950. The medical residence is in the foreground, with the single-storey tuberculosis hospital in front of it and the Rialto Buildings on St James's Walk in the background, just beyond the trees. During Easter Week in 1916, the upper storeys in Rialto Buildings were occupied by British troops. Photograph taken from the Garden Infirmary (Hospital 4). Private collection.

applications so that they could make the appointments. They changed eleven of the names on the original list.[32]

The radiology department at St Kevin's provided services to the hospitals within the institution, to external institutions under the control of the Dublin Board of Assistance and to the dispensaries. It also provided an X-ray service for Dublin Corporation, and this amounted to about 5,000 cases each year. The X-ray equipment was approximately twenty-five years old in 1945. In making the case for new equipment and facilities, attention was drawn to the role St Kevin's Hospital was playing in meeting the demands of the Dublin Hospitals' Bureau.[33] The appeal was successful: new X-ray equipment was installed in the Rialto Hospital and funding was also made available for an operating theatre and a canteen with rest rooms and dining facilities for nurses and medical staff. The first annual dance for the staff took place early in 1941 and was a sign of the growing confidence of the hospital.

The third report of the Dublin Hospitals' Bureau, which was published in 1949, acknowledged the importance of St Kevin's Hospital in meeting the demand for general and medical surgical cases. In 1947, St Kevin's admitted a total of 482 cases from the bed bureau: 268 were medical, 179 were surgical and 35 were maternity admissions. The building of a new operating suite and the appointment of medical and surgical consultants to the hospital were considered to be important factors in overcoming 'the traditional reluctance of the public to accept admission to its hospital beds'.[34] In the first six years of the bed bureau's existence, the voluntary hospitals between them had accepted 9,919 patients and St Kevin's Hospital alone had accepted 3,220. These figures clearly demonstrated that St Kevin's was making a significant contribution to the acute medical and surgical services for the city.

Introduction of acute ambulance service

The introduction of an ambulance service in 1947 for the emergency admission of poor patients favoured further development of the acute services at St Kevin's Hospital. Up to that time, patients for admission had to make their own transport arrangements and fund the cost of a taxi or ambulance if required. This created a problem for very poor patients. The Catholic Social Service Conference introduced a new scheme in March 1947, under which the referring doctor informed the bed bureau if his patient was too poor to secure transport. The bureau would inform the ambulance service, which would then collect and transport the patient to a hospital, and the cost would be met by the Catholic Social Service Conference. This arrangement made it easier to admit acutely ill poor patients to St Kevin's.[35]

The commissioners propose a strategy

In 1944, after two years of very close investigation of the institution, the three commissioners produced their report, which began with the following general impression:

> After prolonged examination and detailed practical experience of the housing and administrative problems at St Kevin's Institution we are convinced that in the long run the most satisfactory solution will be found in the evacuation and demolition of the buildings in the chronic and infirm section (Homes), and in the extension and development of the present acute hospital as a fully equipped hospital for the acutely sick poor and their children.[36]

The commissioners found that not only were the buildings those of the old workhouse but that the administration was still largely based on the workhouse system, with the RMS endeavouring to deal with a vast institution practically single-handedly. There

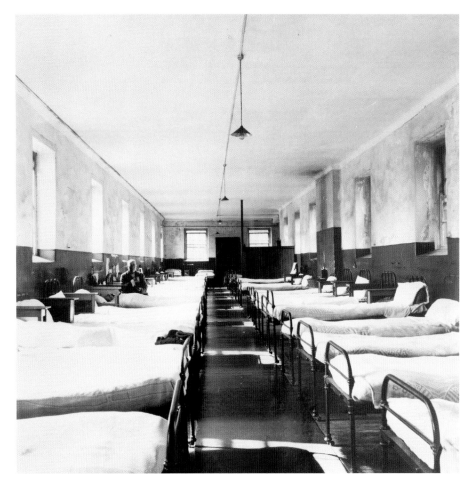

10.13   A ward for ambulant males c.1945. Private collection.

was no proper chain of authority or administrative structure and, as a consequence, the wardmasters and the wardmistresses in charge of different sections of the institution were virtually independent in their actions and were very reluctant to take direction. There were also marked inefficiencies and great laxity within the system and the commissioners found that many patients admitted to the institution stayed, often for a number of years, without good reason.

'Planned disintegration'

The commissioners knew that the building of a new infrastructure for St Kevin's was highly unlikely, so they made several practical recommendations to improve the staffing and the existing buildings. They accepted that their solution might appear to be

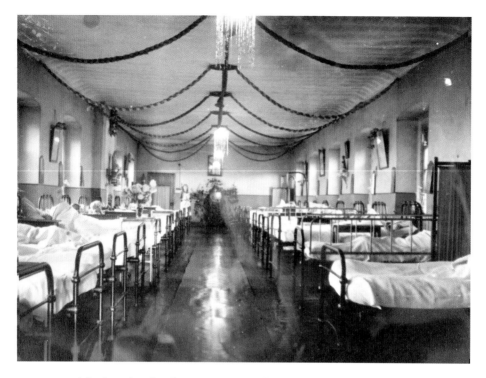

10.14   A ward for dependent females c.1945. Private collection.

drastic to many in the existing climate. They argued that considerable progress could be made by what they termed a policy of 'planned disintegration'. This entailed the gradual removal of the chronic and infirm patients and casuals from the site, the extension of the acute hospital and an increase in nursing and other staff. The commissioners were adamant that, no matter how many new nurses were appointed and no matter how well motivated the staff might be, no progress could be made until there was a significant programme of demolition, refurbishment and the building of new facilities:

> We feel that no impression can be made on those grey forbidding walls; they dominate everything about them and suggest the character of the worst type of a soldiers' barracks. Within the walls, with little exception, the impression is the same and no amount of orderliness which we can introduce can ever have a lasting existence while there remains in the buildings, in their shape, conditions and appearance the sordid reminder of an old and rotten tradition.
>
> Evacuation to other premises must inevitably produce better conditions in staff and administration. Opportunity is opened up to get away finally from a bad old order and to mould the new institution for the aged, chronic & infirm in

decent lines. To say the least of it, the existing accommodation for and service to those classes are not a credit to the State or the local authority, in particular as regards the chief city of Eire.

We feel the time has come – if it be not overdue – to tackle this problem in a big way and with the vision it requires; and that if it be done, lasting benefit will result to the state, the local authority and the poor.[37]

The report of the commissioners also sought to reform the existing administrative structure, to rationalize the activity of the institution and to put in place new key appointments that would drive the process of reform. They concurred with the broad division of the institution into a hospital section and a homes section, as recommended by the Board of Assistance in 1936, and the development of the acute hospital (2–3) as the primary focus of the institution:

The hospital is the only building in the institution which is capable of extension & full development. Its development separately is desirable in that to judge by the failure of the voluntary hospitals to provide sufficient accommodation, steps must be taken to ensure that there will be available a hospital for the acutely sick poor; its development must continue so that it may not be allowed to lapse back into a part chronic hospital. Its primary duty is towards the poor and they should be provided with the best treatment and under the most modern conditions.[38]

Practical reforms

During the war years, despite limited resources, significant developments took place within the hospital. A decision was made to develop the surgical treatment of pulmonary and extrapulmonary tuberculosis. In 1943, a total of 601 major operations and 250 minor procedures were performed, which included major abdominal, thoracic, genitourinary and orthopaedic surgery. In the same year, several items of equipment were approved by the minister for local government and public health for use in the acute hospital; these included an electrocardiograph, an oxygen tent, suction apparatus and cystoscopes.[39] A new operating theatre was completed in 1946, the new laboratory was equipped and a telephone switchboard with extensions to each ward was installed. A matron was appointed to run the acute hospital.

Provision was also made for the appointment of more nurses for the male and female chronic sick departments as well as for orderlies and ward attendants to replace existing inmate labour on these wards. The Department of Local Government and Public Health approved the appointment of 78 attendants for this purpose. Many of those who were appointed to these posts were recruited from the Army Medical Service.[40] In 1948 there were 133 nurses in the hospital and 124 hospital attendants. The compounder's department (the hospital pharmacy), which had been situated in very inadequate accommodation, was moved to a better and larger building. A porter was appointed to deliver medicines to the various hospitals, replacing 'the objectionable sight of inmate messengers from each department, cluttering the entrance to the compounder's shop with baskets and bottles'.[41] A well-equipped unit for physiotherapy was established around the same time. The equipment for the unit included a diathermy apparatus, an ultraviolet ray lamp, an infrared lamp and a radiant heat bath. Edith Kiernan took up the position of physiotherapist, replacing Miss Kelly, who had been employed as a masseuse at the hospital since 1907.[42] Two dieticians were employed to take care of special diets in the kitchen and three 'almoners' (social workers) were also appointed.[43] Maureen Murphy was the head almoner and Therese MacDonagh was the catering superintendent. The department of social services was relocated from one of the old buildings scheduled for demolition to a refurbished section of the former children's hospital.

The number of junior doctors in the hospital also increased, and when the nurses moved out of the night nurses' home it was converted into a medical residence. Caoimhghín Breathnach, a professor of physiology in University College Dublin and a medical historian, who was a houseman at that time, recalls the layout of the house:

> The top floor had eight bedrooms and a communal bathroom; the middle floor three bedrooms, a bathroom and dining room. The dining room was furnished with a table, eight chairs, the remnants of an armchair and the sole source of heating, an electric fire. Every morning death certificates with the relevant charts were laid out on the sideboard. Of sitting room there was none. A radio was rented by the housemen who were passing rich on £15 a month, of which £12 went across the road for victuals. The Board of Assistance could only afford to supply two maids and a cook, who ministered from a kitchen on the ground floor, the rest of which was taken up by administrative offices.[44]

Administrative reform

The commissioners made detailed recommendations to improve the administration of the hospital. They queried the continued employment of tailors, shoemakers and tinsmiths in workshops on the site and considered that many of the goods they produced could be bought more cheaply from commercial firms. However, because of the war they did not recommend any change at that time. They also tightened up the admission procedures for inmates. They observed that no proper records were kept in the ambulance section and that the ambulances had been allowed to 'deteriorate to an alarming degree'. They discovered that children who were boarded out were not being followed up on properly and they introduced a new system of monitoring them. They also endeavoured to find new foster mothers and good homes for more children, including 78 new places, 45 of them in Donegal.

A key appointment to the developing institution was made in August 1948 when Charles R. Boland, a surgeon, was appointed to the position of RMS, which had been left vacant since 1943. Boland combined his administrative duties with clinical responsibility for fractures and orthopaedic surgery. He studied medicine at Trinity College, where he graduated BA (gold medal) in 1924, MB in 1926 and MD in 1928. He became FRCSI in 1929. After graduation he took up a post at Salford Royal Infirmary and Ancoats Hospital in Manchester. He subsequently held posts in London hospitals including the Royal National Orthopaedic Hospital and the Hammersmith Hospital. He gained experience of London County Council hospitals and this experience was very useful when planning the development of St Kevin's Hospital.[45] He was appointed surgeon to the county hospital in Cashel, a post he held for a brief period before his appointment to St Kevin's Hospital. Boland was a member of a talented family: his brother Frederick Boland was chairman of the United Nations General Assembly and chancellor of the University of Dublin (Trinity College).[46] In August 1951, Jack Molony was appointed assistant RMS to help Boland with administration and to deputize for him in his absence. Molony was also given responsibility for the clinical management of older patients. He had graduated in medicine from UCD in 1949 and subsequently worked in Philadelphia for a year. He was awarded an MD in 1953. Molony worked in St Kevin's Hospital until 1960, and was appointed as consultant rheumatologist to St Vincent's Hospital in 1961.

A reforming doctor

The appointment of Victoria (Vicki) Coffey to the resident medical staff of St Kevin's Hospital in April 1943 led to major reforms in standards of care. She was born in Dublin in 1911 and graduated in 1936 from the Royal College of Surgeons in Ireland, starting her medical career as a house officer in the Meath Hospital. She subsequently gained experience in obstetrics and children's diseases and obtained the diploma in public health (DPH). On her appointment she was given responsibility for a maternity department with 22 beds, a children's hospital with 74 beds, an infants' ward with 40 cots, as well as the female skin and 'mental' wards. The conditions on these wards were dire and she became a committed advocate on behalf of the patients and staff.

The regular reports she wrote for the RMS give a vivid picture of the difficulties involved in nursing patients outside the acute hospital. The skin and 'mental' departments were housed in the original City Workhouse and Foundling Hospital buildings. Some of the patients were seriously ill, yet there were no nurses in the department at night. Instead, the patients were cared for by unqualified wardmistresses. In her reports, Coffey immediately began to request night nurses for these wards. There was also a constant shortage of hot water and this made it particularly difficult to nurse patients with skin diseases. The patients were not seen regularly by a consultant dermatologist and Coffey could only access such consultations by requesting them through the office of the RMS. Psychiatrists did not consult regularly and young patients with psychiatric problems were mixed with older patients in the wards. Coffey's growing exasperation with the terrible conditions and with the lack of any improvement is apparent in her report of 10 July 1946:

> The general state of repair of this department is deplorable – the walls are really filthy dirty – the plaster is falling off the walls; the nurses have to dress and undress in a room which is also a communal passageway to and from the mental ward. The facilities for treating patients – as reported in March '44 and again in Sept. '45 – are really worse than primitive in their inadequacy. Can something be done to clean this building and make it even temporarily suitable to treat and house the sick and aged?[47]

Sick children

Coffey was also responsible for the children's infirmary, which was situated in a temporary building with corrugated roof and sides. It was converted for the accommodation of children in 1927, having previously been used as an isolation block for the Dublin Union. The children's infirmary was known as the Catholic Children's Hospital or Hospital 10 and was situated towards the Rialto end of the hospital.[48] Coffey faced a daunting task in caring for these children. The accommodation was suitable for about sixty children but there were ninety-seven children in the building. Twenty of these were healthy children and they were housed in the infirmary simply because their families had been admitted to the institution. The remaining children suffered from a variety of illnesses, which she listed: abscesses, blepheritis, bronchitis and other respiratory diseases, burns, cardiac disease, erythema nodosum, marasmus, mental debility, otorrhoea, pertussis, pneumonia, rheumatism, rickets, ringworm skin diseases and tuberculosis.

The building was cold and badly ventilated, and the roof was leaking. There was no running water in the wards. In order to accommodate so many children the cots had to be placed close together and frequently there was no space between them. To make matters worse, there was no isolation facility and children with infectious diseases readily infected others. Sick children had to be taken to another building for X-rays and they had to be carried by an inmate as there was no wheelchair or trolley available. The unit was grossly understaffed and often there were only three nurses on duty. On some afternoons there were only two nurses to care for nearly 100 children.

Healthy children on the wards were often boisterous and there were frequent fights, with resultant injuries. Coffey requested that the practice of admitting healthy children to the infirmary should be stopped, that the number of cots should be reduced to sixty and that staffing levels should be increased. Some children who had recovered from acute illnesses could not be discharged because the parents, despite repeated requests, would not take them. Some of these children were eventually sent

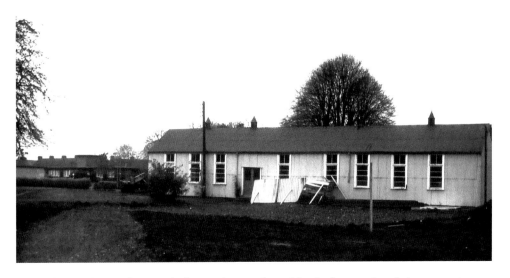

10.15   The Children's Infirmary, which was subsequently used for the first social work department in 1950. The junior doctors' residence can be seen in the background on the left. Photographed in 1978 by Dr Ron Kirkham.

10.16   Sean T. O'Kelly (fourth from left), minister for local government, visits the Children's Infirmary in 1933. Photograph: *Irish Press*, 22 Apr. 1933.

C   THE IRISH PRESS, SATURDAY, APRIL 22, 1933.

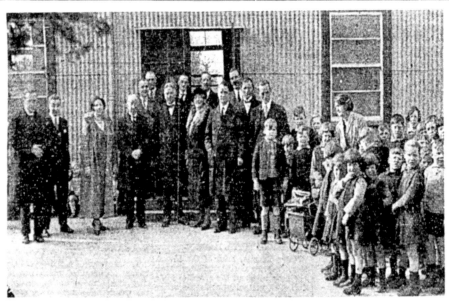

MINISTER'S VISIT to South Dublin Union, in connection with proposed extensions to be carried out.   (L. to R.—Front row)—Rev. Fr. Coffey (Chaplain), Dr. W. Dwyer, Mrs. Fitzsimmons, Mr. S. T. O'Kelly (Minister for Local Government), Mr. MacCarron, Ald. Mrs. Kettle, Dr. Ward, T.D., and Mr. D. Donovan.   (Back)—Ald. T. Lawlor, Mr. Condon (Clerk of Union), Mr. P. Doyle, T.D.; Senator L. O'Neill, Mr. J. Shiels, and Councillor Tunny, photographed at the Children's Hospital

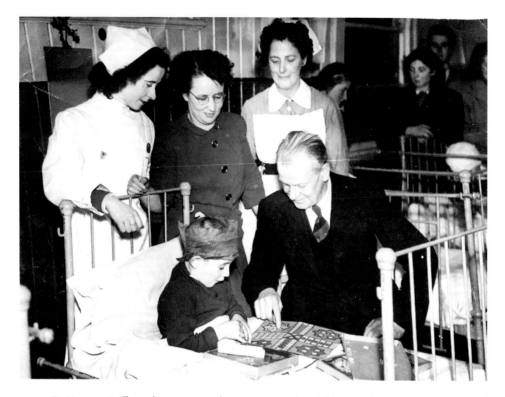

10.17   Dr Victoria Coffey and Séamus Murphy at a party in the Children's Infirmary c.1945. Courtesy of Nessa Rowan.

home accompanied by officials from the institution. Coffey's constant agitation led to improvements on the wards: the number of nurses was increased in the sick infants' ward and piped water was installed. When Coffey took up duty in 1943 the death rate among sick infants (children under 2) was 61.8 per cent (576 admissions, 356 deaths). Over the following six years she managed to get this figure down to 13.5 per cent.[49] Coffey went on to specialize in child health and she developed a neonatal unit and a department of paediatrics in St Kevin's Hospital during the 1950s.

In 1954, Coffey read a paper to the Royal Academy of Medicine of Ireland in which she remarked that her hospital cared for most of the children in Dublin with hopeless or incurable congenital abnormalities.[50] She began to take a special interest in these children and collaborated with Patrick Moore, head of biochemistry in St Kevin's Hospital and professor of biochemistry in the RCSI, in a study of metabolic disorders in newborn infants. Both became pioneers in this important area of child health and together they established the first laboratory specializing in the diagnosis of inborn errors of metabolism in Ireland. The metabolic unit screened mentally handicapped children living in residential care for phenylketonuria, 'maple-syrup urine' disease, homocystinuria and other amino-acid disorders, and for the mucopolysaccharidoses. In 1955, Coffey contracted poliomyelitis in the course of her duties and this left her with unpleasant sequelae for the rest of her life. Nevertheless, she carried on with her work with characteristic drive and determination. The unit continued to deliver a high-quality service and to conduct important research until its closure in 1989, just two years after Moore's death.

Research on thalidomide-related disability

Coffey received Medical Research Council and Department of Health support in 1962 for her work on thalidomide-related disability among children in Ireland. Thalidomide was a drug used to alleviate morning sickness. The drug, which was first sold in Ireland in early 1959, was linked to severe physical disabilities in babies in 1961, and the German manufacturers, Chemie Grünenthal, suspended its distribution globally in the winter of that year. In a six-month period Coffey visited 174 institutions around the country where children had been born. She examined 86,000 birth records to determine the defects found during two periods, one before thalidomide use and one when it was available in Ireland. This was the first study in Ireland to determine the number of children with congenital anomalies born to mothers who had taken thalidomide. Coffey went on to study the effects of maternal viral infections on newborn infants, and she was an early investigator of sudden infant death syndrome in Ireland. She established a research unit in the hospital, the Foundation for Prevention of Childhood Handicap, and she would remain its director of research until she was over 80.

In 1961, Coffey was appointed lecturer in teratology in Trinity College, and she was awarded a PhD from Trinity in 1965 for her dissertation, 'The incidence and aetiology of congenital defects in Ireland'. She was conferred with the fellowship of the Royal College of Physicians of Ireland (RCPI) in 1979 and was elected an honorary fellow of the American Academy of Pediatrics. Coffey was a founder member of the Irish and American Paediatric Society in 1968 and its president in 1974. She was also a founder fellow of the Irish Faculty of Paediatrics in 1981. She retired from the staff of St James's Hospital in 1976 and the board took the decision to close the children's unit the following year because of its proximity to Our Lady's Hospital for Sick Children in Crumlin. She died in 1999 in the hospital to which she had devoted her professional life.

Priority for government

In the early years following the foundation of the state, health did not have an independent ministry but was linked with local government. In the mid 1940s, the minister for local government and public health, Sean MacEntee, decided that a separate ministry of health should be established as a matter of urgency. A major step was taken in this direction in January 1944, when the cabinet agreed to delegate the functions of the minister relating to health to Dr Conor Ward, MacEntee's parliamentary secretary. Ward was a general practitioner in Monaghan town and, after taking part in the War of Independence, he had joined Fianna Fáil. Ward wished to build an effective health service but he had access to only very limited government resources – although the Irish Hospitals' Sweepstake provided finance to support priority developments, which compensated to some degree for the lack of public resources available for the improvement of hospital and medical services.

The improvement of St Kevin's Hospital was included among a shortlist of urgent issues that Ward proposed to tackle in his new role.[51] In 1945, the embryonic Department of Health produced its first strategy for the development of acute hospital services in Dublin. Four hospitals were envisaged to serve Dublin city: an enlarged Mater Hospital and a second hospital on the north side; a new St Vincent's Hospital at Elm Park and a new hospital on the St Kevin's complex. St Michael's Hospital in Dún Laoghaire and a reconstructed Loughlinstown Hospital would serve south Co. Dublin.[52] High-level support within the civil service facilitated the programme of reform being driven by the commissioners at St Kevin's Hospital.

Reform of the chronic departments

From the time of their initial appointment to St Kevin's Hospital in 1942, the commissioners had placed emphasis on the development of the acute facilities. However, in May 1946 Séamus Murphy turned his attention to the wards for chronically ill patients. At that time there were approximately 1,100 'chronic sick' in the institution and they were accommodated in six departments. Murphy made several proposals in a paper, 'Proposals in respect of chronic departments', and he concluded:

> in respect of medical attention, treatment and supervision … it is utterly inadequate; it is also uneconomic in that by absence of treatment some inmates remain here indefinitely or for very long periods who, if suitable treatment were given, could be discharged. With regard to chronic departments, there are lingering traces of the old workhouse attitude.[53]

There were so many chronically sick patients and so few doctors that it was inevitable that the diagnosis would be missed in some cases. Denis K. (D.K.) O'Donovan, who was professor of medicine at University College Dublin, recalled being asked to review some patients in the wards for the chronic sick. He found six patients with undiagnosed advanced hypothyroidism and he started them on thyroxine. He was struck by the number of post-encephalitic patients there were as a result of the 1918 flu epidemic, with all sorts of abnormal movements, torsions and tremors.[54] The day-to-day medical cover at the time was delivered by three resident medical officers, who reported to the RMS. Murphy proposed that these should be replaced by six house surgeons or physicians who would be under the supervision of visiting physicians and surgeons.

These proposals were broadly supported by James Deeny, the chief medical advisor in the Department of Health. Deeny also proposed that four consulting specialists should be appointed because of the range of chronic diseases. He recommended the appointment of a cardiologist, a respiratory physician, a rheumatologist and a urologist. The proposals were accepted and four specialists took up duty on temporary contracts in 1947: Patrick T. O'Farrell, cardiologist; Gerard T. O'Brien, respiratory physician; Thomas J. O'Reilly, rheumatologist; and Thomas J.D. (Tom) Lane, urologist. O'Farrell, a pioneer in cardiology, was a consultant on the staff of St Vincent's Hospital and head of the electrocardiographic department when he was appointed as visiting cardiologist to St Kevin's Hospital.[55] O'Brien was a consultant physician with a special interest in respiratory diseases who worked at the Richmond Hospital. Lane worked in the Meath Hospital, where he served first as pathologist, then as radiologist and finally as urological surgeon. He was the first to specialize full-time in urology in Ireland.[56] The provision of such a range of medical and surgical expertise, to treat patients with chronic disabilities so that they could be discharged home, was a remarkable initiative for its time.

An arthritis unit

The rheumatologist, Thomas J. O'Reilly, received his specialist training in several rheumatology centres in London. He published in leading journals including *The Lancet* and the *British Medical Journal*. At his interview in May 1946 for the position in St Kevin's Hospital, he suggested that an arthritis unit should be developed in the hospital, and after his appointment he pursued this goal. The main purpose of the unit was to accommodate very disabled patients from the country who could benefit medically from treatment if they had somewhere to stay. The types of disease from which they suffered included rheumatoid arthritis with deformities, osteoarthritis of the hips and knees, and ankylosing spondylitis. These patients were poor and could not afford hotel accommodation in Dublin. O'Reilly, whose manner has been described as 'friendly and unhurried', was prepared to undertake the function of medical director to the unit.[57] The proposal was supported by the commissioner, Séamus Murphy, who allocated twenty-four beds in the chronic section of the hospital for the arthritis unit and obtained the necessary financial support from the Department of Local Government and Public Health.[58]

A courageous surgeon

James Hanlon, a graduate of University College Dublin, was appointed visiting eye and ear specialist in January 1947. Hanlon was considered an excellent eye and ear surgeon and had studied the specialty in Vienna. He introduced the operating microscope for middle-ear surgery to Dublin.[59] Hanlon was also an outstanding sportsman, a champion diver and golfer. In 1950, his world was shattered at the age of 42. His problems started when a patient he was examining coughed into his eyes. As a consequence he developed a resistant infection in his left eye. After an unsuccessful operation in London, he also lost the sight in his right eye due to sympathetic ophthalmia. His doctors, in a desperate attempt to save his eyesight, treated him with high doses of streptomycin, a new antibiotic at the time, which could cause deafness as a side effect. Tragically, Hanlon lost his hearing and, within a few months of the onset of the infection, became totally blind and deaf.[60] He was a man of great courage and went on to study physiotherapy in London before joining the staff of the Central Remedial Clinic in Dublin, becoming one of the original staff when the clinic was founded in 1952.[61] John McAuliffe Curtin was appointed visiting ear, nose and throat specialist to replace Hanlon at St Kevin's.

Other visiting staff appointed at this time included John P. Conroy as anaesthetist, Robert Steen as paediatrician and Alan Mooney as ophthalmologist. Edward Keelan was appointed as visiting obstetrician and gynaecologist in 1950. Keelan graduated from University College Dublin in 1916 and subsequently studied in Vienna for two years. He is credited with being the first to perform a vaginal hysterectomy in Dublin.[62] Keelan was a consultant to the Coombe Hospital (and its master from 1942 to 1949), where he was in advance of his time in his efforts to foster the relationship between mother and child.

Development of the acute hospital

The medical patients in the hospital were under the care of the visiting physicians: Philip (Phil) Brennan, who was also on the staff of St Vincent's Hospital, and William O. (Billy) Cremin. These physicians did medical rounds every morning. Brennan was appointed as visiting medical officer to St Kevin's Hospital in 1948. He was highly regarded for his skill at bedside diagnosis and had a special interest in diseases of the chest.[63] The general surgical patients were under the care of Patrick (Paddy) Fitzgerald, who had worked at Johns Hopkins Hospital, Baltimore. He was assistant surgeon in St Vincent's Hospital and in the Incorporated Orthopaedic Hospital in 1947 when he was appointed as acting surgeon to St Kevin's Hospital, where he carried out major surgical procedures such as gastrectomy and sympathectomy (for hypertension). He was appointed consultant surgeon to St Vincent's Hospital in 1952 and professor of surgery at University College Dublin in 1954.

The patients were admitted by two medical officers in the admission unit, which was situated near the main entrance. Between thirty and fifty patients were admitted every day. As Caoimhghín Breathnach recalls:

> The admitting officer examined the patient, wrote up the chart, made an inscribed provisional diagnosis, directed the destination (acute or chronic, medical or surgi-

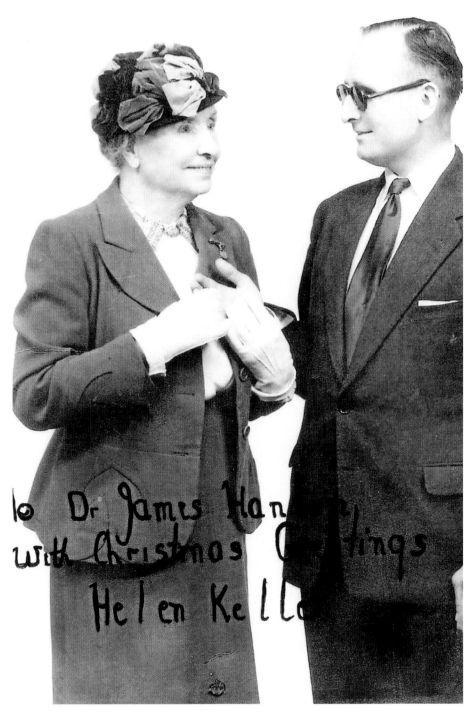

To Dr James Han...
with Christmas Greetings
Helen Kello

10.18   Mr James Hanlon and Helen Keller, the American writer and humanitarian, in 1954. Despite being blind and deaf from infancy, she became a champion of human rights and was one of the founders of the American Civil Liberties Union (ACLU). Courtesy of Dr John Hanlon.

cal) and recommended the next step (to be seen immediately or later by the man on duty). Every prescription or subsequent contact had to be noted and initialled on the chart.[64]

Most of the admissions were by ticket from the dispensary medical officers and the internal staff had little control over the numbers admitted. Breathnach also remembered the excellence of nursing standards: 'Nursing standards were high and in some cases excellent to the level of today's "Nurse of the Year" standard.'[65] If a transfusion of blood was required before 1950–1, donors came in on demand, most of them being young soldiers.

The Rialto Chest Hospital and the treatment of tuberculosis

Known as 'consumption', tuberculosis has been described as 'the scourge of the tenements'. It was responsible for 45 per cent of all deaths between the ages of 15 and 45 in the new Irish state.[66] The rate of tuberculosis was substantially higher in Dublin than in any other city in Britain or Ireland and entire families were wiped out by it.[67] Sickness and early death were an accepted part of life in the slums. The minister for local government and public health, Seán T. O'Kelly, wrote to the Dublin Board of Assistance in 1936 suggesting that the 172-bed tuberculosis hospital situated near the Rialto gate in the grounds of the Dublin Union should be transferred to Dublin Corporation. In this way it would be dissociated from the poor law system and would form an integral part of the Dublin Borough Tuberculosis Scheme.[68]

The Board of Assistance agreed in principle to the proposal but there was considerable prevarication and it was not until 1943, in response to agitation by the Royal Academy of Medicine, that Dublin Corporation decided to take over the tuberculosis hospital (the Rialto Hospital) from the Dublin Board of Assistance. It was given the name Rialto Chest Hospital, to give it a more positive image and to make it more attractive to potential patients. The handover took place on 2 April 1943 and the lord mayor, Alderman Peadar S. Doyle, was present to mark the occasion. John Duffy was appointed medical superintendent of the Rialto Chest Hospital. Duffy studied medicine in University College Dublin, graduating in 1922, and he was awarded an MD in 1932. He developed tuberculosis early in his career and spent time in Swiss and Scandinavian sanatoria. Influenced by his experience, he decided to specialize in the management and scientific study of tuberculosis. He gained experience in Wales, Switzerland and New York and as a result he had an unrivalled knowledge of the disease. Duffy was sceptical about the use of artificial pneumothorax, but he was an advocate of thoracic surgery. Patients with persistent positive sputum were often keen to have surgery to convert their sputum and allow their discharge from hospital. Duffy was also one of the first to realize that if thoracic surgery was to reach its full potential, it should be developed as an independent specialty. Young doctors who worked with Duffy benefited from his bedside teaching and also from his teaching file of films and case reports.[69] Duffy placed great emphasis on the importance of prevention and on adequate care after discharge from hospital. Under his guidance the Rialto Chest Hospital became the most progressive hospital for the treatment of tuberculosis in the country.

Noël Browne and his campaign against tuberculosis

John Duffy knew from his American experience that a tuberculosis association could be very effective, provided it was a popular movement and not elitist. He therefore played an active part in the lay and professional anti-tuberculosis campaigns designed to shake the authorities out of their lethargy. He addressed a public meeting in the Mansion House in 1944 and urged people who had suffered from TB to organize. The meeting was attended by a man named Charlie O'Connor, who had spent long periods in a sanatorium. O'Connor took up the challenge and formed the Post-Sanatoria League as a lobby group. O'Connor also played a key role in encouraging a young doctor, Noël Browne, to enter politics.[70] Browne's family had been devastated by tuberculosis: his parents and a number of his siblings died from the disease.

Browne studied medicine in Trinity and after graduation worked in the sanatorium in Newcastle, Co. Wicklow. He was scathing about the standard of medical care in sanatoria in Ireland but he recognized Duffy's talent, describing him as 'gentle, hardworking and talented'.[71] When Browne became minister for health in 1948, he was determined to improve the care of patients with tuberculosis. He began to spend the capital of the Hospitals' Sweepstake on the construction of modern sanatoria around Ireland as opposed to spending only the interest, which had been the practice. This policy brought first-class surgical and radiological suites, a physiotherapy unit and two new wings with verandas to the Rialto Chest Hospital. Two of the old wards were divided to make them suitable for nursing post-operative cases and they became, in effect, intensive care units before the term came into common use. A prefabricated building was erected to accommodate nurses who would study for a post-registration diploma in tuberculosis. The hospital had 273 beds but the turnover was slow because of the nature of the disease. Laurence B. (Larry) Godfrey joined Duffy as medical assistant in 1948. A team of outstanding nurses and ward sisters was also recruited, many of whom had trained in centres of excellence.[72] Unfortunately, Duffy developed rheumatoid arthritis, but despite the pain and joint disfigurement, he continued to work and to see patients. Caoimhghín Breathnach worked for Duffy as a house physician in 1951. He recalled:

> Dr Duffy taught by subterfuge, and a resident did not realise that he was learning
> a way of life rather than the minutiae of a restricted medical specialty ... One after-

noon when I sought his help he was lying, or rather standing, in ambush ... he was now racked by rheumatoid arthritis; he could not walk without the aid of crutches, and when he sat it was only on a high stool or the edge of his desk.[73]

After discussing the patient with the young Breathnach, Duffy took a book from his shelves entitled *Aequanimitas*, by the great Canadian physician, William Osler. He read aloud an inspirational section of Osler's famous essay on work, describing 'work' as the 'master word' responsible for all advances in medicine. Breathnach later recalled:

> Perhaps I was smitten by the lofty sentiments of the passage and realized that he was quietly undermining my ennui, but it was gradually that I came under the spell not so much of Osler's eloquence as of his gentle admirer, barely able to support *Aequanimitas* on his gnarled hands ...[74]

Duffy worked in the Rialto Chest Hospital until his appointment as the first medical superintendent of James Connolly Memorial Hospital in Blanchardstown in 1955.[75] He died unexpectedly in 1957, just two years after taking up his new post. Despite the development of the Rialto Chest Hospital, St Kevin's Hospital continued to care for about 100 patients with tuberculosis, 60 male and 40 female. The average age of the patients was 35 and many were confined to bed because of the severity of their illness.

Cardiothoracic surgery

The development of modern cardiac services in Ireland began with the appointment of Maurice Hickey to the Rialto Chest Hospital as a thoracic surgeon in 1948.[76] Hickey, who graduated from University College Cork in 1941, trained in the London Chest Hospital. He operated in Rialto, Mallow and Castlerea Hospitals on a rotating basis on Tuesdays, Wednesdays and Thursdays, and returned to Dublin at the weekend. He achieved dramatic results, performing cardiac surgery on severely ill patients, and his achievements were reported in the newspapers on a regular basis. He was the first surgeon in Ireland to operate successfully on a patient with mitral stenosis; he carried out the operation in the Rialto Chest Hospital in 1949.[77]

Hickey was thoracic surgeon to the Rialto Chest Hospital from 1948 until he left to take up a post in Cork in 1956.[78] He was succeeded by Desmond Kneafsey who qualified from the RCSI in 1945 and became FRCSI in 1948. After a period in the Rialto Chest Hospital, Kneafsey was appointed to a post in Galway. Brendan O'Neill and Keith Shaw were later appointments to the Rialto Chest Hospital. O'Neill graduated from University College Cork in 1936 and became FRCSI in 1942. He worked at St Mary's Hospital in the Phoenix Park and at the Rialto Chest Hospital. He was highly regarded for his skill at performing lobectomies for tuberculosis and bronchiectasis.[79] Shaw was born in Dublin in 1919, graduated from Trinity College in 1942, and three years later obtained his FRCSI. He held postgraduate posts in a number of hospitals in England and Scotland before working with some of the leading cardiothoracic surgeons of the time in the London Chest Hospital, St George's Hospital and Colindale Hospital. He served with the RAMC between 1947 and 1949, before his appointment to the Rialto Chest Hospital.

Patrick (Pat) O'Toole was appointed in 1949 to provide anaesthesia for the surgery carried out in the Rialto Chest Hospital. He was also anaesthetist to the Richmond Hospital and was the first to use curare in these hospitals. Prior to O'Toole's appointment, the house surgeons used gas-oxygen-ether when administering anaesthetics in St Kevin's. O'Toole trained them in the new art of anaesthesia using pentathol and tubocurarine. O'Toole 'loved the challenge of major surgery which he undertook with great courage and determination at a time when similar procedures were only evolving elsewhere'.[80] The hospital also benefitted from a team of physiotherapists, under the leadership of Marie O'Donoghue, which played a key role in managing patients post-operatively.

The poet Patrick Kavanagh

Patrick Kavanagh was probably the most famous patient to be treated in the Rialto Chest Hospital. Kavanagh was found to have a shadow on his left lung in February 1955 when he attended the chest physician Brendan O'Brien, in the Meath Hospital. O'Brien referred him to Keith Shaw, and he had a bronchoscopy in the Rialto Chest Hospital, which proved inconclusive. He was admitted to the hospital at the beginning of March and was started on anti-tuberculosis treatment. As he had not improved by late March, Shaw decided to operate. The operation was arranged for 31 March and Kavanagh's only stipulation was to ask that the time be changed from 8 a.m., the hanging hour, to 9 a.m. Shaw found an advanced cancer and he removed Kavanagh's left lung. The poet had a prolonged period of convalescence in the Rialto Chest Hospital and later recalled this as one of the happiest periods of his life. According to his biographer, Antoinette Quinn:

> It was the happiness of feeling safe and secure. Once he had adapted to the hospital regimen, he liked the fixed routines. He was protected from all the financial anxieties that had harassed him in recent years, the unpaid bills, the endless cadging, the sometimes dishonest ruses he had resorted to in order to get by. He was delighted to find himself a star performer, the centre of attention. Friends flocked to see him, some of them beautiful women; bottles of whiskey stood on his locker.[81]

Kavanagh gave a talk, entitled 'Hospital notebook', on Radio Éireann just a few months after the operation. He paid special attention to the subject of visiting hours:

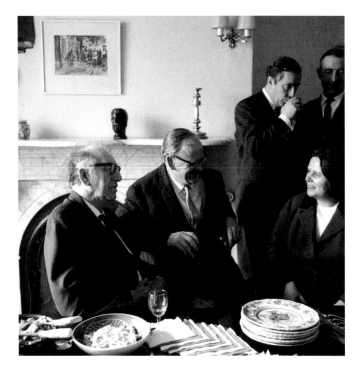

10.19 Patrick Kavanagh's wedding breakfast in April 1967: Patrick Kavanagh (left), Keith Shaw (centre) and the bride, Katherine Moloney (right). Courtesy of the National Library of Ireland.

visiting hours are very necessary to cope with the extraordinary way in which the ordinary Dublin person goes in for visiting friends and acquaintances in hospital ... the crowds coming in the gate were like the crowds going to a football match, thousands of people.

Now, to cater for the visitors outside the hospital gate, there would be on visiting days people with food stalls at the main gate and the principal item was grapes. Some days I received as many as a dozen brown paper bags full of grapes. I could never get any of the other patients to eat any of these grapes ...

When I was going into hospital a well-wisher consoled me with the remark that now I'd have plenty of time to read some good books, and almost all visitors brought me books until in the end I had a fair-sized library. I think a lot of people brought me books which they themselves had been unable to read but which they had heard were good and they wanted me to do the heavy work.

Years later Shaw recalled some of the circumstances surrounding the poet's admission under his care:

When he was admitted to Rialto Hospital for surgery of lung cancer, it became known to the establishments of church, state, and university that Ireland's premier poet might die destitute in a local authority hospital. Before his operation, he received visits from the great and the good, became reconciled to the church, and was promised a post in the department of English at the National University. He was greatly amused by these attentions.

He felt that he had a lot to write before his operation, therefore he asked for a room and a typewriter. These were gladly provided, but never used, as his spare time was spent in the local pub, and short of confiscating his clothes, he could not be kept in the hospital.

Patrick asked that I keep for him the rib removed at operation. I promised this in return for a copy of his novel *Tarry Flynn*, then banned and out of print. He made a good recovery after successful surgery in spite of refusal to stop his heavy smoking. However he was frightened and insecure, and needed a lot of support and reassurance. We would retire to Mooney's, and talk about himself and everything under the sun. He kept asking for his rib, but couldn't find a copy of *Tarry Flynn* until he eventually found a second-hand copy in New York, and we ceremoniously swopped the rib for the book in Mooney's pub.[82]

Kavanagh placed the following inscription in the book:

To Keith Shaw M.D. F.R.C.S.I.

This simple pastoral as a token of remembrance of a curious happiness I knew when in the Rialto Hospital a year ago.

Patrick Kavanagh
Dublin, January 1956

As promised in exchange for a rib—my own rib.[83]

10.20   Kavanagh's inscription on a copy of *Tarry Flynn*, for Keith Shaw. Courtesy of the late Keith Shaw.

Kavanagh wrote a beautiful and mystical sonnet called 'The Hospital' when he was a patient in the Rialto Chest Hospital, which has been described by the poet Brendan Kennelly as the only known love poem to a hospital:[84]

> A year ago I fell in love with the functional ward
> Of a chest hospital: square cubicles in a row
> Plain concrete, wash basins – an art lover's woe,
> Not counting how the fellow in the next bed snored.
> But nothing whatever is by love debarred,
> The common and banal her heat can know.
> The corridor led to a stairway and below
> Was the inexhaustible adventure of a gravelled yard.
>
> This is what love does to things: the Rialto Bridge,
> The main gate that was bent by a heavy lorry,
> The seat at the back of a shed that was a suntrap.
> Naming these things is the love-act and its pledge;
> For we must record love's mystery without claptrap,
> Snatch out of time the passionate transitory.[85]

Kavanagh convalesced after his operation on the banks of the Grand Canal, near Baggot Street. He believed that he was reborn as a poet during this period, which, two years later, he immortalised with two sonnets: 'Canal Bank Walk' and 'Lines Written on a Seat on the Grand Canal, Dublin'.

11

St Kevin's Hospital

I scored out wall after wall – both outer and honey-combing it on the inside – what a pleasure to issue the instruction, 'Get rid of those walls, all of them.' I felt like Nero! (But a benevolent one.)[1]

Dr Noël Browne became minister for health following the general election of 1948. Browne, aged 32, brought a drive and momentum that were unprecedented in the traditions of the Department of Health. One of the projects to which he gave his energetic support was the plan to turn St Kevin's into an acute hospital with a postgraduate medical school.[2] A working group had been established by his predecessor, Dr James Ryan, and it included several leading doctors, academics and health administrators, such as Joseph W. Bigger, William Doolin, Bethel Solomons and James Deeny.[3] The group's recommendations were included in a document entitled 'A report on the development of St Kevin's as a hospital centre', which was released in April 1949.[4]

The development of St Kevin's as a hospital

The first recommendation of the 1949 report was the development of a new hospital at St Kevin's for public assistance patients unable to obtain admission to voluntary hospitals.[5] It recommended the development of the X-ray and pathology departments, a rehabilitation unit, a nursing school and facilities for a postgraduate medical school. It advocated the separation of the acute, convalescent and long-term nursing care facilities from the accommodation for the infirm, casuals and others who did not need nursing. It proposed that two zones should be created by a dividing line drawn east-west immediately south of the Foundling Hospital complex and north of the convent and of the hospitals currently known as Hospitals 1 and 2. All existing structures south of this line would be in the hospital section while all buildings north of the line would be in the welfare section.[6] This recommendation had long-term consequences for the future configuration of St James's Hospital, which now stands south of this line, and for the Trinity Centre for Health Sciences, which occupies the site of the welfare section, north of the line. Séamus Murphy was unhappy with the proposal to house welfare cases in the old buildings north of the line, many of which had been built during the eighteenth century. He stated that he did not want 'a work-house corner' in the institution. There was general agreement that the welfare cases should ultimately be placed in other institutions. This, in effect, is what happened over the following decade.[7] After elections in 1948, a new Dublin Board of Assistance was formed but without the executive powers of previous boards. The Local Government (Dublin) (Temporary) Act 1948 stipulated that a chief executive officer would be appointed by the minister for health to exercise the executive functions of the Dublin Board of Assistance. The post was to be held by the existing commissioner, Séamus Murphy.[8]

Several high-level meetings were held throughout 1949 between representatives of the Department of Health and of the Dublin Board of Assistance to agree on a scheme for the development of St Kevin's Hospital. The potential impact that the two new hospitals under construction at the time – the Coombe Hospital in Donore Avenue and the Hospital for Sick Children in Crumlin – might have on St Kevin's Hospital was discussed at these meetings, as was the desirability of building a nursing school and a student nurses' residence in the grounds of the hospital. The development of a nursing school at St Kevin's would provide nurses for new posts around the country and would raise the standard of nursing in the hospital. A nurses' home would provide accommodation for student probationers in St Kevin's as well as those in the Rialto Chest Hospital. However, these proposals were not implemented and it would be another twenty years before a school of nursing was established in the hospital.[9]

An enthusiastic minister

Noël Browne wished to see an immediate commencement of the developments at St Kevin's and their completion within a seven-year programme. As minister for health, Browne had a policy of visiting hospitals and later recalled his visit to St Kevin's:

> One of the really memorable experiences of my time at the Dept. of Health was on the afternoon of my visit to the sordid and squalid workhouse it then was with its prison walls, to call for the map of the place and the plan of the hospital, with a pencil – Seamus Murphy the commissioner was present – I scored out wall after wall – both outer and honey-combing it on the inside – what a pleasure to issue the instruction, 'Get rid of those walls, all of them.' I felt like Nero! (But a benevolent one.)[10]

Browne also suggested to the Dublin Board of Assistance in 1950 that the Victorian buildings fronting James's Street should be demolished and replaced by 'an attractive frontage' for the hospital.[11]

Browne was unambiguous about his and the department's plans for St Kevin's Hospital. He told his senior civil servants that he wanted the hospital to be equal to, if not better than, any voluntary hospital in Dublin.[12] Browne also gave very strong support to the proposed postgraduate medical school, which would supply continuing education to local-authority medical officers. Eventually there was agreement that St Kevin's would have 1,200 beds, including a new hospital block of 320 beds for acute, semi-acute and long-term nursing care. A new X-ray department would be built on the west side of the acute hospital as a replacement for the existing facility and a hospital laboratory, which could serve as a regional laboratory for the Leinster area, would also be developed. The secretary of the Department of Health, Patrick S. Ó Muireadhaigh, wrote to the Dublin Board of Assistance:

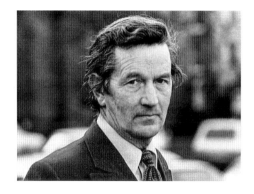

11.1   Dr Noël Browne, minister for health from 1948 to 1951. Reproduced with permission of the photographer, Victor Patterson.

> The minister for health is confident that if the proposals which follow are accepted by your board the standard of diagnosis and treatment in St Kevin's Hospital will be second to none. This upgrade of the institution can be achieved by the provision of a staff of highly trained specialists, a numerically adequate and competent nursing staff and the provision of modern hospital equipment and proper accommodation for patients.[13]

The minister would provide a grant from the Hospitals' Trust Fund, which administered the income from the Irish Hospitals' Sweepstake, to cover 100 per cent of the cost of building the postgraduate centre, and a grant of two-thirds of the cost of the improvements to the hospital section and of the building of a nurses' home. The Dublin Board of Assistance was expected to take out a loan to cover the balance.

Proposal for a postgraduate medical school

The medical establishment in Dublin opposed the Department of Health's aspirations to convert St Kevin's into an efficient municipal hospital with a postgraduate teaching school for medical graduates.[14] These developments were seen as interfering with the rights of the existing medical schools and the profession.[15] The proposal was portrayed in the medical press as the creation of a medical school 'which will be directly and completely controlled by the state'.[16] The plan to introduce salaries for the teaching staff was also unacceptable to the doctors, who claimed it would be unjust 'to pay salaries to the staff while more brilliant men in our voluntary hospitals give their services almost for nothing'.[17]

The Department of Health was prepared to support the medical school and hospital with a generous allocation of staff. Directors were proposed for medicine, surgery and pathology, and these posts would be supported by teams of assistants, subspecialists and house physicians.[18] The concept of a postgraduate school had first been proposed by James Deeny, the chief medical advisor in the Department of Health, and he envisaged residential courses for medical officers working for local authorities:

> They would learn new techniques in treatment, minor surgery and anything new which might add to their ability to serve their patients. This was to ensure that all practitioners would be kept up to date and would not have to rely exclusively for their post-graduate instruction on the representatives of the pharmaceutical companies.[19]

The Department of Health estimated that there were approximately 870 medical officers in the employment of local authorities in the country. The majority were dispensary doctors, many of whom worked in remote areas and found it difficult to keep abreast of new developments in healthcare.[20] It was envisaged that the school would teach throughout the year and that applicants would be able to select a suitable month to attend. The number on each course was to be limited to twenty places 'to ensure satisfactory teaching'.[21] Doctors taking up new appointments under local authorities would sign an undertaking to attend a course in St Kevin's Hospital once every five years. A substitute was to be provided while the doctor was attending the course. The new postgraduate school would be under the direction of a committee representative of the medical schools.[22] Browne sought support from the medical school in University College Dublin to develop St Kevin's Hospital into a teaching institution as he considered that Archbishop John Charles McQuaid would not accept an agreement involving consultants affiliated to the medical school at Trinity College.[23] However, the proposal was not supported by the medical faculty in University College Dublin, and this effectively blocked it as the proposal could not be developed without the support of an academic institution. Browne later recalled:

> [M]y appeals were rejected. What a pity that the people of Ireland had to wait until 1971 when the then minister, with the help of Trinity consultants and medical school, went on to establish today's outstanding success for our Irish health services.[24]

James Deeny, pragmatist and visionary

James Deeny was a man of remarkable foresight matched by equally remarkable energy. In 1946, when attention was being given to the appointment of a new RMS for St Kevin's Hospital, he suggested that the successful candidate should be given a period of advanced training in hospital management in the University of Chicago. At around the same time he wrote a memo on the potential of a redeveloped St Kevin's Hospital that was extraordinarily prophetic in view of the subsequent development of St James's Hospital:

> Rialto Hospital in the grounds of St Kevin's would, with some alteration, make a suitable chest hospital in the re-organised institution. It would be the first of a series of specialised units providing for clinical research, teaching and technical development far in excess of anything existing in this country. Added to this unit would be a cancer institute, ... a neurosurgical institute, a national centre for plastic surgery and other medical specialties requiring a high degree of scientific organisation. Instead of the Lock Hospital a modern venereal disease unit might be added to St Kevin's.[25]

Programme for radical development

Although the postgraduate school was not developed because of opposition, there remained within the Department of Health an aspiration to develop St Kevin's as a municipal teaching hospital. Plans were already being made to appoint two full-time permanent physicians and two full-time surgeons. Visiting consultants were to be retained or appointed in areas such as urology, rheumatology, anaesthetics, ophthalmology, otolaryngology, geriatrics, gynaecology and orthopaedics. Throughout the 1950s, a major programme of radical development began to take shape on the site, which would change St Kevin's into an active general hospital. A scheme setting out in broad terms the plans for the refurbishment of St Kevin's was presented to officials of the Department of Health by Séamus Murphy and Charles Boland, RMS, at a meeting in September 1949. The report was prepared at the instigation of senior officials in the Department of Health. It included plans for the decanting of welfare patients to other institutions and for the demolition or reconstruction of buildings on the site. It also included plans to erect a new block of wards to accommodate 320 patients together with a nurses' home. Subsequently, so much space was made available in existing buildings, as a result of the decanting programme, that it was decided to upgrade the Rialto Chest Hospital as an alternative to building the new 320-bed ward block, thus creating substantial savings. Although the proposed nurses' home never moved beyond the drawing board, Dublin Corporation erected a temporary home near Garden Hill for probationers working in the Rialto Chest Hospital.[26]

Browne resigned as minister for health in April 1951 and a general election soon after returned Fianna Fáil to power. Dr James Ryan was reappointed minister for health and he continued to support and to take an interest in the development of St Kevin's Hospital. He became dissatisfied with the rate of progress being made by the Dublin Board of Assistance and in the summer of 1953 he requested a review of the

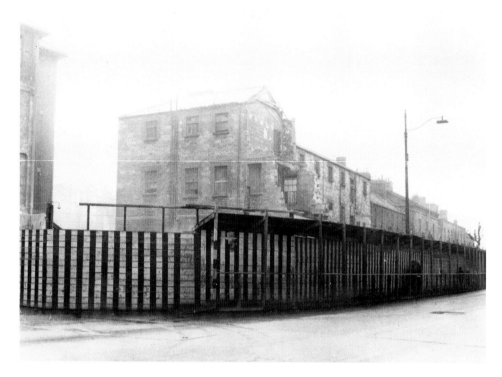

11.2   Demolition of the frontage on James's Street in 1953. Private collection.

overall programme. The minister was prepared to increase the grant for approved works 'with a view to encouraging the local authority to undertake them quickly'.[27]

It was apparent by the autumn of 1953 that most of the welfare cases at St Kevin's would soon be moved to locations outside the hospital. This brought about a reassessment of the need for the buildings north of the line that were being used for welfare cases and the decision was taken to demolish most of the old Foundling Hospital buildings.

The reconstruction of St Kevin's Hospital

The reconstruction of St Kevin's began in June 1951 with the closure of the Protestant hospital. This hospital functioned as a home for ambulant elderly Protestants and there was a small section for the infirm. The work of reconstruction was completed in January 1952 and the building was reopened as Hospital 2, with 150 beds providing acute care and rehabilitation for older patients. The thinking behind the new facility for older patients was very advanced for the time and Hospital 2 was among the first geriatric assessment units in the world.

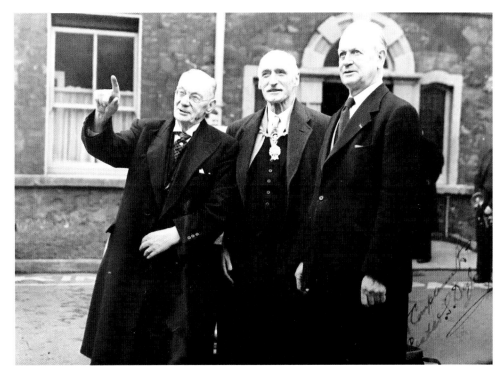

11.3　On the occasion of the demolition of the frontage of St Kevin's Hospital, 4 Dec. 1953: Peadar Doyle (left), the lord mayor, Bernard Butler (centre) and Séamus Murphy (right). Doyle was Éamonn Ceannt's quartermaster during the 1916 Rising, and Murphy commanded the Marrowbone Lane garrison. Courtesy of Nessa Rowan.

11.4　New entrance to St Kevin's Hospital, with the Queen Mary building in the background. This building became the headquarters of the Dublin Health Authority in 1960. Private collection.

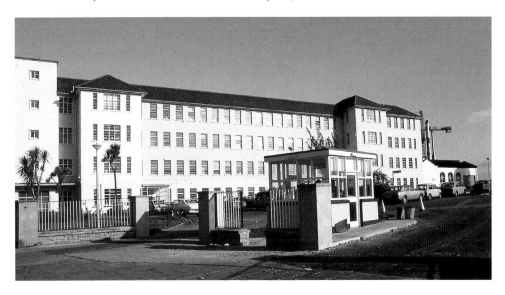

A new building to house forty patients was constructed in early 1952 close to Hospital 3 (previously Hospitals 2–3). This development allowed ward space to be vacated on the ground floor of Hospital 3, which was then refurbished to house the radiology and physiotherapy departments. Later, the new building was used to accommodate children with tuberculosis and, subsequently, in the 1970s and '80s, as a hospital for psychiatric patients (Hospital 6). The Infirmary, which at the time was used for genitourinary patients, non-ambulant infirm patients and patients with cancer, was closed in 1952 for reconstruction. When reopened, as Hospital 1, it had 132 beds, and the wards were used for acute medical admissions for both male and female patients. Prior to reconstruction, Hospital 5 was used to house approximately seventy ambulant inmates. It was closed in 1953 and reopened twelve months later as an acute female medical unit. The refurbished wards were centrally heated, whereas before reconstruction many of them had been

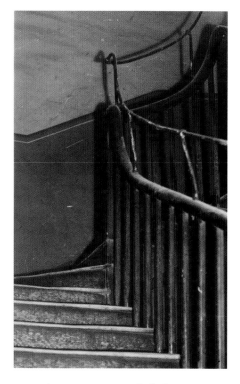

11.5   The stairs in Hospital 2 before refurbishment. Private collection.

heated by open fires. The old Garden Infirmary was refurbished at a cost of £150,000, and was reopened in 1956 by the minister for health, Thomas F. O'Higgins. The hospital had 228 beds for long-stay patients and became known as Hospital 4.[28] Demolition of the frontage facing James's Street began in 1953, and a new entrance replaced the old archway. The Protestant chapel, which was attached to the front of the dining hall of the Foundling Hospital, was demolished and replaced by a new chapel on the southern perimeter near Hospital 3. The new chapel was consecrated by the archbishop of Dublin, Dr Arthur Barton, in March 1955. The dining hall itself was demolished later in the decade but the vaults were preserved. The fine Gothic Catholic church, which was originally constructed by Johnston to serve the needs of the Foundling Hospital, was also demolished and, from then on, Sunday and weekday Masses were celebrated in the church near the Rialto gate, which had been built to serve the spiritual needs of the patients in the tuberculosis hospital.

A new well-equipped maternity unit with eighty-nine beds and a premature infant unit was opened in September 1954 by O'Higgins.[29] The new unit was built as an extension to Hospital 5 and contained an operating theatre. While the old unit had been

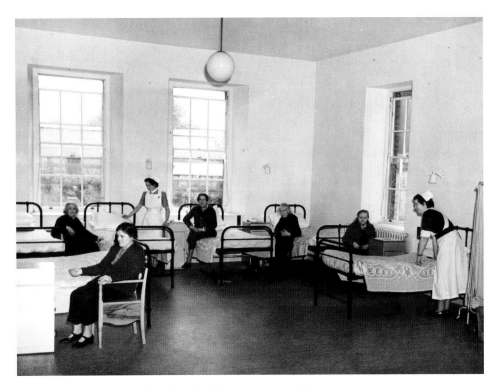

11.6   A ward area in Hospital 2 after refurbishment. Private collection.

staffed by one sister, three nurses, one wardmistress and an attendant, the new unit employed seven sisters, thirty-five nurses, four attendants, eleven ward attendants and two porters. Edward Keelan, who was already a visiting consultant, was appointed consultant obstetrician/gynaecologist with a team of two registrars and two junior house doctors.[30] No provision had been made for an antenatal clinic, so two wards were adapted to provide this service to expectant mothers. The antenatal clinic soon proved inadequate and representations were made to the Dublin Health Authority, which, after a long delay, led to a new purpose-built antenatal clinic, opened by the minister for health, Erskine Childers, in 1971.

Units for short-term male and female welfare dependants were opened at Island-bridge in 1954 and 1956, facilitating the closure of the casual units at St Kevin's. The new Cherry Orchard Fever Hospital, which opened in Ballyfermot in 1955, allowed the vacation of the old fever hospital in Cork Street. The name of this institution was changed to Brú Chaoimhín, and patients were moved there from the old men's infirmary, known as the 'Queen Mary'. After refurbishment, the Queen Mary was reopened in 1956 for long-stay male patients. The ground floor of the building was

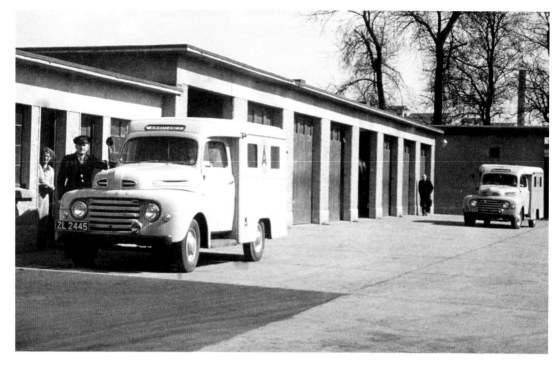

11.7   The new ambulance base, which was built in 1950. Private collection.

refurbished to accommodate an admission unit for the hospital. The long-stay male patients housed on the upper floors were later transferred to St Mary's Hospital in the Phoenix Park, and in 1960 these floors were converted into office accommodation for the newly formed Dublin Health Authority. The transfer of female patients to Brú Chaoimhín commenced in the autumn of 1955, facilitating the demolition of Hospital 8, the female chronic hospital in the welfare section. This building stood directly north of Hospital 1 and housed 556 patients prior to demolition in 1955.

The Rialto Chest Hospital closed in 1955 when the patients were transferred to the new James Connolly Memorial Hospital in Blanchardstown. The vacated building went through major refurbishment and reopened in 1957 as Hospital 7, with 256 fully equipped adult beds, including surgical beds. It also contained a paediatric unit with forty cots and a new surgical section with two new operating theatres. The operating theatre in Hospital 3 was retained for urological operations.

The catering facilities were also enhanced with the opening of a new staff canteen in 1951. Until 1954, the laundry of St Kevin's had been run on unpaid inmate labour with about thirty people working under the supervision of a wardmistress. This arrangement ended in 1954, staff were employed to work in a refurbished laundry, and the use of unpaid inmate labour was stopped throughout the hospital.

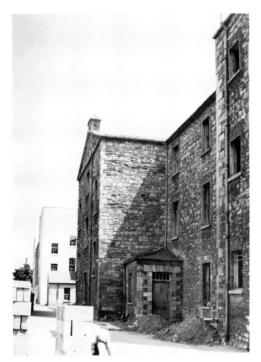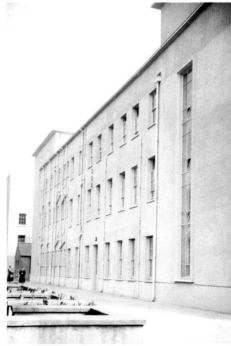

11.8   Hospital 1 (left) before reconstruction, with the already completed Hospital 2 in the background, and (right) after reconstruction. Private collection.

Significant progress

In terms of the capacity of St Kevin's, the net result of the closures and the refurbishment was a loss of approximately 520 beds. Despite the disruption of the extensive programme of works, the turnover rose significantly during the 1950s, from 8,600 admissions in 1952 to 11,916 in 1959.[31] Officials in the Department of Health were happier now that significant progress was being made. The demolition of most of the Foundling Hospital buildings cleared the ground between the Queen Mary building on the east side and the long, low two-storey stone building and the three-storey Georgian house on the west side. This vacant site, fronting James's Street, was considered as a potential location for a new acute hospital.

At around the same time, Denis McCarthy, who had succeeded Boland as RMS in 1954, wrote, 'St Kevin's is now progressing steadily towards the goal of becoming a first-class municipal hospital.'[32] McCarthy graduated in medicine in 1930 from University College Dublin and in the following year he joined the Indian Medical Service. During the Second World War he served in the North Africa campaign. He retired from the Indian Medical Service in 1947 having risen to the rank of Lt. Colonel. He was appointed medical officer to St Patrick's House, Carrick-on-Shannon, in 1950

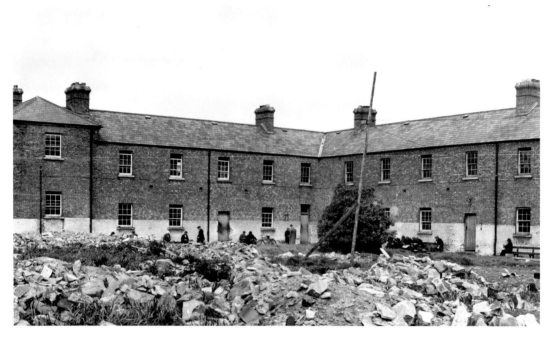

11.9   Hospital 5 (above) before reconstruction and (below) after reconstruction. Private collection.

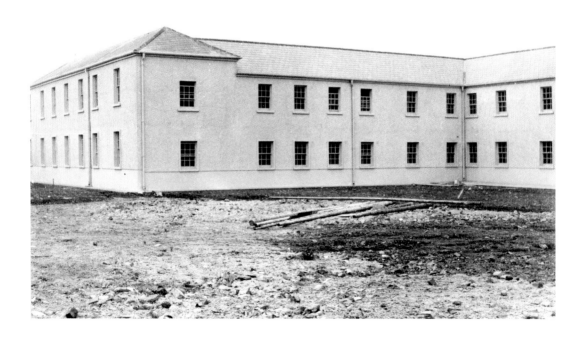

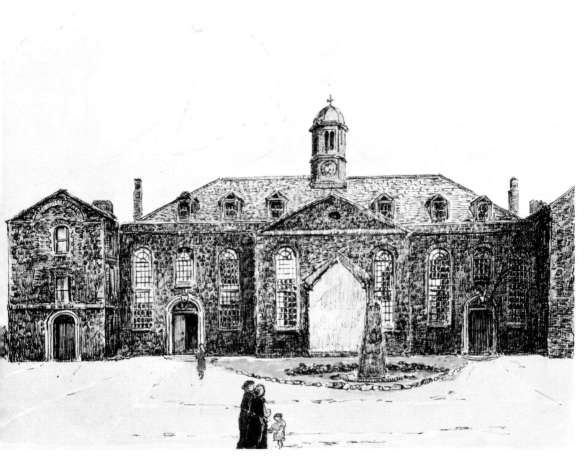

11.10   The dining hall of the Foundling Hospital in 1957, after the demolition of the Church of Ireland chapel, by Flora Mitchell. Private collection.

and in the following year he was appointed RMS to Limerick City Hospital. He was appointed RMS to St Kevin's Hospital four years later. In this position one of his responsibilities was the care of the geriatric patients, and he lectured on geriatric medicine to students from University College Dublin.[33]

At the conclusion of major works in the 1950s, the absence of any medical or surgical outpatient facilities remained unresolved despite repeated requests from St Kevin's Hospital to the Department of Health to provide this essential component of an acute hospital. Facilities were limited to the admission department in the Queen Mary building and a small, congested, return-dressings department attached to it.[34] Eventually, at the end of 1963, a ward on the ground floor of Hospital 7 was converted into an outpatient department.[35]

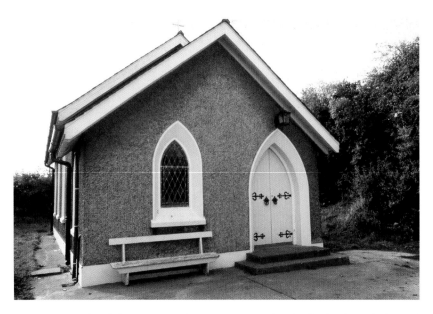

11.11   The new chapel that was erected in 1955 to serve Church of Ireland, Methodist and Presbyterian patients. It stood on the southern perimeter of the hospital, on the site now occupied by the Mercer's Institute for Successful Ageing (MISA). Private collection.

11.12   A vacated ward in one of the old Foundling Hospital buildings. Private collection.

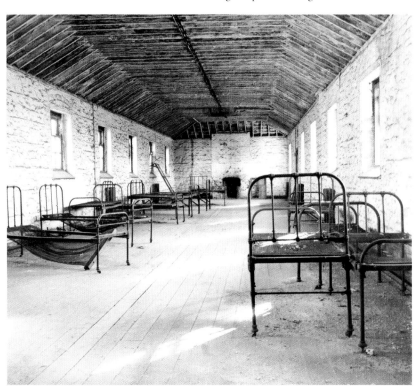

St Kevin's Hospital 1960

11.13   A map of St Kevin's Hospital in 1960 after a decade of demolition and refurbishment showing the positions of Hospitals 1–7. Image: Anthony Edwards.

The nuns cope with new challenges

Unlike the Mater Hospital and St Michael's Hospital, Dún Laoghaire, St Kevin's Hospital was never under the control of the Mercy order. In St Kevin's the nuns were employees, similar to the lay nurses, and did not have the independence of nuns working in a Mercy hospital. From the time of the first arrival of the Sisters of Mercy in the South Dublin Union in 1881 until the 1940s, the mother superior of the convent unofficially acted as the matron of the nursing nuns. Early in the 1940s, Sr M. Carthage Carroll was officially appointed matron of the acute hospital and of the children's hospital. Anne Mannion, who was not a member of the nursing profession, acted as matron of all the other hospitals and was largely responsible for housekeeping tasks.

With the development of St Kevin's Hospital, a decision was made to appoint one matron over the entire complex. The authorities favoured a nun for the position, but the superior general of the order, who was based at Carysfort Park in Blackrock, thought that the duties would be too onerous, and as a consequence Sr M. Carthage Carroll resigned in 1950 and Anne Young, who was the matron of Jervis Street Hospital, was appointed matron of the entire hospital. Two nuns, Sr M. Teresa Fallon and Sr M. John Berchmans Connolly, were appointed assistant matrons and four lay assistant matrons were also appointed. The hospital duties of the nuns now came under the control of Anne Young. In consultation with the mother superior of the convent, Young transferred nuns from ward to ward as necessary and the nuns' hours of duty were brought into line with those of their secular colleagues. At that time, nurses worked a ninety-six-hour fortnight, 8 a.m. to 8 p.m. and 8 a.m. to 2 p.m. on alternate days, with a day off each week. In order to fulfil their religious duties, the nuns required a longer lunch break, and to achieve this they had to forfeit a day off on alternate weeks to ensure they worked their ninety-six-hour fortnight.

Tension between the religious and lay sisters

Tensions began to emerge between the lay administration and the Sisters of Mercy. The nuns did not do night duty and this meant that for secular ward sisters, night duty came around more frequently. Walking from hospital to hospital in the dark was not without risk, and it was considered inappropriate to place the nuns in such danger. The issue had previously been raised in 1938 when plans were first considered to develop St Kevin's as a municipal hospital. Then the minister for local government and public health proposed that lay nurses should run the acute hospital and that the nuns should care for inmates in the chronic wards. The Dublin Board of Assistance did not agree and the nuns remained on the acute wards. The nuns' objection to undertaking night duty was strengthened by letters from the superior general of the order and from Edward Byrne, archbishop of Dublin, who wrote:

> I feel the time has come when I should inform the Board of Assistance that in my considered opinion, the particular circumstances of the Dublin Union make it most undesirable that the Sisters of Mercy there be asked to undertake night duty.[36]

Now the issue had surfaced again. The lay sisters put forward the argument that by reducing the number of religious sisters working on the wards, secular ward sisters, who would be available for night duty, could be employed in their place. The nuns referred the matter to Archbishop John Charles McQuaid and he gave them strong support, as had his predecessor. He wrote to the minister for health, Dr Noël Browne, suggesting that the minister should release the nuns from any obligation to take part in night duty at St Kevin's Hospital. Browne rejected the archbishop's request on the basis that if lay nurses could do night duty, so could the nuns. McQuaid was reportedly very irritated by the minister's response, which was the first disagreement

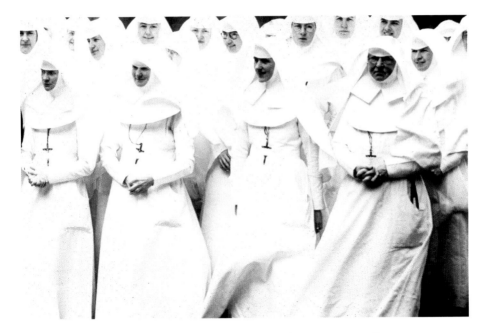

11.14   A group of nuns photographed at St Kevin's Hospital c.1960. Private collection.

11.15   A function in the hospital to mark the departure of Nurse Hanraghan (seated in the front row and wearing white cardigan) for the African missions. Private collection.

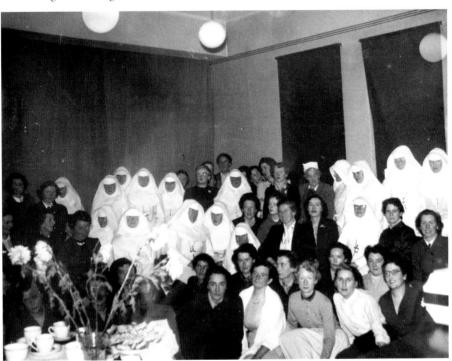

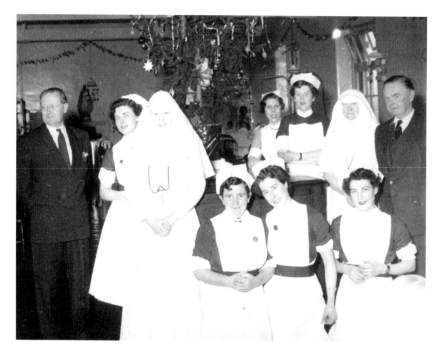

11.16 Celebrating Christmas: Mr Hugh MacCarthy, Sr M. Agnes Therese, Sr M. Celestine, Mr Charles Boland and nursing staff. Reproduced with permission of the Mercy Congregational Archives.

11.17 A nurse in the operating theatre in Hospital 3. Private collection.

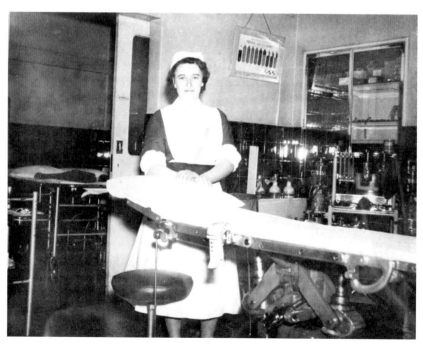

between the two men over matters relating to the health services.[37] It was quickly followed by others and culminated in a major disagreement over Browne's attempts to introduce a mother-and-child scheme to provide universal free medical services to mothers and children.[38] In 1958, after further discussion and deliberation, the nuns agreed to participate in night duty. The sisters adapted well to the new system, but the duties were onerous:

> On night duty, each sister, as night sister, was responsible for two or three hospitals, involving, sometimes, as many as six hundred and thirty patients. She had to do rounds in each hospital assigned to her, starting at 8 p.m. during which she saw all the patients, and checked in the staff in each unit. That round took about two hours to complete. The next began at midnight, when the twenty-four hourly returns were entered on the appropriate sheet. The final round was at 5:30 a.m. These rounds necessitated walking through the grounds during the night, from one hospital to the next. In the morning, she had to write a detailed report, in a journal, for matron, as well as giving a verbal report to the appropriate assistant matron. At 7:30 a.m. she checked in the wardsmaids, and sent telegrams, in the name of the medical superintendent, to the relatives of any patients who may have died during the night. She came off duty, usually, at 8:10 a.m.[39]

Despite the agreement of the nuns to participate in night duty, McQuaid did not forget the alliance between the lay administration and Browne over the issue, and some years later he withdrew the nuns from St Kevin's Hospital.[40]

Controversial medical appointments

In 1952, advertisements were placed in the Dublin newspapers for full-time salaried medical and surgical staff in St Kevin's Hospital, with no commitments to other hospitals. The Irish Medical Association was opposed to the full-time salaried structure of these posts and they discouraged applicants. They placed the following advertisement in the *Irish Times* on 21 April 1952:

> Medical practitioners who may have applied for, or who intend to apply for, recently advertised appointments as surgeons and physicians or for other medical appointments at St Kevin's Hospital, Dublin, or who shall have been invited to sit on a selection board in connection with such appointments, are requested to communicate immediately with the secretary at 10 Fitzwilliam Place, Dublin.

Despite the opposition, the appointments went ahead and staff were recruited through the local appointment commissioners. Two surgeons, Charles Boland, who was then the RMS, and Hugh MacCarthy, were appointed and they commenced their duties in October 1952. Two physicians, Patrick (Paddy) Blaney and James Mahon, were also appointed and they took up duty in January 1953.

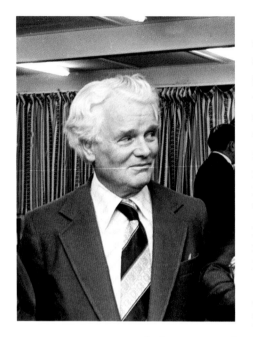

11.18   Dr Patrick Blaney, appointed physician in 1952. Photograph: Bobby Studio.

11.19   Dr James Mahon, appointed physician in 1952. Courtesy of the Mahon family.

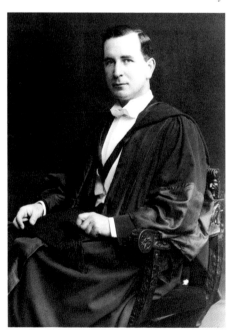

Following his appointment as full-time consultant surgeon, Boland resigned as RMS and concentrated on orthopaedic surgery. His colleague, Hugh MacCarthy, had had an outstanding undergraduate career in the RCSI. He became a member of the Royal College of Physicians of Ireland in 1943, a fellow of the Royal College of Surgeons of both Edinburgh and Ireland in 1944 and a fellow of the American College of Surgeons in 1949. He was appointed as assistant surgeon to the Richmond Hospital in 1945, where he was known as 'the boy surgeon' because of his youth. He performed pioneering chest and mitral-valve surgery in the Richmond Hospital with Patrick O'Toole as anaesthetist.[41] He was appointed surgeon to St Kevin's Hospital in 1951, reputedly applying for the position because he did not like private practice. Barry O'Donnell, in his book, *Irish surgeons and surgery in the twentieth century*, described him as 'a master technician'.[42] Hugh MacCarthy died suddenly in 1978 on his way to a meeting of the medical board in the hospital.

Paddy Blaney graduated from Queen's University Belfast in 1939, became MRCP (London) in 1951 and was awarded an MD in 1952. He did his postgraduate training in the Mater Hospital, Belfast, and in Nottingham General Hospital, where he was appointed senior registrar in 1952. Very highly regarded as a bedside clinician and teacher, he showed an awareness of the importance of social factors in the genesis of disease. His acumen in the diagnosis and treatment of acute illness was matched by his compassion and care for those with chronic disabilities.[43]

James Mahon studied medicine in Trinity, graduating MB in 1938 and MD in 1950. He joined the RAMC in 1940 and during the Second World War he served in Burma and India, where he was the officer commanding the British Military Hospital in Bangalore. After the war he worked in London until he was appointed county physician to Sligo County Hospital in 1950. He took up his post as consultant physician to St Kevin's in 1953. He was awarded a WHO medical

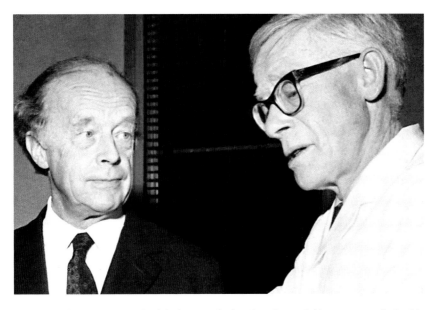

11.20   Dr Thomas Hanratty (right) photographed with Erskine Childers, minister for health. Photograph: Bobby Studio.

fellowship in 1959. Mahon was a greatly respected physician. He was also an excellent golfer, becoming Irish Close Golf champion in 1952 and captain of Portmarnock Golf Club in 1973. He retired from St James's Hospital in 1979.

With the appointment of full-time salaried medical and surgical staff, the role of the specialist temporary consultants appointed in the late 1940s was reviewed. Some of these were converted to 'visiting specialist staff'. The visiting staff would be available to the hospital for consultation but they would not have any inpatient beds. The respiratory consultant Gerard O'Brien accepted the post of visiting specialist, but the cardiologist Patrick O'Farrell was very unhappy with the proposed new arrangements. He had established a cardiology unit in two wards, male and female, and he wished to continue in his position as cardiologist. His request was refused and he was informed that cardiology and chest disease were 'within the routine scope of the work of the general physician'.[44] O'Farrell refused to accept the post of visiting cardiologist and described what was done to him as a 'bitter experience'. In contrast, the rheumatologist Thomas O'Reilly and the urologist Tom Lane were asked to remain on the staff and to continue to be responsible for patients in the hospital. At the time, rheumatology and urology were considered specialist fields, but cardiology was not. Additional medical staff were also recruited in the 1950s for the radiology and anaesthetic departments.

Thomas Hanratty was appointed as obstetrician/gynaecologist in June 1960, succeeding Edward Keelan, who had moved from St Kevin's to the Coombe Hospital in 1956. Hanratty graduated with a first-class honours degree in medicine from

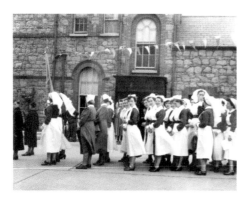 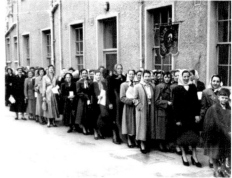

Left 11.21   Nurses take part in the May procession in the hospital grounds. Private collection.

Right 11.22   Domestic staff wait to participate in the May procession in the hospital. Private collection.

University College Dublin in 1942. He was awarded an MD three years later. He worked in Newcastle and Southampton and in Guy's Hospital, London. In 1949, he became MRCP, MRCPI and in 1953 MAO. Hanratty did his specialist training in the National Maternity Hospital and served as its assistant master. He established a very successful private practice in Dún Laoghaire. In 1963, he gave up this practice and other clinical commitments when he was appointed as full-time obstetrician and gynaecologist in St Kevin's. He devoted the rest of his career to developing one of the most outstanding maternity units in the country, with a very low perinatal mortality rate. There were approximately 2,500 births annually at the hospital during this period. His maternity unit was: 'one where the standard benchmark was one of excellence. He had a great rapport with all his patients but he had a particular and abiding concern for the less privileged members of society who came to him.'[45]

Hanratty had exceptional ability as a teacher and hundreds of pupil midwives were taught by him in the school of nursing and midwifery. He retired in 1984, and two years later Pope John Paul II bestowed upon him the Knighthood of St Gregory, which was presented to him at a ceremony in the hospital chapel.[46]

Advances in the care of older patients

James St Laurence O'Dea was appointed assistant RMS to Denis McCarthy in 1954. McCarthy and O'Dea had clinical responsibilities for patients in the long-stay wards. Geriatric medicine was being developed as a specialty in the United Kingdom following the publication of seminal papers by Dr Marjorie Warren in the *British Medical Journal* (1943) and *The Lancet* (1946). Warren worked at the Isleworth Infirmary in London, which took over an adjacent workhouse to form the West Middlesex Hos-

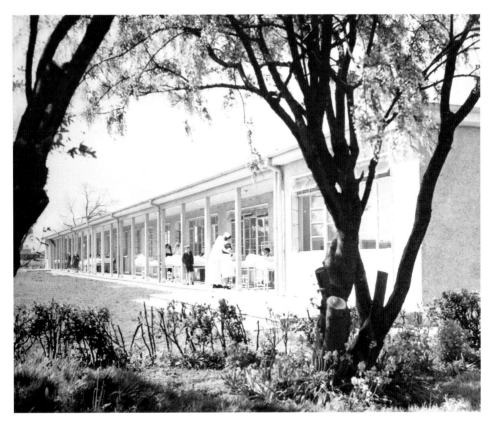

11.23   A hand-tinted photograph of the open-air tuberculosis ward that was built in 1940. It was subsequently converted to an inpatient psychiatric ward. Private collection.

pital in 1935. She systematically reviewed several hundred inmates of the workhouse, most of whom were old and infirm, and found that many suffered from untreated diseases. Warren was able to discharge patients after organizing appropriate treatment and rehabilitation and her achievements stimulated the Ministry of Health to appoint the first geriatricians within a few months of the introduction of the NHS in 1948. Warren visited St Kevin's in 1963, on the invitation of McCarthy, to view the progress being made in the care of older patients in the hospital.[47] Denis McCarthy died unexpectedly in 1964, and O'Dea succeeded him as RMS.

A modest man of great integrity and considerable experience, James O'Dea had joined the staff of St Kevin's Hospital in 1954. He served as president of the Irish Medical Association and was a member of the Consultative Council on the General Hospital Services and the Medical Research Council. He was a man of vision and played a very important role in the development of St Kevin's Hospital. He was appointed medical administrator of St James's Hospital in 1971. The coordination and rationalization of Irish hospital services and their integration with the community health services was one of his lifelong ambitions. On his retirement in 1979, he became a consultant on the design and planning team of the new hospital.

J.J. (Jack) Flanagan was appointed deputy RMS to St Kevin's Hospital in 1964, with responsibility for the geriatric service. Flanagan graduated from University College Dublin in 1943. He did his postgraduate training in London and returned to Dublin in 1949 to take up the position of chest physician at St Mary's Hospital in the Phoenix Park. He was awarded an MD in 1954 for a thesis on tuberculosis. Following the decline in the incidence of tuberculosis, Flanagan decided to enter the developing specialty of geriatric medicine. In 1967 he was awarded a WHO fellowship that enabled him to visit leading geriatric units in Great Britain, the Netherlands and Belgium.

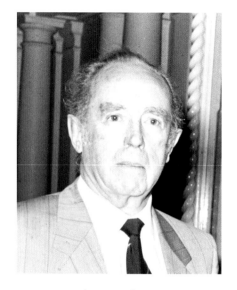

11.24   Dr J.J. Flanagan, who was appointed as the first consultant geriatrician to the hospital. Photograph: Bobby Studio.

Flanagan introduced a day hospital service for older patients in 1968, and this facilitated earlier discharge of older patients from hospital and the continuation of their rehabilitation at the day hospital. He was appointed as physician in geriatric medicine in 1971, becoming the first full-time consultant in the specialty in Ireland. A speech therapist and two additional physiotherapists were also recruited. Gradually the different paramedical disciplines that form the multidisciplinary team were established in the hospital.

There was dire poverty in Dublin in the 1950s and 1960s and a study undertaken in 1959 on 193 patients aged over 65 and admitted to St Kevin's Hospital found that 170 had a totally inadequate diet. Lassitude, depression and mental apathy were frequently observed in the under-nourished patients. Anaemia was common due to iron and vitamin deficiency, and some patients had swollen legs as a result of low protein levels in the blood due to poor nutrition. Many of the patients suffered from osteoporosis and osteomalacia due to deficiencies of calcium and vitamin D. Malnutrition also resulted in increasing levels of tuberculosis among the poor. Good food and vitamin therapy often brought about a marked improvement in these patients. The hospital had central heating and was a welcome haven for older people who lived in cold tenement flats. When speaking about these issues, Maureen Murphy, the chief social worker in St Kevin's, stated that it was a scandal that so many old people suffered from malnutrition in an agricultural country.[48]

Largest general hospital in the state

During the 1950s, the activity of the hospital increased significantly. By 1959, the average length of stay, which had been 83.7 days in 1952, had fallen to 44.5 days. When the refurbishment was completed at the end of the 1960s, St Kevin's Hospital was the largest general hospital in Ireland, with specialties of surgery, medicine, rheumatology, genitourinary medicine, gynaecology, paediatrics, obstetrics, geriatric medicine, radiology and pathology. There was an outpatient department, a day hospital, physiotherapy, speech therapy, occupational therapy and a school of nursing. Séamus Murphy retired as CEO of the Dublin Board of Assistance in 1957, and he was succeeded by Eugene O'Keeffe; James J. Nolan was appointed general secretary of the board. Séamus Murphy was a remarkable man of vision and tenacity whose work throughout the first half of the twentieth century led to the development of St Kevin's Hospital. In 1960, the Dublin Board of Assistance was replaced by the Dublin Health Authority, the membership of which was composed of local councillors nominated by Dublin County Council, Dublin Corporation and Dún Laoghaire Corporation. As a result, St Kevin's became a local-authority hospital.[49]

At this time, formal teaching sessions for junior doctors did not exist, but registrars organized weekly clinical meetings, which were chaired by either of the two physicians, James Mahon or Paddy Blaney. The range of conditions from which the patients suffered was very wide, and the doctors became very skilled at clinical examination and diagnosis. As a result, there was a high success rate among the registrars at professional examinations such as membership of the RCPI and fellowship of the RCSI. Many of the registrars went on to become leading members of the medical profession in Ireland and abroad. Because of the breadth of the experience gained at St Kevin's Hospital, the Local Appointments Commission favoured candidates who had worked in the hospital when appointing county physicians and county surgeons.[50]

The hospital began to provide teaching sessions for medical students from the RCSI and University College Dublin in 1964, and for a time UCD psychiatry professor Ivor Browne and his department were based in Garden Hill, the former residence of the master of the South Dublin Union. Browne was the founder and director of the Irish Foundation for Human Development, which was also based in Garden Hill. The foundation concentrated on three main areas: 'the environment and society, the essential nature of the person, and human groups and relationships between people'.[51] Garden Hill also housed the first day centre for emotionally disturbed children, which was established in 1966. The centre was administered by St Loman's Hospital and it had a staff of two psychologists and three teachers and a capacity to treat thirty children.[52] Two other units were developed in the vicinity of Garden Hill: a psychosomatic unit, which was directed by Dr John Cullen, and a psycho-endocrine unit, which was directed by Professor Austin Darragh.[53] The Eastern Health Board continued to hold the lease of the Garden Hill site for a number of years after the establishment of St James's Hospital.

The 1960s was a period of consolidation at the hospital. There were staff changes but these were relatively modest. Francis (Frank) Ward succeeded Boland as surgeon and two more physicians, Peter Faul and Joseph Timoney, joined the staff. A venereologist, Francis M. Lanigan-O'Keeffe, joined the visiting staff in 1959. He was subsequently appointed consultant venereologist to the Coventry and Warwickshire Hospital. There were two consultant radiologists in the hospital, Michael G. Magan and Edward Malone, and four assistant radiologists. Kibon Aboud was appointed assistant medical superintendent to James O'Dea. A number of changes and additions were made to the visiting medical staff including the appointment of Maurice Fenton as ophthalmic surgeon, Walter Verling as venereologist, Maurice F.A. O'Connor as ear, nose and throat specialist, and Dermot Flynn and Victor Lane as urologists. The medical staff included 13 registrars: 5 in medicine, 2 in obstetrics, 2 in surgery, 2 in anaesthesia, and one each in pathology and paediatrics. There were 24 house officers, 48 ward sisters, 280 nurses and 98 student nurses. Four physiotherapists were employed in the 1960s, with Edith Kiernan as the senior physiotherapist and five radiographers, with Margaret O'Neill as the senior radiographer. In the same period there was one occupational therapist, Anne E. Sedgewick, and one speech therapist, Miriam O'Connor, on the staff.

Development of pathology services

The activity of the pathology services in the hospital grew as St Kevin's expanded. A new pathology department was established on a regional basis in 1955 and John Harman was appointed as director of pathology. Harman graduated from UCD in 1939 and subsequently trained in pathology in the United States. He was appointed associate professor of pathology at Wisconsin Medical School in 1950. His research at Wisconsin evaluated the effects of radiation on tissue cells, and when he returned to Dublin his funding for research transferred with him.[54] He was very interested in research and teaching and some contemporaries commented that he was 'never entirely at home in a hospital environment'.[55] Harman was appointed professor of pathology in University College Dublin in 1958 and pathologist to the Richmond Hospital in the same year. He resigned as director of pathology in

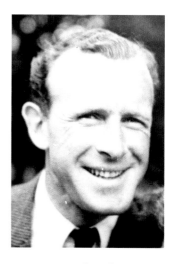

11.25   Dr Patrick Mullaney, consultant pathologist. Courtesy of Dr Susan Mullaney.

St Kevin's in 1959 and was succeeded by the assistant pathologist, Patrick J. Mullaney. Mullaney had graduated from Trinity College Dublin in 1937 and was awarded an MD in 1949. He spent time in Barbados, where he worked as government pathologist and bacteriologist before joining the staff of St Kevin's Hospital. He became a fellow of the College of Pathology in 1965. Mullaney's appointment was followed by others, including biochemist Patrick Moore and haematologist Kim Ryder. Mullaney complained about the unsatisfactory arrangements for the laboratory service: the laboratories were situated in inadequate accommodation, subspecialties were housed in five different buildings and the biochemistry department had expanded into ward accommodation in Hospital 7.[56] During the next decade the number of staff in the pathology department rose to twenty, and a quarter of a million examinations were processed each year despite the very cramped conditions.

The accommodation crisis in the pathology services at St Kevin's Hospital was brought to the attention of the Dáil in February 1968 by Richie Ryan, chairman of the Dublin Health Authority. Ryan emphasized the inappropriate use of wards for laboratory space and the impact the crisis was having on other services. He declared that senior consultants should have adequate accommodation for their work and that there were other consultants who would be prepared to work in the hospital but who were not willing to join the staff because 'of the slum conditions imposed on them in St Kevin's'.[57] Ryan went on to say:

> We were told by the minister that the conditions in St Kevin's were far superior to the laboratories in most of the voluntary hospitals. We do not know whether this is true or not, but I am prepared to accept it if the minister says so. But, if that is so, it highlights the deplorable conditions in which laboratory work is being done in this city.[58]

In his reply, the minister for health, Seán Flanagan, said that he had appointed a committee, the Consultative Council on the General Hospital Services, to examine the issues involved and to make recommendations on the future configuration of the acute hospital and pathology services in the country. The minister was anticipating that the committee would recommend the development of St Kevin's Hospital so that it could play a pivotal role in providing pathological services to both voluntary and public hospitals. Under these circumstances the minister said that it would be prudent to wait for the report of the consultative body.[59] The report, which became known as the 'Fitzgerald Report', did recommend the development of laboratory services at St Kevin's Hospital.

The Sisters of Mercy leave

In 1962, a meeting between the archbishop of Dublin, John Charles McQuaid, and the superior general of the Mercy order resulted in the withdrawal of the nuns from St Kevin's Hospital. McQuaid claimed that they were needed in other houses of the Mercy order, and he also wished to send some of the nursing sisters to a new Mater Hospital in Nairobi. Three nuns left St Kevin's for Nairobi in 1961 and four were transferred to the Mater Hospital in Dublin. Early the following year,

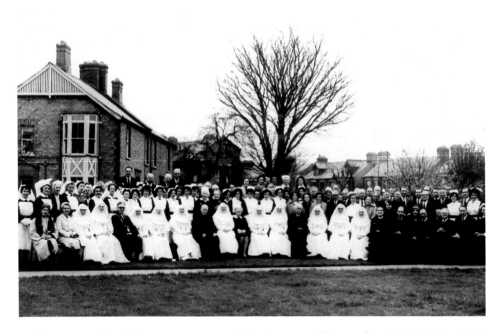

11.26   A group gathered after a ceremony to mark the departure of the nuns from St Kevin's Hospital in 1963. Private collection.

11.27   Dr Denis McCarthy makes a presentation to Mother M. Celestine Rock, the mother superior of the community. Private collection.

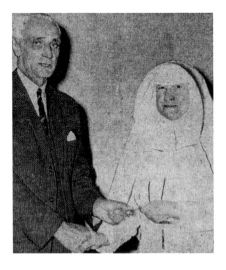

six more were withdrawn and dispersed to convents around Ireland and one of them went to Nairobi. Before the end of the year, a decision was made to withdraw the twelve remaining nuns from St Kevin's. To mark this event, in April 1963 a presentation was made to the mother superior, Mother M. Celestine Rock, and the remaining nuns, by the RMS, Denis McCarthy. The Mercy order had acquired new premises in Newtownpark Avenue, Blackrock, which they developed as a private psychiatric hospital (Cluain Mhuire). This was to be the destination of the remaining nuns, and the furniture and effects belonging to the Sisters of Mercy at St Kevin's were transferred there a few days before the departure of the last five nuns. The nuns finally left the convent on 4 July 1963, ending the 124-year association of the Mercy nuns with the South Dublin Union and, subsequently, St Kevin's Hospital.

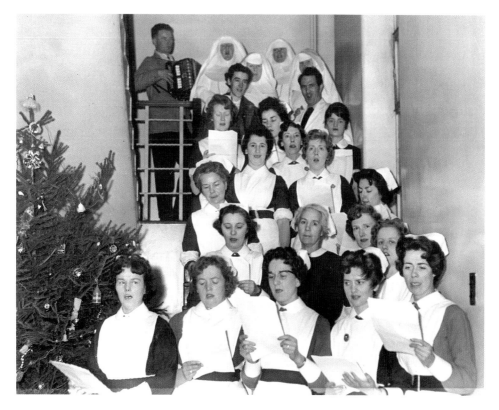

11.28   Anne Young (centre of second row) with a group of carol singers c.1960. Mercy Congregational
Archives.

Anne Young and nursing education

Anne Young, who was born in Rathcabin, Co. Tipperary in 1907, played a key role
in the transformation of St Kevin's into a major municipal hospital and in the development of nursing education. Young had trained at Yarmouth Hospital in England,
qualifying as a nurse in 1930 and as a midwife two years later. Between 1933 and 1935,
she worked as a sister at Great Yarmouth Hospital, Norfolk, and in 1935 she obtained
a diploma in nursing from Leeds University. In 1936, Young became a nurse tutor in
Maidstone. She returned to Ireland in 1937 to work as a nurse tutor in Sir Patrick
Dun's Hospital. Two years later, she was appointed assistant matron and remained in
the post until 1945, when she was appointed matron of Jervis Street Hospital, where
she worked for five years. She was appointed matron of St Kevin's Hospital in 1950,
just before the major reconstruction of the hospital took place, and she held the position throughout the whole period of development. Two of her major achievements
were the establishment of a nursing school at the hospital in 1967 and a midwifery
school in 1970. The nursing school had an intake of forty students per year at that

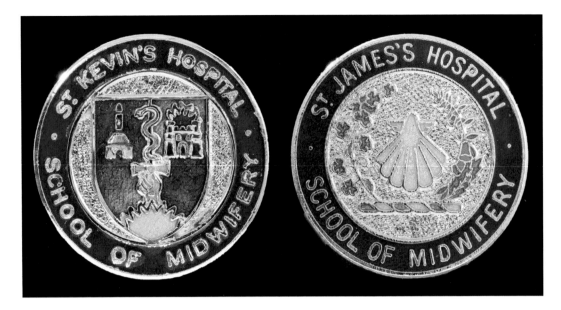

11.29   Midwifery nurses' badges for St Kevin's and St James's Hospitals. Photograph: Anthony Edwards.

11.30   Third-year student nurses, who had entered the nursing school in Jan. 1967. Courtesy of St James's Hospital.

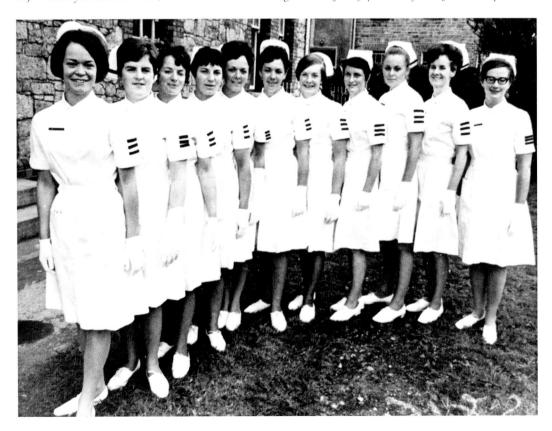

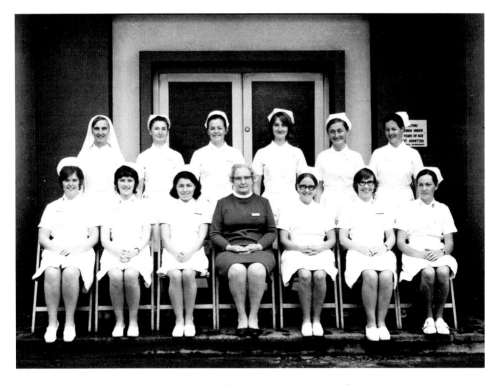

11.31   The first students to receive their midwifery diplomas. Courtesy of St James's Hospital.

time and they lived in the vacated convent building where the school of nursing was also located.

In 1968, Anne Young was appointed director of nurse education for the Dublin Health Authority, in addition to her duties as matron of St Kevin's Hospital. Among her achievements was the creation of a training syllabus for registered nurses for the intellectually impaired and the organization of 'back to nursing' courses, particularly for married women who wished to re-enter nursing. Young also initiated management courses for nurses in conjunction with the College of Commerce in Rathmines. She became president of the Irish Matrons' Association and represented Irish nursing at many international meetings and conferences. Young went on to become the first matron of St James's Hospital. She retired from this position due to ill health in 1972 and died four years later. She was succeeded as matron by Nora McCarthy, who had served as her deputy for a number of years.

Brídín Tierney was the first principal nurse tutor in the school of nursing. After graduating with a BA (hons) in languages from University College Dublin, she studied nursing at St Vincent's Hospital, where she later became a nurse tutor in the nursing school. Tierney was invited to spend time in Nigeria as a nurse tutor by the Medical Missionaries of Mary. She returned to Ireland in 1966 to steer the development of the nursing school at St Kevin's Hospital, which she did successfully. She was highly regarded by her colleagues throughout the country and was appointed as chairperson of the group which produced the *Working Party Report on General Nursing* (Tierney Report). Published in 1980, the report had a major influence on the development of Irish nursing. One of its recommendations was the establishment of a degree course in nursing. Tierney encouraged nursing research and she was the first research officer at An Bord Altranais, between 1981 and 1985. When Tierney retired in 1990, she was succeeded by her former deputy, Ita Leydon.

Challenging external developments, which would have major consequences for the future of St Kevin's Hospital, began to emerge during the 1960s. These included the desire of the small voluntary teaching hospitals in Dublin to amalgamate, and the imperative for the medical school of Trinity College to be associated with a major teaching hospital. These two factors, together with the long-held ambition in the Department of Health to form a major municipal teaching hospital, would result in the development of St James's Hospital.

12

The Federated Hospitals and the establishment of St James's Hospital

The [Federated] Group now faces the exciting challenge of developing, in conjunction with St James's Hospital and on the St James's site, a great new hospital.[1]

In 1953, the Irish Medical Association invited the American Medical Association to assess the standard of instruction given in Irish medical schools compared to that given in medical schools in the United States. A group from the American Council on Medical Education and the Association of American Colleges was appointed to inspect the Irish schools.[2] The resultant report was very negative and for a time Irish medical qualifications were not accepted in the greater part of the United States. This was a significant setback for Irish medical schools and urgent action was needed, in particular to deal with a major criticism in the report, which was of the lack of integration between the medical schools and the hospitals. A subsequent report of a joint inspection of Irish medical teaching by the General Medical Council (London) and the Medical Registration Council of Ireland, carried out in 1955, was also highly critical and again stressed the lack of cooperation between the hospitals and the medical schools, and the poor laboratory facilities.

The negative findings of these reports could not be ignored and each medical school had to devise a strategy which would secure its survival. J.W.E. (Jerry) Jessop, professor of social medicine, was appointed dean of the medical school in Trinity College in 1959 and he set out on a major programme of reform. Jessop's vision and energy played a key role in developments in both the medical school and the teaching hospitals and he was very committed to the concept of amalgamating the smaller voluntary hospitals into a major teaching hospital on one site. Consultants in these hospitals also realized that federation of the voluntary hospitals was urgently needed due to the rapid growth in expensive technology. Another concern, not committed to paper, was the increasing dominance of the Mater and St Vincent's hospitals and the growth in size and influence of the medical school of University College Dublin.[3] The amalgamation of the smaller Dublin teaching hospitals had been discussed in various forums from the beginning of the twentieth century. The case for amalgamation was based on economics, rationalization of the clinical services and the enhancement of research and teaching. Plans to amalgamate Mercer's, Sir Patrick Dun's and the Royal City of Dublin (Baggot Street) hospitals were at an advanced stage just before the onset of the Second World War. However, the momentum was lost during the war years and the planned amalgamation did not happen.[4]

Moves towards federation

The move towards federation began in earnest in 1957, when four influential doctors met informally to discuss a strategy to bring together the small voluntary hospitals in Dublin. They were Peter Gatenby from the Meath Hospital, George Fegan from Sir Patrick Dun's Hospital, and Stanley McCollum and John Sugars, both from the Adelaide Hospital.[5] After their initial discussions, the group approached the governing boards of seven hospitals: the Adelaide (154 beds), the National Children's (91 beds), the Royal City of Dublin (193 beds), Sir Patrick Dun's (168 beds), the Meath (282 beds), Mercer's (124 beds) and Dr Steevens' (203 beds). A joint committee of lay members and medical consultants was established to consider the proposal and it met on several occasions over the following two years under the chairman-

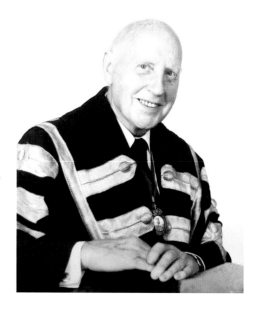

12.1 J.W.E. Jessop, dean of medicine (1959–73). Reproduced with permission of the Royal College of Physicians in Ireland.

12.2 Professor Peter Gatenby, professor of medicine. Medical School Archive.

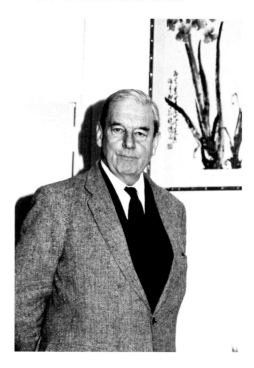

ship of Robert Woods, ear, nose and throat surgeon to Sir Patrick Dun's Hospital. The committee decided that the hospitals should amalgamate ultimately in one or more buildings and, in the interim, that there should be cooperation between the hospitals in the development of medical specialties, professorial units and a coordinated laboratory service. After further discussions, the hospitals agreed to form an associated group and to consider a closer union later. An approach was made to the minister for health, who agreed to provide enabling legislation. The Hospital Federation and Amalgamation Act became law on 8 July 1961, establishing a federation and providing a procedure for ultimate amalgamation of two or more hospitals as might later be desired. All the hospitals involved were situated south of the Liffey and, although the number of beds in each was modest, the federation as a whole had 1,215 beds.[6]

Administrative structure

A central council was established to coordinate and eventually to administer the amalgamated hospitals, and 6 November 1961 was designated as establishment day. Each hospital had five representatives on the central council and five were appointed by the Dublin Health Authority. Provision was also made for two representatives from any university that might make an agreement with the central council for the education of medical students. Arthur Chance, surgeon to Dr Steevens' Hospital, was the first chairman of the central council and he served in this office until 1964. The principal legal powers of the central council were the control of capital expenditure and the appointment of all consultants throughout the federation.

The central council met monthly and had two principal subcommittees: the medical committee and the finance and administration committee. The finances of the central council were provided mainly by a levy on the constituent hospitals. Neville Dowling was appointed as chief executive/planning officer and Desmond Dempsey as deputy chief executive officer. The central office of the Federated Hospitals was located at 82 Ranelagh Road, Dublin 6. The administrative staff transferred from there to accommodation in St James's Hospital in 1975.

Teaching agreement with Trinity College

For most of the twentieth century there were ten separate general teaching hospitals in Dublin. In the early years medical students in Dublin paid fees to one general teaching hospital but had access to all. As part of the reform process in the 1950s, hospitals and medical schools were aligned with each other. Sir Patrick Dun's Hospital, the Royal City of Dublin Hospital, Dr Steevens' Hospital and the Adelaide Hospital were the general hospitals linked with the school of physic (medical school) of Trinity College. Initially Mercer's Hospital joined the Charitable Infirmary, Jervis Street, and the Richmond Hospital in an association with the RCSI. However, in 1969, Mercer's

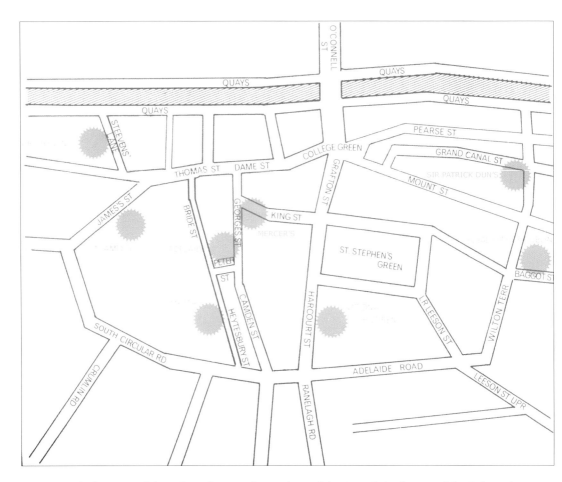

12.3 The locations of the Federated Hospitals. Brochure of the Annual Conference of the Federated Dublin Voluntary Hospitals and St James's Hospital 1975.

changed its teaching affiliation to the school of physic at Trinity College. The Mater Hospital and St Vincent's Hospital were associated with the medical school of University College Dublin.

Since its origins in the middle of the seventeenth century, the clinical teaching in the school of physic had been organized and delivered in the teaching hospitals by consultants who were not members of Trinity College's full-time academic staff. It was not until 1960 that a department of clinical medicine was formed in Trinity with the appointment of Peter Brontë Gatenby to the chair of clinical medicine. Gatenby, who was a member of the Irish branch of the famous Brontë literary family, had graduated from Trinity College where his father, James Brontë Gatenby, was a professor of zoology. Peter Gatenby taught and practised medicine at the Meath Hospital and Dr Steevens' Hospital and gradually developed a successful research base in temporary accommodation at the Meath Hospital. He was also a consultant at the Rotunda Hospital and had an international reputation for work on the anaemia of pregnancy. His unit in the Meath Hospital attracted young, highly motivated researchers, many of whom subsequently made significant contributions to the development of medical research and teaching. Donald Weir and Ian Temperley, both of whom would play major roles in the development of St James's Hospital, were among Gatenby's first researchers. The teaching and research programme of the medical school was further developed by the evolution of specialist units throughout the Federated Hospitals.

The development of the federation made it much easier for Trinity College to organize clinical teaching. It also allowed the university to enter into an agreement in 1970 with the federation as a whole, rather than with individual hospitals, for the purpose of developing clinical teaching. This agreement made provision for the participation of hospital representatives on appointment committees for full-time academic clinical staff, and Trinity College was to be represented on all hospital consultant appointment committees. The agreement also made it possible for the university to proceed with the establishment of whole-time departments in all the major clinical subjects for the first time. This helped to overcome the impasse created by the fact that the minister for health, who was primarily responsible for hospitals, could not allocate funds for clinical teaching, and the minister for education could only give funds to the university, which had no formal rights in the hospitals.[7] Under the new arrangement, essential core staff in the new academic departments held whole-time, joint contracts with the board of the university and with the central council of the federation. As a consequence, the university could request funds from the minister for education for the support of teaching and research in the new clinical departments and it could accept responsibility for these departments as it did for departments on the university campus.[8]

Rationalization of specialties

Rationalization of clinical laboratory services was seen as a priority for the new federated group. Before federation each hospital had its own small laboratory. Consequently, pathologists and technicians felt isolated and the small laboratories were not able to cope with expanding demands. Over a period of time histopathology, cytology, haematology, biochemistry, microbiology and immunology laboratories were concentrated in certain hospitals, and in the pathology department in Trinity College. A similar concentration of particular expertise in areas of medicine and surgery in individual hospitals promoted the development of specialty units. The disciplines of cardiology, gastroenterology, neurology, respiratory disease, haematology/haemophilia, dermatology and nephrology were developed as specialties within medicine. Similar changes took place in surgery, with specialist units in orthopaedics, vascular surgery, maxillofacial and plastic surgery, genitourinary surgery, thoracic surgery and gastrointestinal surgery developing in different hospitals.

Plans for amalgamation

One of the major objectives of the new central council was to bring the smaller hospitals together in a single hospital, and a planning committee was established for this purpose in 1962. Two years later a plan emerged that proposed the merger of five hospitals on the site of Sir Patrick Dun's Hospital. It was envisaged that Dr Steevens' Hospital would continue to function as an orthopaedic centre and the Meath Hospital as a centre for genitourinary and gynaecological surgery.[9] The Department of Health was quite prepared to back this plan and allocated £43,000 for the acquisition of property around Sir Patrick Dun's Hospital. However, a year later it came to light that there was a proposal to build a major road that would run through the hospital site. The plan had to be abandoned and, as none of the other Federated Hospitals sites was large enough to accommodate a new hospital, the committee began to look for other sites.

A six-acre site at Tullamaine on Burlington Road was considered, but subsequently the city manager suggested a 16-acre site at the fever hospital in Clonskeagh. Donogh O'Malley, minister for health, did not favour this suggestion and proposed the use of a 60-acre site at Cherry Orchard Hospital in Ballyfermot as an alternative. The central council reacted to this suggestion with enthusiasm, and planning consultants Llewelyn-Davies, Weeks and Partners were commissioned to report on the proposed development. Their report, which was received in March 1967, approved the site and included an outline plan to develop a hospital of 1,244 beds. The following June, the Department of Health agreed to the appointment of a project team to commence more detailed planning. Shortly after this, further development was stopped when the minister for health decided to establish a group, the Consultative Council on the General Hospital Services, under the chairmanship of Patrick Fitzgerald, professor of surgery at University College Dublin, to report on hospital planning for the whole country. This decision was greeted with considerable dismay by the central council.[10]

The Fitzgerald Report

The Consultative Council on the General Hospital Services was given a nationwide remit to report on the future planning of hospital services. The professors of medicine and surgery at Trinity College, Peter Gatenby and George Fegan, were both members of the review body. There was a growing recognition of the fact that hospital services throughout the country were poorly organized and were being developed on an ad hoc basis. With regard to the voluntary hospitals, the report pointed out that, although they were receiving state funding, the Department of Health had little influence on their policies and practices. There was unnecessary duplication of services, which was, in part, the result of competition between the individual hospitals. The Fitzgerald Report, published in 1968, advocated that the hospital system in the country should be reorganized into regions. It also proposed the establishment of a central professional body that would plan and coordinate all specialist developments throughout the country, both in the health boards and in the voluntary hospitals.[11] The overall message of the report was that a limited number of high-calibre and well-resourced hospitals would produce far better services than those delivered by the plethora of small hospitals that existed at the time. There was a need for a radical review of the organization, funding and staffing of hospitals throughout Ireland which would bring the system in line with established services in other countries.

The Fitzgerald Report recommended that there should be four major hospitals in Dublin, two regional and two general. Under this plan the activities of the Federated Hospitals would be divided between new hospital developments, one at St Vincent's Hospital and one at St Kevin's Hospital. It was proposed that a hospital of over 1,000 beds should be built adjacent to the new 450-bed St Vincent's Hospital at Elm Park, but it would remain under the management of the federation. A proposed 500-bed hospital at St Kevin's would also be under the control of the federation, while the rest of the hospital would remain under the Dublin Health Authority. The proposals were accepted by the minister for health, Seán Flanagan, and he asked the hospital authorities to meet and discuss their implementation. While there was support within the Federated Hospitals for the optimization of specialty resources, there was scepticism about the practicality of two independent hospital management systems operating at both Elm Park and St Kevin's Hospital. The consultants of the Federated Hospitals met at Sir Patrick Dun's Hospital to discuss the issue and they were addressed by two surgeons, Brandon Stephens from the Meath Hospital and Stanley McCollum from the Adelaide and the National Children's Hospital. There was vigorous opposition to the proposal to split the Federated Hospitals between the St Vincent's and St Kevin's sites and it was argued that the strength of the Federated Hospitals would be greatly diminished if they were not all on the same site.[12]

At this time, discussions were taking place about a proposed merger of Trinity College and University College Dublin, and the suggested location of part of the federation on the Elm Park campus was viewed with suspicion. There were also reservations about the St Kevin's proposal, as Ian Howie, former chairman of St James's Hospital board, recalled: 'The grim history of St Kevin's and a lack of appreciation, and possibly ignorance, of the work at the public hospital for the poorest sections of the community, made these proposals additionally unattractive to the federation.'[13] The central council requested Llewelyn-Davies, Weeks and Partners to advise on the future siting of the Federated Hospitals in light of the Fitzgerald Report. They examined the potential of sites at Elm Park, St Kevin's and Cherry Orchard and they again produced a report favouring Cherry Orchard Hospital as the first option, placing St Kevin's Hospital second. However, the Department of Health rejected Cherry Orchard and maintained that St Kevin's Hospital was the preferable option. Erskine Childers, minister for health, was particularly keen on a development at St Kevin's Hospital. In a symbolic and dramatic gesture, Childers signalled the new beginning

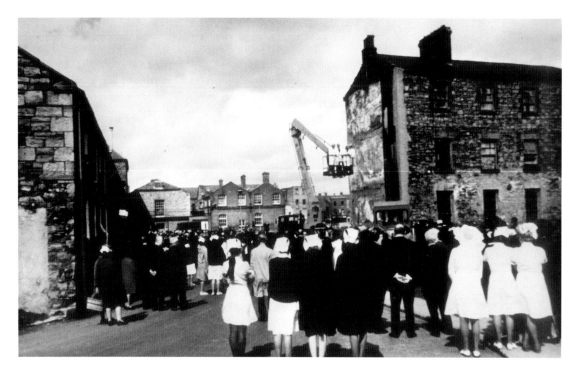

12.4   The minister for health, Erskine Childers, with a small group of dignitaries, on an elevated platform in St James's in 1971. The minister knocked a brick off one of the Foundling Hospital buildings scheduled for demolition, in a ceremony to mark the establishment of St James's Hospital. Courtesy of Moloney O'Beirne Architects.

by initiating the demolition of some of the remaining Foundling Hospital buildings in April 1970. It was Childers who suggested that the new hospital should be called St James's Hospital because of its location in St James's parish.

The Meath Hospital and the Adelaide Hospital remained opposed to the move to St Kevin's Hospital. In 1996, these two hospitals merged with the National Children's Hospital to form the Adelaide and Meath Hospital incorporating the National Children's Hospital (AMNCH). Two years later these hospitals moved to a new hospital in Tallaght, which also became a teaching hospital for Trinity College Dublin.[14]

Formation of St James's Hospital

Minchin Clarke, the third chairman of the central council, led the council in exploring options for progress with the Dublin Health Authority. In 1970, a joint negotiating body, which consisted of representatives of the Federated Hospitals and the Dublin Health Authority, was formed to discuss the future development of St Kevin's Hospital. Negotiations between this group and the Department of Health finally led to an establishment order, on 11 June 1971, for a new hospital, which would be known as St James's Hospital. The structure of the board of the new hospital drew on the public service tradition of St Kevin's Hospital and the voluntary tradition of the Federated Hospitals. The establishment order stated that the board would be appointed by the minister, and that there would be equal numbers of members from the central council and the Eastern Health Board. The chairman was to be elected by the members, alternating annually between the two groups forming the board. The minister gave a written commitment to build a new 350-bed hospital, with the required support services and teaching facilities, at St Kevin's. He formally

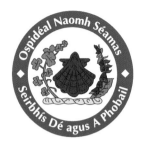

12.5   The logo of St James's Hospital. Courtesy of St James's Hospital.

renamed the hospital St James's Hospital on 29 November 1972 and installed the new autonomous hospital board. A joint medical committee, representative of the consultant staff of St James's Hospital and the Federated Hospitals, was formed to review and develop the medical and associated services of the hospital. Although the first board of St James's Hospital was composed of representatives of both the Health Board and the Federated Hospitals, the latter anticipated that the new hospital, when constructed, would be under the management of the Federated Hospitals.[15]

The name of the apostle James has been associated with the locality of the hospital for hundreds of years. The parish of St James covered a large area situated immediately outside the walls of the city and stretching west as far as Kilmainham. The original St James's parish church was probably built in the late twelfth century. The church stood on the north side of James's Street, east of Steevens' Lane. The church gave its name to St James's Gate, a tower that straddled James's Street and which controlled access to the walled city on its western boundary. The gate is shown on the old maps of Dublin at the junction of Watling Street and Thomas Street. St James's Gate survived into the early eighteenth century and it was still standing when the City Workhouse opened its doors in 1706.

The parish has historical associations with the shrine of St James the Apostle in Santiago de Compostela.[16] Santiago was a very popular destination for Irish pilgrims in the Middle Ages and these pilgrims are said to have gathered at the church of St James in Dublin en route to the Spanish shrine.[17] There was also a hostel to accommodate pilgrims just outside the city walls at St James's Gate. According to tradition, there was a pilgrims' shrine in the same vicinity.[18] It became customary for pilgrims to wear a badge, and from the very early years the scallop shell became the badge of the pilgrimage to Santiago. It was for this reason that the scallop shell was incorporated into the design of the logo of the new St James's Hospital. The shell is flanked by a sprig of shamrock and a stem of foxglove (digitalis) to give Irish and medical dimensions to the logo.

First meeting of the board of St James's Hospital

The Eastern Health Board (EHB), formed as a consequence of the Fitzgerald Report, took over the responsibilities of the Dublin Area Health Authority on 1 April 1971.[19] Its headquarters was in the Queen Mary, which stood on the left, inside the main entrance to St James's Hospital. A lease of the former St Kevin's Hospital was granted to the board of the new hospital by the Eastern Health Board. James McCormick, chairman of the Eastern Health Board and professor of general practice and community health in Trinity College Dublin, welcomed the creation of the hospital:

> The [Federated] Group now faces the exciting challenge of developing, in conjunction with St James's Hospital and on the St James's site, a great new hospital. This must be a new hospital not only in structure but in concept. It must develop with a full appreciation of the changing role of the hospital. Hospitals, originally founded as hospices to care for the sick, have become increasingly concerned with the more dramatic, curative and scientific aspects of medicine, and the problems of caring for the old, the infirm and the chronically disabled have suffered relative neglect. The conquest of infectious disease has improved life expectancy and has dramatically altered the pattern of hospital admissions. Most new hospitals have failed to grasp the implications of this change and are merely updated old hospitals.[20]

The new St James's Hospital board met for the first time on 2 July 1971. Patrick J. Burke TD, the nominee of the Eastern Health Board, was appointed as the first chairman. Ian Howie, a professor of zoology in Trinity College, was the nominee of the Federated Hospitals and he was appointed as chairman the following year. Howie was born in Edinburgh and studied zoology at the University of St Andrew's, Aberdeen. He came to Dublin when he was appointed lecturer in zoology at Trinity in 1953. Subsequently, he held several senior positions in the college administration and was registrar of the college when he was appointed to the board of St James's Hospital. He was a very able administrator and was vice provost of Trinity College from 1974 to 1981.

Trinity College did not have a right to representation on the board of St James's Hospital even though the university had representatives on the central council of the federation. However, the central council ensured university representation on the board by including two representatives from Trinity among its nominees. This situation lasted until 1984, when the university was granted direct representation. The new board of St James's began negotiations with Trinity College, with the intention of developing the hospital as a major teaching hospital for the university. A teaching agreement was signed by both institutions in December 1972, beginning an era of close cooperation between the university and the hospital that has had a significant impact on the health services and on health education and research in Ireland.

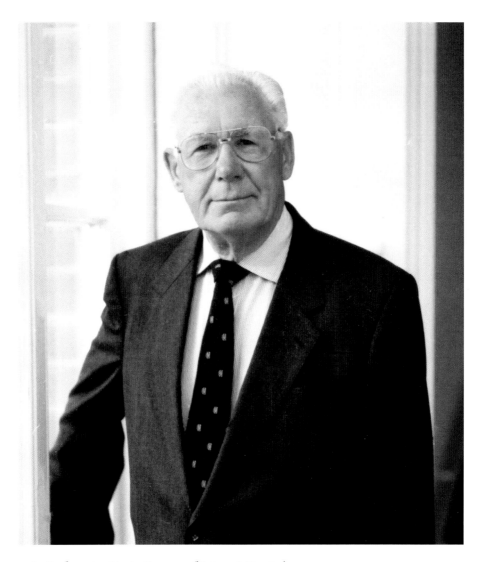

12.6   Professor Ian Howie. Courtesy of St James's Hospital.

Comhairle proposals

Following the establishment of St James's Hospital in 1971, the boards of Mercer's, the Royal City of Dublin Hospital and Sir Patrick Dun's agreed in principle to the amalgamation of their hospitals in a new hospital to be erected at the St James's Hospital site. Comhairle na nOspidéal, led by its chairman, Professor Basil Chubb, presented new proposals in a report outlining a hospital strategy for south Dublin to the minister for health in 1973. Comhairle was the statutory body responsible for advising the minister for health on the organization and operation of hospital services. The report suggested that south Dublin should be served by three hospitals: St James's, St Vincent's and another, which would be developed in the Newlands Cross area. It recommended that the new St James's Hospital should have between 500 and 600 beds and it also recommended that there should be both regional and national specialties at St James's and St Vincent's. The specialties were allocated to individual hospitals at subsequent negotiations involving the south-city hospitals.

The designated hospitals

Mercer's, Sir Patrick Dun's and the Royal City of Dublin Hospital became known as the designated hospitals, as they had agreed to transfer to a new hospital on the St James's site. Representatives of the designated hospitals and St James's formed a committee to plan the new hospital. Dr Steevens' Hospital, although not one of the original designated hospitals, would also close, and its services, apart from orthopaedics, would move to St James's Hospital. These hospitals had made a major contribution to the development of medicine and to the healthcare of the sick poor of Dublin. Each of these old voluntary hospitals had its own unique history, culture and traditions, which would greatly enhance and enrich the new St James's Hospital. Histories of these hospitals have already been written, so what follows is a short description of each hospital.[21]

Mercer's Hospital

Mercer's Hospital was established in 1734. It was built on a site with a tradition of healthcare and service to the poor stretching back several hundred years. The earlier foundation was known as St Stephen's Hospital and it was associated with the Abbey of St Stephen, which was founded in 1220. The abbey received an endowment in 1394 to establish a hospital for people suffering from leprosy. Although the monastery was suppressed by Henry VIII, the hospital continued to function until the middle of the seventeenth century. The buildings were finally demolished around 1680. Mary Mercer acquired the ground in Stephen Street in 1724 with the intention of building a house for the maintenance of poor women. She later abandoned this project and instead transferred the house to a group of trustees to develop a hospital 'for the reception and accommodation of such poor sick and diseased persons as might happen to labour under diseases of a tedious and hazardous cure'.[22] She enlisted the aid of Jonathan Swift to implement her plans and later he became a governor of the hospital.[23] Mary Mercer died in 1734 just a few months before the opening of the hospital. She bequeathed £6,000 to establish a charity school but she did not endow the hospital. In the early years of its existence, the hospital was largely dependent on charitable donations to meet its recurring costs. Regular charity concerts were arranged and the hospital was one of three institutions to benefit from the first performance of Handel's *Messiah* on 13 April 1742 in the Musick Hall on Fishamble Street.

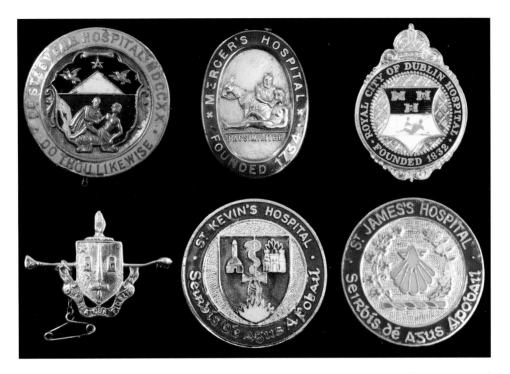

12.7 The nurses' badges of Dr Steevens' Hospital, Mercer's Hospital, Royal City of Dublin Hospital (Baggot Street), Sir Patrick Dun's Hospital, St Kevin's Hospital and St James's Hospital. Courtesy of the director of nursing, St James's Hospital.

12.8 Mercer's Hospital around 1900. Private collection.

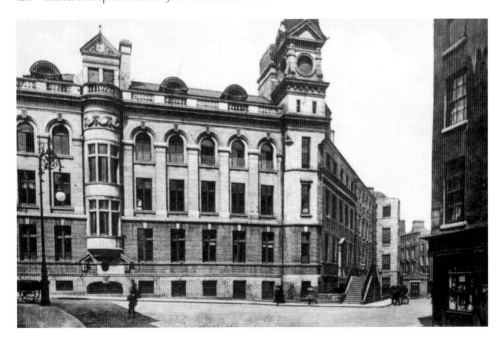

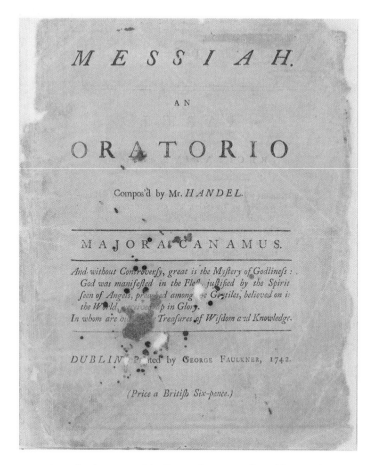

12.9   Cover for the music of the first performance of *Handel's Messiah* in 1742.
By permission of the Board of Trinity College, the University of Dublin.

Over the past 300 years, this oratorio has been heard by more people than any other sung musical work and it has raised more money for charity than any other piece of classical music in history.[24]

The physicians, William Stephens and Francis Le Hunte, and the surgeons, Hannibal Hall, William Dobbs and John Stone, formed the early visiting consultant staff of the hospital.[25] The hospital had ten beds when it opened. Piped water was installed in 1735 and a 'bagnio and fluxing room' was provided. The original house was replaced in 1757 with a larger building containing fifty beds. In the early 1880s, a new wing was constructed with a distinctive façade facing King Street. In June 1904, a new operating theatre and an X-ray department were built. Mercer's Hospital was the first hospital in Dublin in which clinical lectures for medical students were delivered.[26] A new residential block for students and a modern laboratory were erected in the 1960s. This laboratory provided the immunological services for the Federated Hospital group.[27]

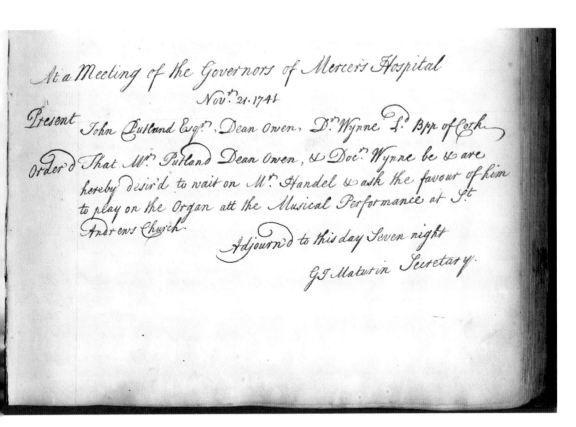

At a Meeting of the Governors of Mercer's Hospital
Nov.r 21. 1741

Present John Putland Esqr., Dean Owen, Dr. Wynne Ld Bpp of Cork

Order'd That Mr. Putland Dean Owen, & Docr. Wynne be & are hereby desir'd to wait on Mr. Handel & ask the favour of him to play on the Organ att the Musical Performance at St Andrews Church.

Adjourn'd to this day Seven night

GT Maturin Secretary.

12.10 A resolution of the board of governors of Mercer's Hospital to invite George Frideric Handel to play the organ at a musical performance at St Andrew's on 21 November 1741. National Archives of Ireland.

12.11 A ticket for a state lottery in 1751 for the benefit of a number of Dublin hospitals, including Mercer's Hospital. Private collection.

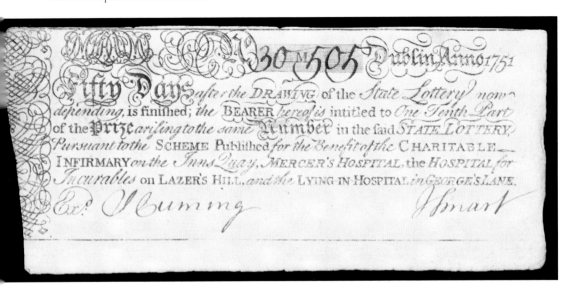

Sir Patrick Dun's Hospital

Sir Patrick Dun was born in Aberdeen and came to Dublin in 1676 in the service of the duke of Ormond. He was physician-general to the army and played a very prominent part in Irish medicine of the period, being president of the College of Physicians on four occasions. On his death in 1711, he left his property to his wife for her lifetime – after her death it was to be used to establish a number of professorships in the College of Physicians.[28] The bequest was subjected to repeated litigation and it was eventually decided to use some of the estate to establish a hospital with the primary purpose of providing clinical instruction for the medical students of the school of physic, a medical school linked to both the College of Physicians of Ireland and Trinity College.[29] The foundation stone of the hospital was laid in 1803 and the first patients were admitted in 1809. The hospital, built specifically as a teaching hospital,

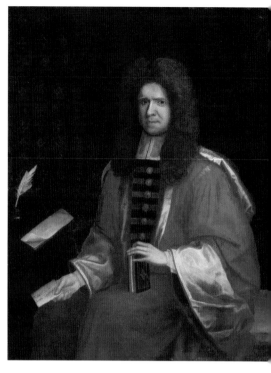

12.12   Sir Patrick Dun by Sir Godfrey Kneller. Reproduced with permission of the Royal College of Physicians of Ireland.

was a major innovation for its time.[30] During the early years of its existence, the hospital concentrated purely on medical cases and it was not until 1868 that a surgeon was appointed.

There were excellent teachers associated with the hospital from the very beginning. Many of these gained international reputations and fame. Robert Graves, as King's professor of the institutes of medicine, gave lectures at the hospital between 1827 and 1841. Graves was a great advocate of bedside clinical teaching and was the first to use a stethoscope in Ireland. His name is remembered in the eponym 'Graves' disease of the thyroid gland'.[31] Robert Smith was appointed as professor of surgery in Trinity College in 1849 and taught in Sir Patrick Dun's until 1873, when he was succeeded by Edward Halloran Bennett.[32] The names of these men are still familiar in medical schools and teaching hospitals throughout the world, as they are linked with a fracture of the wrist, known as Smith's fracture, and a fracture of the thumb, known as Bennett's fracture.[33] William Steele Haughton introduced the first clinical X-ray equipment in Ireland at Sir Patrick Dun's early in 1896. This was remarkable, as X-rays had only been discovered by Roentgen during the previous year.

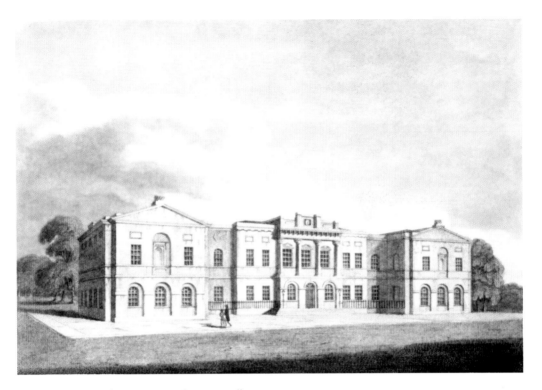

12.13   Sir Patrick Dun's Hospital. Private collection.

In the second half of the twentieth century, the hospital began to develop a number of specialized areas, including facilities for the investigation and treatment of venous ulcers and vascular diseases. The vascular services at the hospital were developed by George Fegan. He worked at the hospital from 1950 and served as professor of clinical surgery at Trinity College between 1967 and 1972. He had an international reputation for the treatment of varicose veins using a technique known as compression sclerotherapy. Although Fegan held a part-time professorship, he began to develop the nucleus of a department of surgery, appointing lecturers, research fellows and technical staff.[34] Otolaryngology and gastroenterology were also strong specialties in the hospital. The otolaryngology service was developed by Sir Robert Henry Woods, who joined the staff of Sir Patrick Dun's Hospital in 1906 on his return from specialist training in Vienna. A skilful surgeon, he invented surgical equipment and he replaced the standard white drapes used during operations with green drapes to reduce glare.[35] Gradually the use of green drapes spread to other hospitals and is now universal practice. He retired in 1933 and was succeeded by his son Robert (Bobbie) Rowan Woods, who had also studied in Vienna. Bobbie

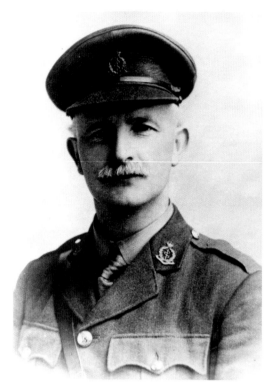
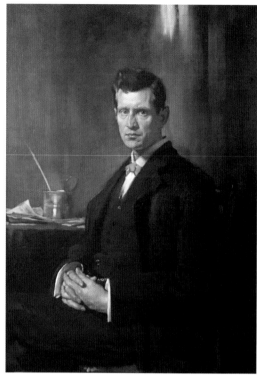

Left 12.14   William Steele Haughton. Private collection.

Right 12.15   Sir Robert Henry Woods by William Orpen. Photograph: Robert Woods. Courtesy of the Woods family.

Woods became renowned for his development of the technique of stapedectomy of the middle ear and was one of the first Irish surgeons to carryout a laryngo-oesophagectomy.[36] Woods' commitment to uniting the small voluntary hospitals was a key factor in the formation of the Federated Dublin Voluntary Hospitals.

Donald Weir, who was appointed Regius professor of physic in 1978, established the Federated Dublin Voluntary Hospitals' gastroenterology unit at Sir Patrick Dun's Hospital in 1967. He introduced the first endoscopy day ward in Ireland when he was awarded a grant to refurbish two rooms in the basement of the hospital.[37] The gastroenterology unit was supported on the surgical side by the skills of Thomas (Tom) O'Neill and David Lane. Lane was also a musician who played the oboe to a professional standard and in the occasional lull between operations, Weir recalls, 'he would find an isolated part of the hospital where he practised his oboe, an instrument he played with great artistic ability. Indeed, as he played, it gave everyone the comforting feeling that everything was under control in the hospital.'[38]

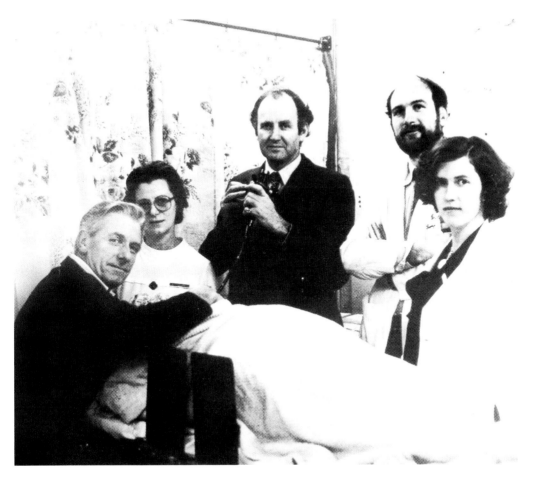

12.16   Prof. Donald Weir performing an endoscopy, assisted by his registrar, Dr Conleth Feighery. Left to
right: Gerry Byrne, Anne Dixon (first nurse endoscopist), Weir, Feighery and Dr Catriona Little. Brochure
of the Annual Conference of the Federated Dublin Voluntary Hospitals and St James's Hospital 1980.

The governors of Sir Patrick Dun's entered into an agreement with Trinity
College to provide an integrated teaching centre and library at the hospital in
1969. This was an embryonic clinical-sciences centre and the forerunner of the later
development at St James's Hospital.

Royal City of Dublin (Baggot Street) Hospital

The Royal City of Dublin Hospital, commonly known as Baggot Street Hospital, was
founded in 1832. It initially had fifty-two beds, and all of the original medical staff
were associated with the RCSI. It started as a general hospital but soon introduced
specialist facilities: an ophthalmology ward in 1836, a children's ward in 1838 and a

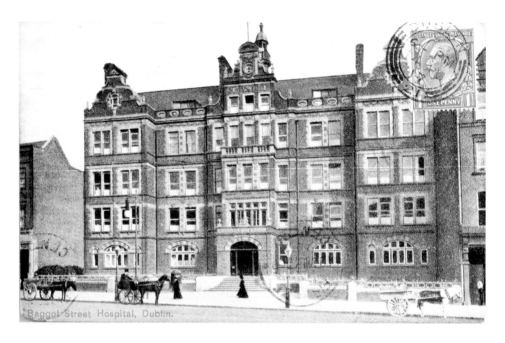

12.17   Postcard image of the Royal City of Dublin Hospital, Baggot Street. Private collection.

gynaecological ward in 1842. Arthur Jacob was the most famous surgeon of the founders of the hospital. While working in the anatomy department of Trinity College he
identified the layer of the retina (Jacob's membrane) that contains the light-sensitive
cells known as rods and cones. Later he also wrote the first description of a rodent
ulcer on the face, and this condition was known for many years as Jacob's ulcer.[39] Jacob
worked as an eye specialist in the hospital. John Houston, another founder, gained
eponymous fame for his description of the 'valves' or permanent folds of the wall of
the rectum known as Houston's valves. He introduced the microscope to Irish medicine and was one of the first to use the instrument to examine cancer cells.[40]

Despite constant financial headaches, the services of the hospital grew and the
number of beds rose to 100 by 1867. Special accommodation, known as the 'Drummond Wing', for patients suffering from infectious diseases, played a major part
in coping with an outbreak of smallpox in Dublin in 1872.[41] The Drummond Wing
was used as a unit for the treatment of tuberculosis in the first half of the twentieth
century. Extensive refurbishment of the hospital was undertaken towards the end of
the nineteenth century. The whole front of the old hospital was removed and a new
façade of decorative brick and terracotta was added.

A radiology department was established in 1902 and a deep X-ray therapy department for cancer treatment, the first of its kind in the country, was opened in 1927.
The treatment of cardiac and respiratory diseases emerged as great strengths of the

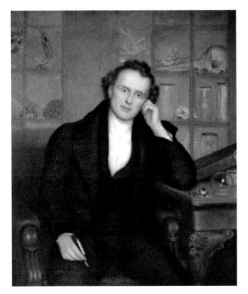
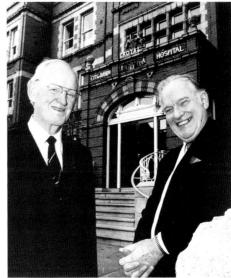

Left 12.18   Arthur Jacob by Henry Mallin. Courtesy of Jasper Jacob.

Right 12.19   Mr Keith Shaw and Dr Gerard Gearty. Reproduced from Davis Coakley, *Baggot Street: a short history of the Royal City of Dublin Hospital* (Dublin, 1995).

hospital in the latter half of the twentieth century. Respiratory medicine was introduced to the hospital by Terence Chapman, who joined the staff in 1954. Thoracic and cardiac surgery were developed following the appointment of Keith Shaw in 1958 and a year later a cardiopulmonary laboratory was established in a large basement room of the hospital. Shaw also set up a laboratory for experimental surgery in Trinity College and worked on the development of cardiac bypass surgery before doing the first successful open-heart operation in Ireland in 1960. He subsequently joined Professor Eoin O'Malley to form a national cardiac surgery unit in the Mater Hospital. Shaw was supported by David Hogan, a very able anaesthetist. The cardiology facilities at the hospital were developed initially by Rory Childers, son of the novelist and revolutionary Erskine Childers and brother of Erskine Childers who served as president of Ireland. Gerard (Gerry) Gearty succeeded Rory Childers in 1963 when the latter accepted a position in Chicago.[42] Gearty was born in Longford and studied medicine at University College Dublin. In 1956, he obtained a post as senior house officer in the Alder Hey Children's Hospital in Liverpool and in the following year he was appointed senior registrar in paediatric cardiology, a post he held for four years before completing his training at Sefton Hospital, where he worked in adult cardiology. Following his appointment to Baggot Street Hospital, Gearty established an intensive coronary care unit and shortly afterwards he set up a coronary care ambulance service with the support of the Irish Heart Foundation.

The results of this initiative were published in the *British Medical Journal* in 1971. He introduced coronary angiography in Baggot Street Hospital in 1972 and percutaneous transluminal coronary angioplasty a decade later.[43] When Baggot Street closed as an acute hospital and moved to St James's Hospital in 1988, Gearty, although he was nearly 60 at the time, embraced the new development with enthusiasm. He continued to teach medical students in St James's Hospital for many years after his retirement and was awarded an honorary DSc by the University of Dublin in 1991.[44]

Dr Steevens' Hospital

Dr Steevens' Hospital was the oldest of the Federated Hospitals. It was the second voluntary hospital in Dublin, the first being the Charitable Infirmary in Jervis Street.[45] It was built with funding from a bequest of Dr Richard Steevens, who was president of the College of Physicians and professor of medicine at Trinity College. His sister, Grizel, oversaw the building of the hospital, which was designed by Thomas Burgh, who was also the architect of the Old Library in Trinity College and of the City Workhouse. Dr

12.20   Dr Steevens' Hospital by Thomas Wilson. Courtesy of his son, Tom Wilson.

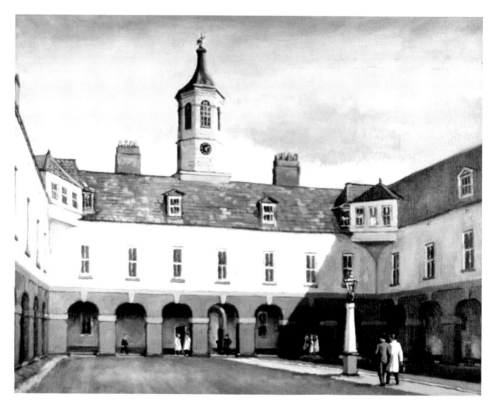

Steevens' Hospital admitted its first patients on Monday, 23 July 1733. Grizel Steevens lived in the hospital and acted as its treasurer until her death in 1747 at the age of 93. Jonathan Swift was one of its first governors. Esther Johnston, Swift's 'Stella', left £1,000 to maintain an Anglican chaplain in the hospital when she died in 1728 and one of the wards was named 'Stella's ward' in her honour.

A number of very distinguished doctors were on the original staff of Dr Steevens' Hospital. Thomas Molyneux, who was a fellow of the Royal Society and professor of medicine at Trinity College, was one of the original trustees of the hospital. Richard Helsham, a friend of Jonathan Swift and his physician, was also on the staff. He was appointed to the chair of natural and experimental philosophy at Trinity and later succeeded Molyneux in the chair of medicine. His book, *Lectures on natural philosophy*, was a standard textbook for over a hundred years. Bryan Robinson, who took the degree of MD at Trinity in 1711, served as physician to Dr Steevens' Hospital. He wrote a book, *Animal economy*, in which he used mathematical models to explain biological mechanisms. William Stephens joined the staff of the hospital in 1749, and he was also on the staff of Mercer's Hospital. He had studied in Leiden under Herman Boerhaave, one of the most famous physicians of his time. He was president of the College of Physicians of Ireland three times and in June 1731 he presided over a meeting in the rooms of the Philosophical Society in Trinity College at which the Royal Dublin Society was founded.

Stephens invited Samuel Clossy, a young Dublin doctor, to carry out post-mortem examinations on patients who died at Dr Steevens' Hospital. Clossy published the

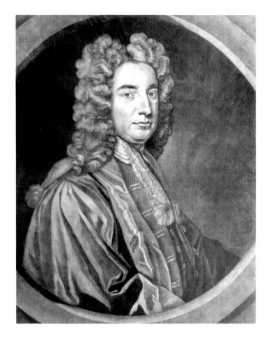

12.21 Richard Helsham, artist unknown. Reproduced by permission of the Worth Library.

12.22 William Stephens, artist unknown. Reproduced by permission of the Worth Library.

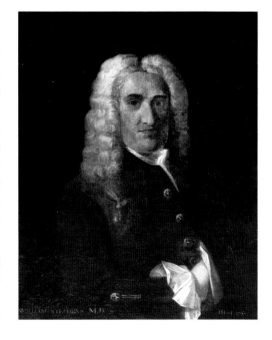

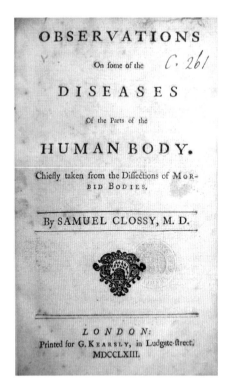

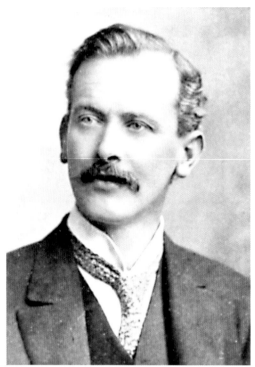

12.23   Title page of Samuel Clossy, MD, *Observations on some of the diseases of the parts of the human body* (London, 1763).

12.24   Walter Clegg Stevenson. Courtesy of the Stevenson family.

results of his findings in *Observations on some of the diseases of the parts of the human body* in 1763. His method of correlating clinical and pathological observations was a remarkable achievement and his book is now recognized as a classic in its field. Clossy emigrated to New York where he became one of the founders of King's College, a precursor of the medical school of Columbia University.[46] Abraham Colles was the most famous surgeon to work in the hospital. As a young man he was apprenticed to Philip Woodroffe, surgeon to Dr Steevens' Hospital and to the Dublin Foundling Hospital. After a further period of study in Edinburgh, Colles returned to Dublin and took up duties at Dr Steevens' Hospital. In 1814 he described a fracture of the wrist that has been known as 'Colles' fracture' ever since.[47] Colles was also an expert on the treatment of syphilis and published a book on the subject. Another surgeon, Walter Clegg Stevenson, appointed to the hospital in 1904, pioneered the use of radioactive radon gas for cancer treatment. He worked closely with John Joly, FRS, professor of geology at Trinity College. Together they developed a safer and more effective method of giving radiotherapy, which became known as the

'Dublin method'.[48] Percy Kirkpatrick, the first consultant anaesthetist in Dublin, was appointed to Dr Steevens' Hospital in 1899 and served in the post for over fifty years. Kirkpatrick was also a prolific writer and medical historian and wrote definitive histories of Dr Steevens' Hospital and of the medical school in Trinity College.

In the twentieth century, Dr Steevens' Hospital developed a strong orthopaedic and trauma unit where total prosthetic replacement of the hip was pioneered in Ireland. Brendan Prendiville, who was appointed to the hospital in 1957, developed a department that ultimately evolved into a very successful plastic surgery and burns unit.[49] Maxillofacial surgery was also developed at the hospital.[50] Dr Steevens' Hospital was one of the five Dublin hospitals that cooperated to form an accident and emergency service for the city in 1967, and it remained an active member of the group until its closure.[51] It was anticipated that following the transfer of most of its activities to St James's Hospital, Dr Steevens' would stay open to continue providing orthopaedic services. According to the original plan, the designated hospitals would close on completion of the new hospital at St James's and the patients and staff of each hospital would transfer to it in an orderly manner. These careful plans were thrown into disarray by the emergence of the Irish economic crisis of the 1980s and the resultant radical corrective measures that were taken by the government.

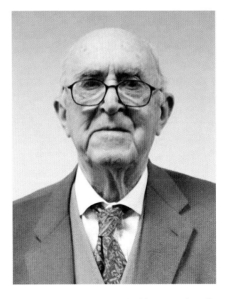

12.25   Mr Brendan Prendiville. Reproduced by permission of the Worth Library.

St James's Hospital and the National Children's Hospital

In 1969, the minister for health, Seán Flanagan, established the Study Group on Children's Hospitals Services, with a remit to advise on the future development and rationalization of paediatric services throughout Ireland, and especially in Dublin. 'I am particularly concerned', the minister wrote, 'to have the position clarified in relation to Dublin because the paediatric hospitals are physically separated from the general hospitals ...'[52] The study group was chaired by Conor Ward, who was at the time special lecturer in paediatrics at University College Dublin and paediatrician to Our Lady's Hospital for Sick Children, Crumlin. The vice chairman was Eric Doyle, who was senior lecturer in paediatrics at Trinity College and paediatrician to the National Children's Hospital, Harcourt Street. In their report, which was published in 1970, the

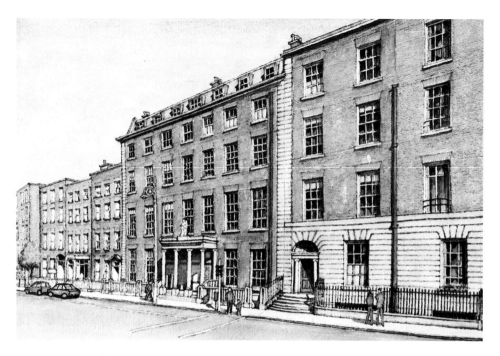

12.26   The National Children's Hospital, Harcourt Street, by Muriel Morgan. Reproduced with permission of the Tallaght Hospital Board.

group accepted 'that the ideal siting for a paediatric centre is within a large hospital complex associated closely with medical schools'.[53] They concluded that this was not practical at the time due to economic and other considerations. They proposed two regional paediatric centres, one on the north side at Temple Street Hospital and one on the south side at Our Lady's Hospital. They recommended that the national centre should be based at Our Lady's Hospital, which although it was not on a general hospital site, was in close proximity to the proposed general hospital on the St Kevin's site (St James's Hospital).

The group agreed that the National Children's Hospital was too small to survive on its own and two possibilities were suggested for its future: to move it to a new hospital on the St Kevin's site or to merge it with Our Lady's Hospital in Crumlin to form a major children's hospital. The committee opted unanimously for the latter. However, when the report was published in 1970, the suggestion that the National Children's Hospital, which was regarded as a Protestant hospital, should amalgamate with the Catholic Our Lady's Hospital for Sick Children was rejected firmly by John Charles McQuaid, Catholic archbishop of Dublin. He had been the driving force behind the foundation of Our Lady's Hospital for Sick Children in 1956 and served as chairman of the board. He was not willing to grant representatives of the National

Children's Hospital places on the board of Our Lady's Hospital. McQuaid resigned as archbishop a year later and was succeeded by Dermot Ryan as archbishop and chairman of Our Lady's Hospital for Sick Children. Ryan opposed the implementation of the recommendations of the report as steadfastly as his predecessor. As a result, the report gathered dust and the rationalization of hospital services for sick children in Dublin was set back nearly fifty years.[54]

The National Children's Hospital was one of the seven Federated Dublin Voluntary Hospitals. When their discussions failed with Our Lady's Hospital for Sick Children, the consultants in the National Children's Hospital decided to approach their colleagues in the federated group. Following negotiations, the board of St James's Hospital sent a letter to the board of the National Children's Hospital in 1974 supporting a substantial development for children in St James's Hospital. Meetings were also taking place at this time between the medical boards of the National Children's Hospital and of Our Lady's Hospital for Sick Children to explore avenues of possible cooperation that would not involve amalgamation. The board of St James's Hospital decided to await the outcome of these negotiations. Despite prolonged discussions, the medical boards of the children's hospitals did not reach agreement. In 1979, the boards of St James's Hospital and the National Children's Hospital began negotiations with the purpose of moving the National Children's Hospital to the St James's site. These negotiations moved quickly, and four months later there was agreement in principle between the boards of the two hospitals. Trinity College welcomed the agreement and activated procedures to fill the vacant chair of paediatrics in the medical school. The Eastern Health Board also responded positively to the proposal at its meeting in April 1980.[55]

The proposal was gathering considerable momentum, so both hospitals agreed to hold a meeting with senior officials in the Department of Health. Much to the disappointment of the hospital representatives, it became clear during this meeting that the department 'was now favourably disposed to the establishment of a substantial paediatric unit in the new Tallaght Hospital'.[56] The chairman of the St James's Hospital board received a letter soon afterwards from the secretary of the Department of Health instructing St James's Hospital to discontinue negotiations with the National Children's Hospital. No reasons were given for the change of policy but it is thought that costs and proximity to Our Lady's Hospital in Crumlin were among the deciding factors.

13

St James's Hospital

St James's Hospital should not be regarded as just another voluntary hospital. It was, and should continue to be, part of the community service.[1]

St James's – early beginnings

At the time of its establishment in 1971, there were 1,270 beds in St James's Hospital. These were housed in seven distinct hospital buildings on a 60-acre site. Most of the buildings were old and separated from each other by open spaces containing fine trees. Cherry trees and well-maintained garden areas brightened the institution in spring and summer. However, during the bleak winter days, it was far from an ideal arrangement as staff hurried between buildings and patients were ferried around the site in ambulances for different procedures. The Guinness brewery was a short distance away and the aroma of hops pervaded the hospital on a regular basis.

The accommodation for patients included 380 acute medical and surgical beds, 450 special beds and 440 long-stay beds. Departments such as maternity, geriatric, psychiatric, urology, paediatric, rheumatology, ENT and gynaecology were in the special beds. A small number of full-time and visiting consultants were responsible for the care of all the patients in these beds. They included two physicians, Paddy Blaney and James Mahon, supported by two younger physicians, Joseph (Joe) Timoney and Michael Buckley. Two general surgeons, Hugh MacCarthy and Frank Ward, were responsible for the surgical beds. Jack Flanagan was the consultant geriatrician and Tom Hanratty was the obstetrician. All of these clinicians, who had worked in St Kevin's, continued in their posts, becoming consultants in St James's Hospital. There were over fifty beds under the urologists, Victor Lane and Dermot Flynn, both of whom also had commitments to the urological department in the Meath Hospital.[2] A number of these consultants, including the physicians Paddy Blaney and James Mahon, the radiologist Edward (Ned) Malone and the medical administrator James O'Dea, became deeply involved in supporting the new developments.

Ned Malone, the director of radiology, played a key role in the metamorphosis of St Kevin's Hospital into St James's Hospital. Malone had studied medicine in the RCSI and after graduation in 1950 he moved to Yorkshire, where he worked in general practice and in the NHS tuberculosis service.[3] In the early 1950s he moved to Newfoundland, where he worked as a radiologist and where he became a fellow of the Royal College of Physicians of Canada. He was appointed as radiologist to St Kevin's Hospital in 1969, becoming one of two consultant radiologists on the staff. Following the establishment of St James's Hospital, Malone redesigned the X-ray department and introduced ultrasound and radionuclide imaging. He appreciated the growing importance of highly sophisticated technology in radiology and worked hard to ensure that a CT scanner would be included in the radiology department of the new hospital.

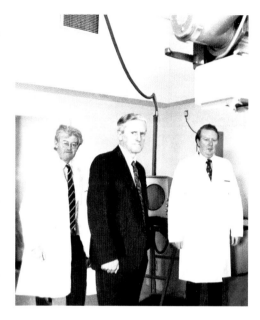

13.1   In the radiology department, Hospital 7: Dr Michael Magan, consultant radiologist (left); Brendan Hensey, secretary of the Department of Health (centre); and Dr Edward Malone, consultant radiologist (right). Courtesy of Ms Bernadette Moran.

In 1975 he led the formation of a medical board and was elected the first chairman, with Blaney as vice chairman. Two years later, after negotiations with the board of the hospital, the name of the medical board was changed to the medical advisory committee and it was formally established as a subcommittee of the board of the hospital. Since then this committee, which meets every month, has played a pivotal role in the development of the hospital and its chairman presents the views of the consultants at the hospital board.

Malone was elected a fellow of the Faculty of Radiologists at the RCSI in 1973. Subsequently he was elected to the board of the faculty and was appointed honorary treasurer. After his sudden death in 1986, the faculty established the Edward Malone Medal, which is awarded annually to an outstanding trainee in radiology. Patrick (Pat) Freyne succeeded Malone as head of department. He introduced a system of rapid or 'hot' reporting of X-rays, initially from the emergency department. This proved successful as it eliminated delays and optimized clinical decision making. Hot reporting was then introduced to all inpatient and outpatient departments. In the early 1980s, a programme for training radiologists was introduced and this contributed significantly to the growing reputation of the department.

A man of vision

Peter Beckett was appointed as the first full-time professor of psychiatry in Trinity College Dublin in 1969. Beckett, who was a cousin of the writer Samuel Beckett, was a graduate of Trinity College. He did his internship in Sir Patrick Dun's Hospital and then joined the RAMC in 1946 and served as captain for two years. He subsequently did a fellowship in psychiatry in the Mayo Clinic. It was while in the Mayo Clinic that he met his wife Victoria Ling Kuo Fan, who had fled from China in 1941. She trained in internal medicine and rheumatology. They married in 1954 and they were both on the staff of the Mayo Clinic. In 1960, Beckett was appointed as professor of psychiatry at Wayne State University in Detroit. On taking up his post in Dublin in 1969, Beckett opened an inpatient psychiatric unit for public patients in a refurbished unit originally built for patients with tuberculosis at St Kevin's Hospital. This unit, which became known as Hospital 6, served as a professorial unit

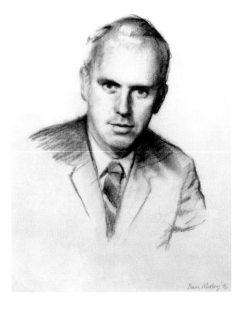

13.2 Prof. Peter Beckett by Berni Markey. Trinity Art Collection. By permission of the artist.

for psychiatry. He succeeded Jerry Jessop as dean of medicine in 1972 and worked enthusiastically to develop the medical school and the new hospital. He found the vested interests that impeded progress very frustrating.[4] His sudden death in 1974 was a major setback for both St James's Hospital and Trinity College.

James McCormick succeeded Beckett as dean and pledged to continue the work of his predecessor in developing St James's Hospital as a major teaching hospital. The board of the hospital received further assurance of the commitment of Trinity College in a letter from the provost, Francis S.L. Lyons, in May 1977:

> The board of the university had resolved that it should add its weight to the impetus behind the developments at St James's by re-stating its aim to press forward with the developments at St James's site to support its role as the primary teaching hospital of the Trinity Medical School.[5]

Steps towards a teaching hospital

In 1973, when speaking at the opening of a three-day conference organized by the Federated Dublin Voluntary Hospitals and St James's Hospital, the minister for health, Erskine Childers, departed from his prepared script and said that it would

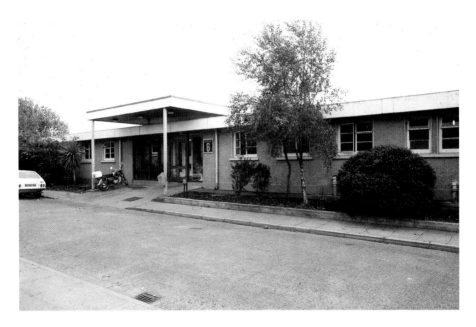

13.3   Psychiatry Unit (Hospital 6). Photograph: Bobby Studio.

be very desirable if the board of St James's would form an expert group to plan the new hospital and would invite architectural and other officers from his department to join it. Ian Howie, the chairman of the hospital board, responded by thanking the minister very warmly for what he saw as an invitation to start the planning process for the new hospital.[6]

In July 1974, the minister for health, Brendan Corish, confirmed the intention of the Department of Health to build a new hospital of between 350 and 500 beds at St James's, depending on the catchment area, which had yet to be defined. Three major new hospitals were planned for Dublin but the development of St James's would receive priority. The board of St James's Hospital was also assured by the Department of Health that the hospital would enjoy the degree of autonomy common to the major voluntary hospitals in the country. The management of the Eastern Health Board, initially led by the deputy CEO, James J. Nolan, and subsequently by the CEO, Kieran Hickey, played a key role in ensuring the success of the new hospital. Both Nolan and Hickey served on the board of the hospital for extended periods.

Comhairle na nOspidéal adopted a policy of jointly appointing all new consultants to both the designated hospitals and to St James's Hospital. This development facilitated the whole process of integration and ensured that 'the legacy represented by the specialties located in the designated hospitals would transfer successfully to St James's Hospital'.[7] There were excellent administrators in the federation such as the CEO, Desmond Dempsey, the HR manager, Patrick Corcoran and the head of finance, Timothy Lyne. Their skill in structuring appointments between the designated hospitals, St James's Hospital and the university allowed the process of amalgamation in the 1980s to occur in an almost seamless fashion.

Some progress was also made in consolidating services between the Federated Hospitals and St James's Hospital at this time. Peter Gatenby, professor of medicine, was appointed as honorary consultant to St James's Hospital in 1973 and was given the clinical care of a unit of fifty long-stay beds in Hospital 4. A number of consultants who worked in the Federated Dublin Voluntary Hospitals began providing services in St James's Hospital; these included Gerard Gearty, cardiologist in Baggot Street Hospital, Donald Weir, gastroenterologist in Sir Patrick Dun's Hospital and Michael Cullen, endocrinologist in the Meath Hospital. The board of St James's Hospital was determined to see teaching and research facilities develop on the hospital campus. This would remain an abiding commitment and it was a very important factor in the ultimate evolution of the hospital into a major centre for clinical teaching and research. The commitment was evident as early as 1972, when the hospital made land available to Trinity College to erect a temporary teaching centre. This provided facil-

13.4   Ambulance leaving the hospital through the Rialto gate on the South Circular Road. Private collection.

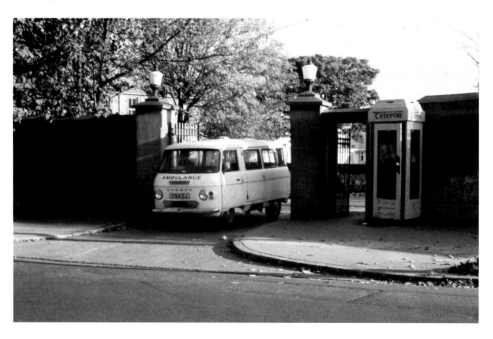

ities for academic staff, laboratory teaching space, lecture rooms and a library, in a single-storey structure that was transferred from Trinity College. This building was supposed to be a short-term measure but it was in use for over twenty years. Also in 1972 the first medical students from Trinity took up residence in St James's Hospital.

There were further plans and negotiations between St James's Hospital and the Department of Health over the following years and, in July 1981, the minister for health, Dr Michael Woods, approved provision of 693 beds in the new hospital. This number would provide generous accommodation for general medicine and surgery and a wide range of specialties. No firm date was given for the commencement of the new hospital and because of the economic climate there was some pessimism.

The School of Physiotherapy

The relocation of the Dublin School of Physiotherapy from Hume Street to St James's Hospital in 1973 was a significant landmark in the development of the new teaching hospital.[8] The school was founded in 1905 at 86 Leeson Street by Amelia Hogg and was originally known as the Irish School of Massage. The school moved from Leeson Street to 12 Hume Street in 1914. Students attended lectures at Trinity College that included anatomy, medical electricity, physics, chemistry and physiology. It became known

13.5   First medical school building at St James's Hospital. Private collection.

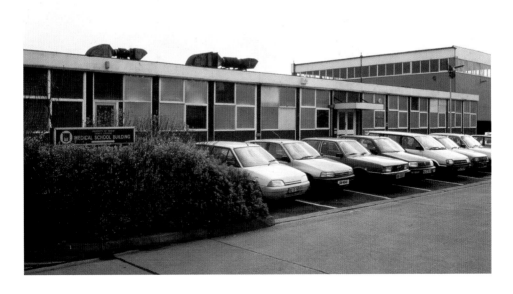

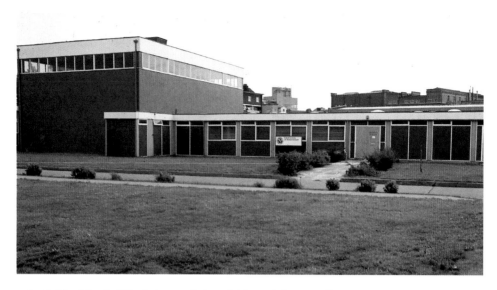

13.6   Dublin School of Physiotherapy, St James's Hospital. Private collection.

as the Dublin School of Physiotherapy in 1942 and, from 1957, students received a diploma from Trinity College on completion of the course. The school came under the auspices of the Federated Dublin Voluntary Hospitals in 1968 and moved to St James's Hospital five years later. It was housed in a purpose-built facility that contained teaching and office accommodation and a large gymnasium. John (Jack) Stockton was appointed director of the school in 1972 and a year later it was officially opened by the minister for health, Brendan Corish. The school was incorporated into the university in 1983, becoming a school within the Faculty of Health Sciences, and a four-year honours degree course was initiated. These academic developments were led by Paul Wagstaff, who was a dynamic head of school from 1980 until his untimely death in 1989. He was an innovative figure who developed postgraduate initiatives as well as consolidating the undergraduate degree course and co-authoring a book, *Physiotherapy and the elderly patient*, with Davis Coakley in 1988.[9]

Eoin Casey supported the development of the physiotherapy department in St James's Hospital. He was appointed as consultant in

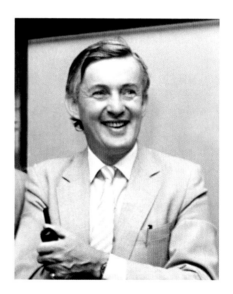

13.7   Dr Eoin Casey, consultant rheumatologist. Photograph: Bobby Studio.

rheumatology and rehabilitation to St James's Hospital and the Federated Hospitals in 1974, succeeding Thomas O'Reilly. A graduate of University College Cork, he initially trained in neurology in London and was awarded an MD in clinical electrophysiology. He subsequently changed the direction of his career and spent several years gaining experience in rheumatology and rehabilitation and developing a particular interest in disorders of the musculoskeletal system. Casey enjoyed teaching and was well-known for his pre-MRCPI tutorials for senior house officers, which took place in his home several times a year.[10] He retired from the staff of St James's Hospital in 2003.

Postgraduate education

In order to provide good general medical training for young doctors wishing to pursue a career in medicine, a rotation scheme was organized for senior house officers by the department of clinical medicine in Trinity College, in cooperation with the Federated Dublin Voluntary Hospitals in 1972. The first of its kind in Ireland, the initial rotation involved four hospitals and consisted of haematology and nephrology in the Meath, general medicine in Dr Steevens', general medicine and gastroenterology in Sir Patrick Dun's and cardiology in Baggot Street. The senior house officers rotated every six months. Victoria Beckett was appointed as the first postgraduate director in 1973. Shaun McCann, Peter Daly and Davis Coakley, all of whom later became consultants at St James's Hospital, were among the first doctors to rotate through the programme. Over the next twenty years, this scheme developed into the largest postgraduate training scheme in the country, with doctors rotating to hospitals outside Dublin and also to hospitals abroad. A pre-fellowship training scheme in surgery was also organized in the Federated Dublin Voluntary Hospitals. The purpose of this scheme was to provide candidates who had the primary fellowship with a good grounding in general surgery, together with experience in some specialized branches. It was a three-year rotation and was designed to prepare candidates for the fellowship examination of the RCSI.

In 1978, the first medical postgraduate centre in Ireland was established in temporary accommodation on a site provided by the Eastern Health Board at the Rialto end of St James's Hospital. It was a joint venture between the Federated Dublin Voluntary Hospitals and St James's, and the centre would become a focus and resource for continuing education for general practitioners in the hospital's catchment area as well as for the medical staff of the hospital. The William Stokes Faculty of the Royal College of General Practitioners was based at the centre and the Vocational Training Scheme for General Practice used it on a regular basis. The centre was enlarged in 1986 to cope with increasing demands and was named the William Stokes Postgraduate Centre at a ceremony attended by several descendants of William Stokes. Stokes, who was Regius professor of physic in Trinity College, was one of the founders, in 1838, of the Dublin Pathological Society, the first society of its kind in the Western world. Every Saturday, Stokes and his colleagues met to share their knowledge about clinical cases

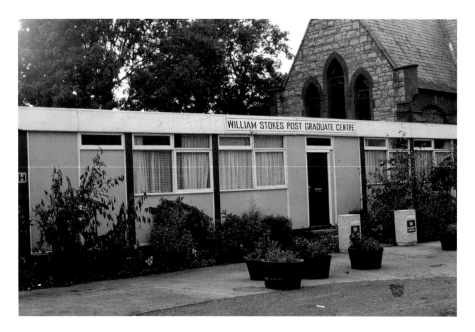

13.8   The William Stokes Postgraduate Centre in 1986. Private collection.

and to discuss post-mortem findings. This pioneering postgraduate society became the prototype for similar societies on both sides of the Atlantic.

In 1988, the steering committee of the postgraduate centre decided to replace the existing centre because of increased use and the high cost of maintaining the old building. Following a fundraising campaign, the centre was demolished and replaced by a new, larger, semi-permanent structure on the same site. The facility was officially opened in November 1988 by Dr Maeve Hillery, wife of the Irish president, Patrick Hillery. This was particularly appropriate as she had worked in St Kevin's Hospital as an anaesthetist.

A significant number of postgraduate programmes were developed in the hospital and medical school in the 1990s. These included an MSc in medical physics, developed by Jim Malone, head of medical physics, and an MSc course in cardiology, developed by Michael Walsh, consultant cardiologist, which attracted both Irish and overseas doctors. As the decade advanced, several other very successful MSc programmes, linked to clinical departments in the hospital, were also developed.

Academic department of medicine moves to St James's Hospital

Peter Gatenby resigned the chair of medicine in 1974 to take up a position with the United Nations. His academic unit was based in the Meath Hospital, with some nominal beds in St James's Hospital. Following discussions between representatives

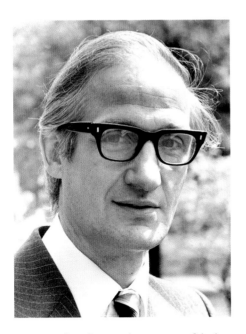

13.9   Prof. Graham Neale. Courtesy of the late Prof. Graham Neale.

of the hospitals and the medical school, the department of clinical medicine was moved to St James's Hospital at the request of the Meath Hospital.[11] Graham Neale, gastroenterologist and consultant at the Hammersmith Hospital, London, was appointed to fill the chair of medicine in 1975. Neale had studied medicine at Bristol University, graduating with many distinctions in 1960. He subsequently worked in Stockholm, the Bristol Royal Infirmary and at the Royal Postgraduate Medical School, Hammersmith Hospital, London.

In Dublin he worked with considerable dedication to establish an ethos of teaching and research within the hospitals associated with the medical school, with the ultimate goal of developing a single hospital for Trinity at St James's.[12] It was an uphill task. As Neale later commented, 'the power of politicians, priests and senior doctors knew no bounds'.[13] Progress on the planning and construction of the new hospital was delayed. This was a source of frustration for the staff in St James's Hospital. However, Neale was not discouraged, 'It is not buildings that matter,' he told an interviewer, 'it's people and that's the name of the game as far as I am concerned.'[14] When the minister for health, Charles Haughey, attended an open day in St James's Hospital in 1977, he was expected to announce plans for a new hospital to be built on its grounds. Instead the staff heard Haughey announce plans to establish a new hospital in Beaumont, in the heart of his own constituency.

Neale had a strong social conscience and his vision of developing a teaching hospital that would give first-class services to patients from all walks of life made an impact during the formative years of St James's Hospital. Five months after he took up his post he was interviewed by Mavis Arnold for the *Irish Medical Times*. The interview was published under the title 'Prof. Neale, a dynamo of endless energy':

He gave no impression of an Englishman faced with a traditional Irish muddle. His determined intention is to build up a medical school which meets modern requirements and to create a university hospital at St James's Hospital which will not only attract the best doctors to come and work there but will continue its long-standing tradition of serving the community.[15]

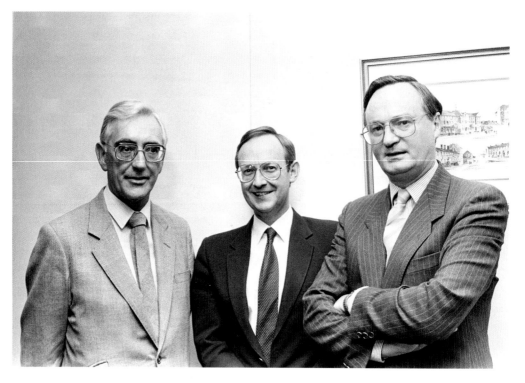

13.10   Desmond Dempsey (left), Prof. John Prichard (centre) and Prof. Conor Keane (right). Photograph: Bobby Studio.

Graham Neale made a major effort to hasten the transfer of clinical departments from the Federated Hospitals to St James's Hospital. He persuaded the university to appoint a senior lecturer, who would be based at St James's Hospital, to the department of clinical medicine. John Prichard was appointed to this post in 1977. He was an Oxford scholar with an international reputation in respiratory disease. Prichard continued his clinical research in Dublin and was awarded a substantial grant from the Wellcome Trust to establish a laboratory for the study of biochemical problems in pulmonary disease. His research was published in leading international journals including *Nature*, *The Lancet*, the *British Medical Journal*, *Thorax* and the *European Journal of Cardiology*. His book, *Edema and the lung*, was regarded as the standard textbook on the subject for many years. Prichard was one of the first consultants appointed to St James's Hospital in the 1970s and he played a key role in developing it as a major teaching hospital for Trinity College. He made a significant contribution to teaching and patient care until his untimely death in 1996. Neale resigned his professorship in 1980 to take up a position at Addenbrooke's Hospital in Cambridge where he developed a pioneering method of intravenous feeding.

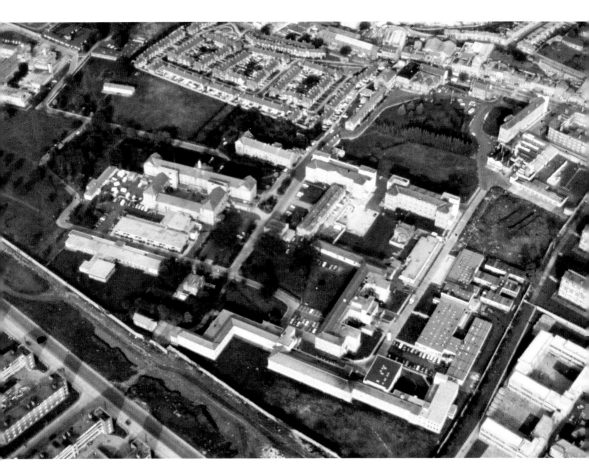

13.11   St James's Hospital in the mid 1970s, as it was before the new development. Private collection.

Project team for the new hospital

The project team for the new St James's Hospital met for the first time in October 1975 under the chairmanship of Ian Howie. The team faced a major challenge as the new hospital was to be built on an extensive site already occupied by buildings, some of which were very old and some comparatively new. Moreover, the new hospital was to be built without compromising the work of the existing hospital. Frank Jackman, the chief architect of the Department of Health, was a member of the project team and he played a key role in the early stages of planning. He continued his commitment to the development of the hospital over subsequent decades. The first task for the project team was to write a brief or plan for the development. The brief envisaged a teaching hospital of 750 beds, together with a clinical science facility, which would provide teaching accommodation for the medical, dental, nursing and physio-

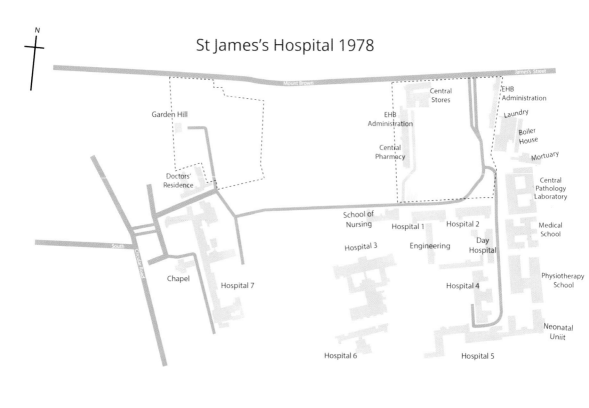

13.12   Map of St James's Hospital in 1978, showing the campus before the new hospital was developed.
Image: Anthony Edwards

therapy schools as well as for clinical research and postgraduate education. Moloney O'Beirne Guy, and Hutchison Locke and Monk, were appointed as architects in 1976. The former were based in Dublin and the latter in Richmond, Surrey. James O'Beirne and David Hutchison were identified as the principal architects for the project. The development control plan of the new hospital was finished in 1978. This plan envisaged that the new hospital would be built in three overlapping phases because of the complexities of building a new hospital on the site of an already existing large and busy hospital.

The first phase was divided into three sub-sections: (1A) a new entrance at the Rialto end of the hospital and a communication centre; (1B) a boiler house, engineering workshops and the Eastern Health Board's ambulance centre; and (1C) a major part of the actual hospital building, including an outpatient department, an accident and emergency (A & E) department, a radiology department, an intensive care unit, operating theatres, nine inpatient wards to accommodate 279 patients, a new psychi-

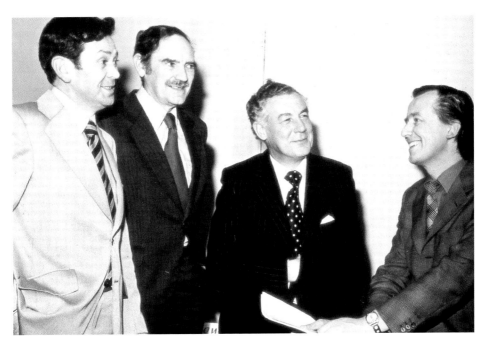

13.13   Left to right: James O'Beirne, architect; Dr James O'Dea, hospital planning and former medical administrator; Prof. Ian Howie; and David Hutchison, architect. Courtesy of Moloney O'Beirne Architects.

13.14   Cover of the development control plan for St James's Hospital. Private collection.

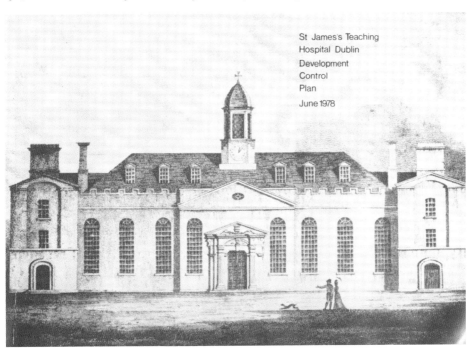

St James's Teaching
Hospital Dublin
Development
Control
Plan
June 1978

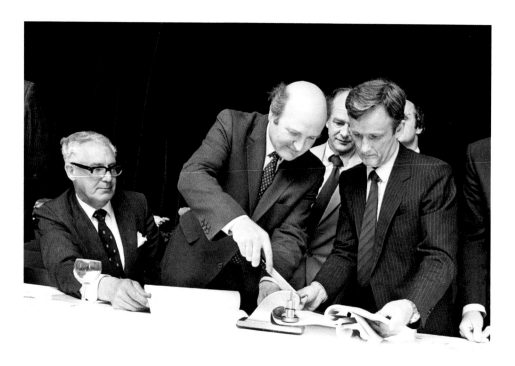

13.15 The minister for health, Barry Desmond, imprints the seal of the Department of Health on the contract to build the new hospital. Left to right: Prof. Ian Howie, chairman of the project team; Desmond; Lorcan Hogan, hospital secretary; and Dr James Behan, chairman of the hospital board. Photograph: Bobby Studio.

atry unit and a day hospital for the treatment and rehabilitation of older patients. Haughey, the minister for health, approved the development control plan for the new St James's Hospital at a ceremony in the staff restaurant held on 5 October 1978. Construction work began on phase 1A in November 1980.

Surgical developments

George Fegan, who was based at Sir Patrick Dun's Hospital, resigned as clinical professor of surgery in 1972 and was replaced three years later by Thomas (Tom) Hennessy, who joined the staff of St James's Hospital and Baggot Street Hospital as the first full-time professor of surgery. Hennessy trained in surgical research in Minneapolis with the world-famous Owen Wangenstein, who invented the gastric suction system that revolutionized the care of patients suffering from intestinal obstruction. Hennessy established a high volume centre for oesophageal diseases, in particular oesophageal cancer, at St James's Hospital. During the 1980s, it became one of the top-tier oesophageal centres in Europe because of its clinical and academic

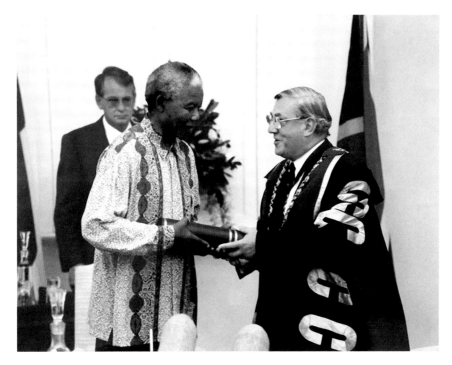

13.16 Prof. Thomas Hennessy, president of the Royal College of Surgeons in Ireland, presenting an honorary fellowship to President of South Africa Nelson Mandela. Photograph: Bobby Studio.

13.17 Dr Maria Paula Colgan and Mr Gregor (Greg) Shanik in the vascular laboratory. Photograph: Bobby Studio.

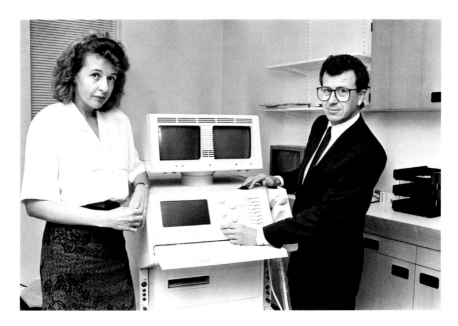

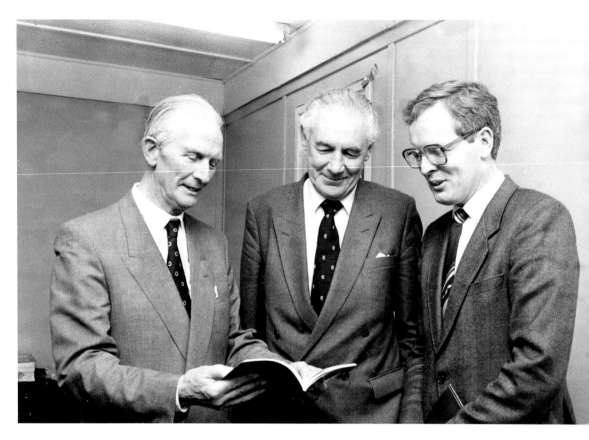

13.18   Mr Frank Ward, consultant orthopaedic surgeon (left), Prof. Ian Howie (centre), and Dr Peter O'Connor (right), former director of postgraduate education, at the launch in the postgraduate centre of *Emergencies in Clinical Practice* (1985) edited by Dr Michael Buckley. Photograph: Bobby Studio.

excellence. Hennessy set up a gastrointestinal physiology laboratory at St James's Hospital with his chief technologist, Dr Patrick (Paddy) Byrne, and this also developed an international reputation. Hennessy's most important clinical study, and one of the most cited Irish medical papers, was published in the *New England Journal of Medicine* in 1996. This research compared the outcomes of surgery alone, which was the existing standard of care for oesophageal cancer, with multimodal therapy, where patients received a combination of chemotherapy and radiation therapy prior to surgery. Hennessy's approach led to a far better outcome and became the internationally accepted standard of care for local advanced cancer. He also made a fundamental contribution to the understanding of Barrett's oesophagus, a precancerous condition that affects the lower end of the oesophagus. Hennessy was the co-author and co-editor of a number of successful textbooks on surgery and he was one of the principal architects of surgical training in Ireland. He helped to develop the careers of many surgeons who subsequently went on to make significant contributions to surgery in their own specialist fields. He was elected president of the RCSI in 1994. Robert (Bobby) Quill was appointed as senior lecturer and consultant in surgery in 1975. Quill had a special interest in surgery of the parathyroid gland.

The academic department of surgery was based in temporary accommodation, originally provided for a microbiology laboratory in St Kevin's Hospital, near the Rialto entrance of the hospital. Among Hennessy's first priorities at St James's Hospital were the establishment of an A & E department and a department of vascular surgery.[16] Gregor (Greg) Shanik was appointed as vascular surgeon in 1977 and he was joined by Dermot Moore in 1984. They went on to develop a leading vascular surgery department with a reputation for high-quality service and research.[17]

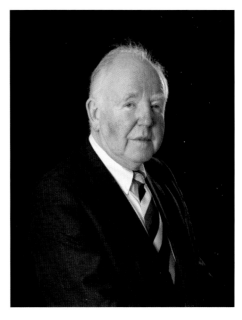

13.19   Mr Richard Stephens, consultant surgeon. Courtesy of Mr Richard Stephens.

An A & E department was established in 1978 and a new consultant post, director of accident and emergency, was created. Frank Ward, who had worked as a general and orthopaedic surgeon in the hospital since 1961, became its director and he held the post until his retirement in 1988. The A & E department was based in Hospital 7, where the accommodation was very limited. The attendances increased by over 8 per cent in the first few years, putting a great strain on space. The establishment of the A & E department was very important as it increased surgical throughput and turnover. With the opening of the A & E, the pressure on the general surgeons was increased significantly. Richard Stephens was appointed in 1980 as a general surgeon and it soon became apparent that he was very able and highly motivated. He made a considerable contribution to the development of the hospital. As his own career evolved, he took a special interest in colorectal surgery and set up a colorectal cancer programme supported by a multidisciplinary team. Over subsequent years other surgical specialties were developed including breast, endocrine, urology and ENT.

Anaesthesia and intensive care

The increase in activity in both general and specialized surgery at St James's Hospital created a demand for an expanded anaesthetic service. This was first achieved by creating a joint department of anaesthesia between St James's and Sir Patrick Dun's Hospitals. This development meant that two consultants from Dun's Hospital, John Goodbody and Brendan Lawless, would share sessions and one would be present each day in St James's Hospital. The commencement of major vascular surgery at the hospital placed great pressure on the anaesthetic services and this led to the appointment of three consultant anaesthetists in 1979. The increasing number of patients having major surgical procedures, both elective and emergency, necessitated the provision of significant monitoring and organ support such as positive pressure ventilation. Specially trained and experienced nurses were also required.

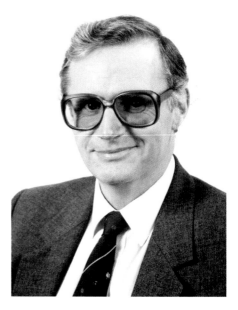

13.20   Dr Ron Kirkham, consultant anaesthetist. Photograph courtesy of Dr Ron Kirkham.

Ron Kirkham, one of the anaesthetists appointed in 1979, had dual qualifications in medicine and engineering. He had a special interest in intensive care and established the first intensive care unit in the hospital. This had four beds, oxygen and suction supplies, adequate lighting and sufficient space to permit access for equipment and personnel if resuscitation were necessary. Emphasis was placed on appointing and training good junior anaesthetists to work in the department. This led to formal recognition of the department for training purposes by the Faculty of Anaesthesia of the Royal College of Surgeons in Ireland, which made anaesthesia at St James's attractive to aspiring non-consultant hospital doctors who would receive a standard of training comparable to the standards of existing teaching hospitals. The development of an intensive care unit, where anaesthetists played a major role in the management of patients and in the day-to-day running of the unit, was an innovation that some clinicians found difficult to accept. Kirkham approached the issue diplomatically:

> The solution to this problem lay in better communication between the individuals involved. Some surgeons worked in other hospitals where anaesthetists already ran the ICUs and they soon accepted the arrangement, however some were reluctant to have clinical decisions, other than those relating to ventilation,

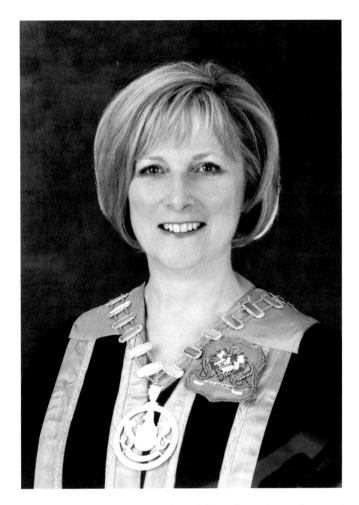

13.21   Dr Jeanne Moriarty, president of the College of Anaesthetists of
Ireland 2009–12. Courtesy of the College of Anaesthetists of Ireland.

made by anyone who was not a member of their team. When this occurred it was
necessary for the anaesthetist involved to politely show that they understood the
problem and were experienced and able to manage it. Tact and sensitivity were
required.[18]

Kirkham went on to lead the planning and development of the intensive care unit in
the new hospital.

The department of anaesthesia continued to expand over succeeding years, and by
2016 it had more than thirty consultants and thirty trainee anaesthetists on its staff.
Two of the consultants were elected president of the College of Anaesthetists of Ireland:
Jeanne Moriarty (2009–12) and Ellen O'Sullivan (2012–15).

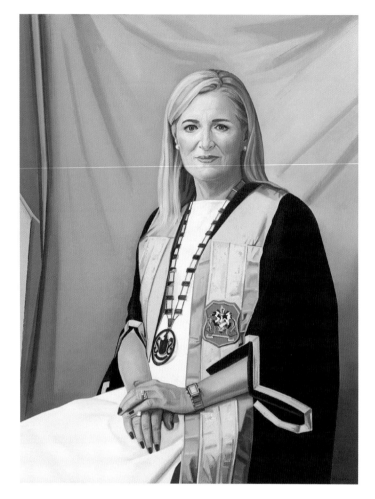

13.22   Prof. Ellen O'Sullivan, president of the College of Anaesthetists of
Ireland 2012–15. Courtesy of the College of Anaesthetists of Ireland.

The laboratory sciences

The foundation of the Royal College of Pathologists in London in 1961 led to the
sub-division of general pathology into a number of separate disciplines. As a consequence, the pathology services in the federated system were reorganized. Clinical
microbiology was developed in the Adelaide Hospital, with the sub-section of serol-
ogy in Mercer's Hospital. The latter would subsequently develop into a department
of immunology.[19] Biochemistry was based at Sir Patrick Dun's Hospital and haematology at the Meath Hospital. Morbid anatomy and histopathology were located
in the school of pathology on the campus of Trinity College where the professorial
department of pathology was based. The distribution of these departments in so

many different locations was an unsatisfactory arrangement and plans were
made to centralize these disciplines in
a new purpose-built laboratory at St
James's Hospital.

Dermot Hourihane was appointed to
the chair of histopathology and morbid
anatomy in 1973. He had graduated
in medicine from University College
Dublin in 1955. Subsequently, he decided
to specialize in pathology, with histopathology as his subspecialty. He trained
in London at the Royal Postgraduate
Medical School and the Royal London
Hospital. Hourihane returned to Dublin
in 1966 when he was appointed reader in
pathology at Trinity College. He was a

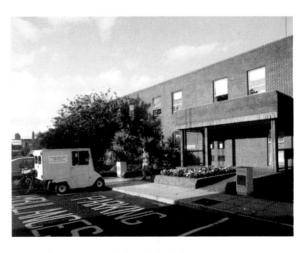

13.23   The new Central Pathology Laboratory.
Private collection.

founder fellow of the Faculty of Pathology in the Royal College of Physicians of
Ireland in 1976. He was dean of the Faculty of Medicine and Dentistry between 1979
and 1983. He was very committed to the development of a central pathology laboratory and believed that building one at St James's Hospital would put pressure on
the Federated Hospitals to move on to the St James's campus. He also anticipated
that the creation of a strong central laboratory would stimulate research both in the
laboratory and in the hospital. Hourihane was appointed by the minister for health
to Comhairle na nOspidéal, the body that shaped and approved all consultant posts
in the country, and this placed him in a very strong position to support the development of consultant positions in the Federated Hospitals and St James's Hospital.

The opening of the Central Pathology Laboratory in October 1981 was a major step
forward for both clinical and academic pathology. It created a critical mass for further
significant progress in both service provision and research. The building provided
centralized facilities for histopathology, haematology, clinical biochemistry, microbiology and immunology. The creation of this laboratory, at a time when the hospital
was beginning a period of rapid expansion of its clinical staff, greatly facilitated the
remarkable advances in research activity that took place at St James's Hospital in
the 1980s. A number of key academics and clinicians who transferred to St James's
Hospital at that time, subsequently made major contributions to their disciplines and
to the development of the hospital. Under the leadership of Conor Keane, associate
professor of clinical microbiology, the department of microbiology established an
international reputation in the battle against hospital acquired infections, in particular infections caused by methicillin-resistant *Staphylococcus aureus* (MRSA).[20] Its
work would eventually lead to the establishment on the St James's campus in 2002 of

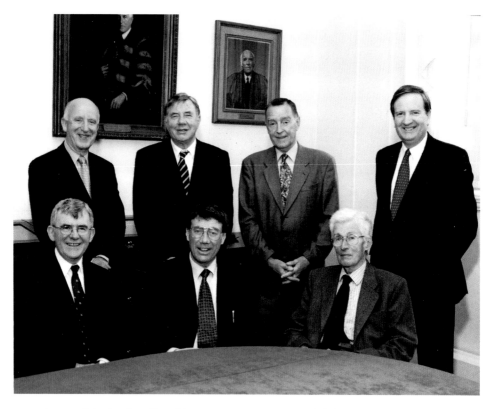

13.24 Deans of the Faculty of Health Sciences 1974–2005. Seated, left to right: Professors Diarmuid (Derry) Shanley (2002–6), Jim Malone (1999–2002) and James McCormick (1974–9). Standing, left to right: Professors John Bonnar (1983–7), Ian Temperley (1987–93), Dermot Hourihane (1979–83) and Davis Coakley (1993–9). Courtesy of the Medical School, Trinity College Dublin.

the National MRSA Reference Laboratory, which provides a national service for the laboratory investigation of MRSA, identifying virulent strains and performing epidemiological studies.

Sir Patrick Dun's Research Laboratory

The attitude of academics, clinicians and the Department of Health towards clinical laboratory research in Ireland had been very negative for many years. The reasons put forward to justify this defeatist approach included a lack of finance and small and divided hospitals. This attitude began to change with the reorganization of the hospitals, the centralization of the clinical laboratories and the appointment of consultants with a significant track record in research at an international level. In 1983, this new impetus was reflected in the decision made by the governors of Sir Patrick Dun's Hospital, encouraged by the professor of medicine, Donald Weir, to fund the construction of a new research laboratory attached to the Central Pathology Laboratory. The £420,000 used to support this development came from the sale of the hospital's nurses' home.[21] The new development became known as the Sir Patrick Dun's Research Laboratory. It was the first research laboratory in a hospital setting in Ireland and was a significant indication of the hospital's commitment to medical research. This facility was a great resource for clinical researchers, whose work resulted in a stream of first-class publications in international journals.

Developments in clinical medicine

Donald Weir succeeded Graham Neale as professor of medicine in 1982, and was the first research fellow and lecturer to work with Peter Gatenby in the Meath Hospital when the department of clinical medicine was established. He went on to work in the Hammersmith Hospital in London and in the Edinburgh Royal Infirmary. He was appointed consultant physician and gastroenterologist to Sir Patrick Dun's Hospital in 1967. A healthcare centre for day patients was built in Hospital 5, St James's Hospital, in 1982, at the request of Weir, following his appointment as professor of medicine. It was fully equipped to perform all the modern forms of gastroenterological and pulmonary endoscopic investigations. The Health Care Centre was also used as a day care centre for diabetic, oncology and haematology patients. The development of this unit meant that many patients, who previously could only have been treated by hospital admission, could now be treated as day patients. From this base, Weir, with his colleague Napoleon (Nap) Keeling, would develop a comprehensive gastroenterology service that eventually became one of the busiest in Europe. Keeling was a pioneer in developing new endoscopic techniques. He perfected the use of stents to relieve the obstruction of bile ducts blocked by malignant growths. This is now the standard treatment for this condition.[22]

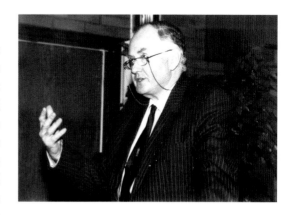

13.25   Donald Weir, Regius professor of medicine. Photograph: Bobby Studio.

13.26   Prof. Napoleon Keeling, consultant gastroenterologist. Photograph: Bobby Studio.

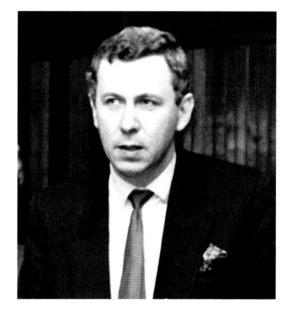

Weir was one of the key figures who inspired the research ethos that permeated St James's Hospital in the 1980s and 1990s. During this period of extreme financial stringency, he kept the academic flag flying with his weekly research seminars, held at lunchtime every Monday. When John Scott returned to Dublin from the United States, he drew Weir's attention to the potential of biochemistry as a tool with which to investigate unresolved problems of clinical medicine. Scott was a biochemist who, on completion of his PhD in Trinity, had worked as a postdoctoral research fellow in Berkeley, California, where he studied folate metabolism. Weir was interested in this approach, and a partnership was formed that would become one of the most productive in modern Irish clinical research. Weir, Scott and their research team, which included Anne Molloy and Joseph (Joe) McPartlin, found that maternal deficiency of folic acid was strongly associated with spina bifida at birth. They demonstrated that if mothers took supplements containing folic acid before and during pregnancy the defect could be prevented. Conleth (Con) Feighery, consultant immunologist, and researchers Cliona O'Farrelly and Alex Whelan, were interested in the pathogenesis of coeliac disease, which often presents with a deficiency of folic acid. Since Weir was already working with John Scott on folate research, it seemed logical that both teams should work together. This research collaboration resulted in the publication of over 300 papers in international journals. On one occasion, when Weir was asked why research was so important in medical care, he replied:

> Research is essential if we are to improve the standards of our disciplines. If we don't continually ask why something occurs we stagnate and tend to move backwards. This is especially true of clinical practice where research is closely associated with standards of clinical practice.[23]

Weir and Scott made very significant contributions to the general development of St James's Hospital as they both served on the board of the hospital for many years. Scott was professor of experimental nutrition at Trinity College Dublin, and he served as bursar of the college between 1977 and 1980. His research was recognized internationally, and he was the first non-American to be awarded the Lederle Award from the American Society of Nutritional Science. He played a key role in building and cementing the comprehensive relationship between St James's Hospital and Trinity College, remaining interested and involved until his death in 2013.[24]

The development of the haematology service

Ian Temperley, a graduate of Trinity College, was appointed consultant haematologist to the Federated Dublin Voluntary Hospitals in 1966 and associate professor of haematology at Trinity College in 1969. He pioneered the development of comprehensive haematology services in Ireland and represented the last of a cadre of 'all-round' haematologists who dealt with both adult and paediatric diseases, clinical and laboratory work, haematological malignancy and coagulation. The establishment by Temperley, in 1971, of the National Haemophilia Treatment Centre in the Meath Hospital represents one of his most important contributions to Irish haematology. Until 1971, the haemophiliac community was largely neglected by medicine and by society in general. When the centre was established, the average life expectancy of 110 patients suffering from severe haemophilia on the centre's register was fifteen years and only eleven patients were over the age of 30.[25] Temperley established a comprehensive multidisciplinary care programme for both adults and children with haemophilia, irrespective of ability to pay, which brought together clinical expertise and support services and implemented novel coagulation treatments as they became available.

The departure of Peter Gatenby for the United Nations in 1974 left Temperley in a vulnerable position, as Gatenby had been his main supporter and had given him access to beds in the Meath Hospital for the treatment of adults with leukaemia. Patients with haemophilia had been pressing the hospital for a purpose-built haemophilia centre. The hospital agreed to accommodate the centre provided that the Department of Health would build two floors above the centre to accommodate private patients. The Department of Health refused to build the extra floors and the hospital withdrew its support for the haemophilia centre. Temperley's position became untenable in the Meath when the hospital requested that the university should move the haematology unit with the medical professorial unit to St James's Hospital because of the significant expenditure involved in supporting them.[26] The adult haematology service and the National Haemophilia Centre moved to St James's Hospital in 1976 and they were accommodated in the medical professorial unit on the top floor of Hospital 1.

Unexpected tragedy

Entering the 1980s, the availability of clotting factor concentrates, such as factor VIII, prepared from pooled blood donations, and their introduction via the National Haemophilia Treatment Centre to Irish patients, appeared to herald a new era. Individuals with haemophilia could, for the first time, expect to live a normal lifespan and lifestyle. Within a few years, the emergence of acquired immunodeficiency syndrome (AIDS) in patients with haemophilia who had received contaminated factor VIII converted this promising development into a catastrophe of global proportions. No individual doctor or healthcare worker involved in the care of these patients would emerge from this unaffected. AIDS is caused by infection with the human immunodeficiency virus (HIV). The virus attacks the immune system and eventually removes the ability of infected individuals to protect themselves against other life-threatening infections and diseases. The first case of AIDS in the National Haemophilia Treatment Centre was diagnosed in November 1984. Following the introduction of testing for HIV early in 1985, it became apparent that a large number of patients with severe haemophilia A were infected with the virus. By September of that year, a new case was being diagnosed every month. Subsequently, over half of these patients developed AIDS and died from the condition.

In 1999, a tribunal of inquiry was established by the government, with Judge Alison Lindsay as the sole member, to inquire into the infection of patients with HIV and hepatitis C as a result of receiving contaminated blood products. The country listened as the harrowing stories of those who had developed HIV unfolded on television and radio over several months. The personal toll on patients, their families and healthcare workers was enormous.[27] Temperley was in the witness box for twenty-four days, of which six concentrated on the Blood Transfusion Service Board and the rest on the National Haemophilia Treatment Centre. In her report, Judge Alison Lindsay praised Temperley for his honesty, for his understanding of his patients and their families, and for his commitment throughout his life to improving the lives of patients with haemophilia. The service for patients with coagulation disorders continued to develop significantly at St James's Hospital in the last decade of the twentieth century. The National Centre for Hereditary Coagulation Disorders was opened in the hospital in August 2000.

Bone marrow transplantation

Temperley recognized the importance of bone marrow transplantation as a therapeutic option for patients with leukaemia even though it was perceived as a radical treatment and was viewed negatively by many clinical colleagues in Ireland. The programme was expensive and initially received no support or encouragement from official sources. Working with the friends and families of affected patients, Temperley took the initiative to establish the Bone Marrow for Leukaemia Trust in 1980, a charitable foundation that has played a crucial role in developing the bone marrow transplantation programme.[28]

Shaun McCann, senior lecturer in haematology, spent three months in 1981 in the Fred Hutchinson Cancer Research Centre in Seattle, where bone marrow transplantation had been developed by Edward Donnall Thomas, who was subsequently awarded the Nobel Prize. McCann was appointed consultant haematologist to St James's Hospital with a special interest in bone marrow transplantation in 1983. A bone marrow transplant unit was established in the hospital in 1984 and McCann performed the unit's first transplant in the same year. The Bone Marrow for Leukaemia Trust supplied financial support

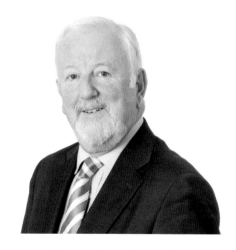

13.27   Shaun McCann, George Gabriel Stokes professor of haematology. Photograph: Anthony Edwards.

for staff training and education, and for the remodelling of the existing ward. The transplant unit developed into the National Centre for Adult Bone Marrow Transplantation under the direction of McCann, who also pioneered the development of molecular biological research in haematology. His commitment to research and teaching was recognized in 1995, when he was appointed George Gabriel Stokes professor of haematology. In 2005, he was the author of a very successful textbook, *Case-based Haematology*, and he wrote another authoritative work, *A history of haematology from Herodotus to HIV*, which was published by Oxford University Press in 2016.

Treating cancer – a new specialty

In April 2008, the taoiseach, Bertie Ahern, launched 'A vision of the cancer network 5 years on' in the National Museum of Ireland, Collins Barracks. During his speech he took the opportunity to pay tribute to Peter Daly, who had retired as consultant oncologist at St James's Hospital. Acknowledging that in 2006 St James's Hospital alone undertook the treatment of 2,300 new cancer patients, he went on to say:

> Professor Daly was one of the first consultants in the field of cancer medicine and made an enormous contribution to the development of oncology services, oncology research and oncology training. His crusading zeal in the cause of developing medical oncology in Ireland and his commitment to his patients were exemplary and I was delighted to hear that last year, he received the Cancer Strategic Development Award. It was richly deserved.[29]

Daly had been appointed as physician, with an interest in malignant diseases, to Mercer's Hospital and St James's Hospital in 1979. He initially shared facilities in the top floor of Hospital 1 with the haematology department and Graham Neale. Following Neale's departure, refurbishment of the top floor was undertaken and the haematology and oncology services moved to Mercer's Hospital as an interim measure. With the closure of Mercer's Hospital in 1983, the joint department of clinical haematology and oncology was established at St James's Hospital, supported by a major inflow of medical, nursing, paramedical and administrative staff from Mercer's Hospital. The post held by Daly was redefined as consultant physician and medical oncologist by Comhairle na nOspidéal in 1983. Haematology and oncology expanded, and by 1993 both specialties were sharing a day ward on the ground floor of Hospital 1.

Barry Breslin was appointed in 1980 as the first consultant in radiotherapy and clinical oncology. He did not have a long career in St James's due to ill health and, having served his patients with great dedication, he retired prematurely in 1992. He was replaced in 1994 by Donal Hollywood, who was also appointed to fill the vacant Marie Curie chair in clinical oncology. Meanwhile, there were also developments in cancer care in the surgical and gynaecological areas as new appointments were made and surgeons transferred from the hospitals that were closing.

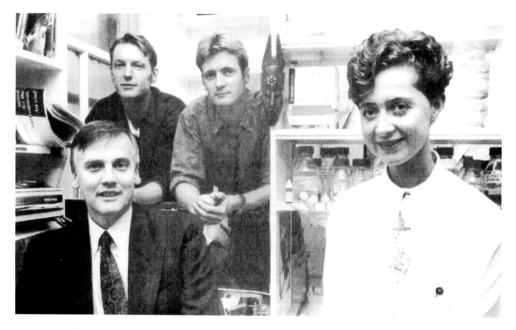

13.28   Prof. Peter Daly and his research team, Dr Richard Hagan, Dr Ross McManus and Nurse Wilma Ormiston. Photograph: *Sunday Business Post*, 2 October 1994.

Specialist nursing care, a key component of the management of haematology and oncology patients, had to be developed nationally at the outset, and St James's Hospital played a leading role in this. Initially nurses travelled to hospitals such as the Royal Marsden in London to gain the necessary training and experience but, with the development of specialist training courses in Trinity College Dublin and University College Dublin, the unit in St James's hospital became the pre-eminent location for gaining nursing skills and knowledge in this field.

In a paper published in *Science* in 1994, an international group led by Dr Mike Stratton of the Institute of Cancer Research at Sutton in Surrey made a very significant contribution to the search for cancer susceptibility genes. A team based in the Sir Patrick Dun's Research Laboratory and led by Peter Daly was among the nine collaborating groups, which were based in Britain, the United States, Ireland, Canada, France and the Netherlands. The researchers identified the gene BRCA-2, located on chromosome 13, which particularly increases the susceptibility of women to breast and ovarian cancer.

John Kennedy joined the department of oncology in 1998. He has a major interest in breast cancer and, prior to his return to Ireland, he was associate professor at the Johns Hopkins Center in Baltimore, Maryland, where he worked on the breast cancer programme. He developed a profile internationally in therapies for breast cancer, and he became lead clinician of the multidisciplinary breast cancer team in St James's Hospital.

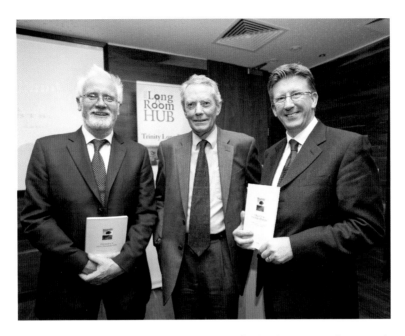

13.29   Prof. Marcus Webb (centre) at the launch of his book *Trinity's psychiatrists* with Michael Gill, professor of psychiatry (left), and Prof. James Lucey, medical director of St Patrick's University Hospital (right). Courtesy of the Trinity Foundation.

Psychiatry: research and development

Marcus Webb was appointed to the chair of psychiatry in 1977, three years after the death of Peter Beckett. Webb trained as a psychiatrist at St Patrick's Hospital in Dublin and subsequently at the Bethlem Royal Hospital and at the Maudsley Hospital in London. His research concentrated on bipolar disorder and alcohol dependence. He contributed significantly to education in psychiatry and to the development of subspecialization in the discipline. During his tenure, Michael Fitzgerald, an acknowledged international leader in the diagnosis and management of Asperger's syndrome, was appointed as the Henry Marsh professor of adolescent psychiatry and Brian Lawlor was appointed as the Conolly Norman professor of old age psychiatry. Lawlor went on to develop a large department that included a memory clinic in the Mercer's Institute for Research on Ageing at St James's Hospital. He became a prolific researcher into Alzheimer's disease and depression in old age. In 2015, together with Ian Robertson, professor of psychology in Trinity College Dublin, he obtained a grant of €150 million to work with partners in the University of California, San Francisco. It was the largest individual research grant in the history of Trinity College. Anthony (Tony) Bates, clinical psychologist at St James's Hospital, pioneered cognitive behavioural psychotherapy, having worked with Aaron T. Beck, one of the originators of the technique in the University of

Pennsylvania. Bates championed the use of mindfulness and wrote several books on mindfulness and depression.[30]

Marcus Webb retired in 2001 and was succeeded as professor of psychiatry by Michael Gill. Gill's research examines the relationship between phenotype and genotype in three key neuropsychiatric disorders: psychoses, autism and ADHD. He is the author of numerous research papers in leading international journals such as *Nature, Nature Genetics, Archives of General Psychiatry*, the *British Journal of Psychiatry* and the *American Journal of Psychiatry*. He was the first director of the Wellcome Trust/HRB Clinical Research Facility at St James's Hospital.

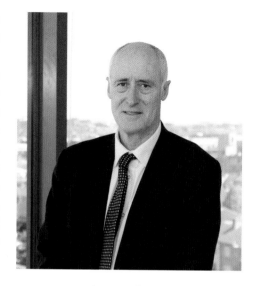

13.30   Brian Lawlor, Conolly Norman professor of old age psychiatry. Photograph: Anthony Edwards.

Obstetrics and gynaecology

Thomas (Tom) Hanratty, who had been appointed as an obstetrician and gynaecologist to St Kevin's Hospital in 1960, continued to run an excellent obstetric service in St James's Hospital until his retirement in 1984. The professorial unit in obstetrics and gynaecology transferred from the Rotunda Hospital to St James's Hospital in 1985, bringing further strength to the teaching and research profile of the hospital. John Bonnar, who was appointed professor of obstetrics and gynaecology in Trinity College in 1975, came to Dublin from Oxford where he was a consultant to the John Radcliffe Hospital and reader in obstetrics and gynaecology at the University of Oxford. Bonnar had a firm belief in the importance of research as an essential requirement for the improvement of clinical practice in obstetrics and gynaecology.[31] He and his colleague, Brian Sheppard, carried out numerous studies on bleeding and clotting related to pregnancy, hormone therapy, oral contraceptives and menstrual bleeding. This research led to new forms of treatment in many of these conditions and Bonnar went on to become a world leader in the field. He served as dean of the Faculty of Health Sciences between 1983 and 1987.

Robert Harrison, an acknowledged expert in the field of fertility studies, also moved to St James's Hospital from the Rotunda Hospital in 1985. He had worked at the Royal Postgraduate School in London, where he developed an interest in fertility, which at that time was emerging as a subspecialty. Harrison returned to Dublin in 1976 as consultant to the Rotunda Hospital and as a senior lecturer in Trinity College. He began working with consultant urologist Michael Butler at St James's

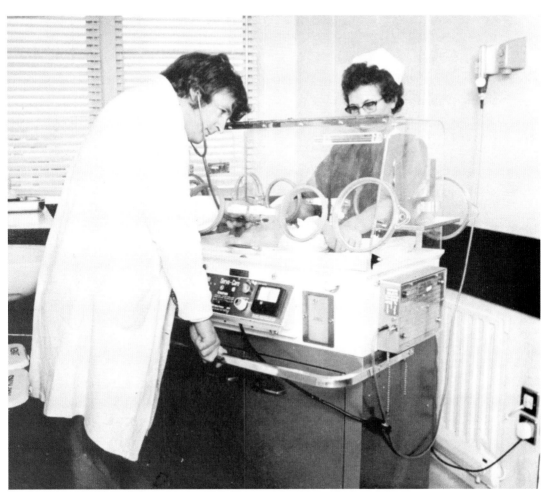

13.31　A doctor and nurse examine an infant in an incubator in the neonatal unit of the maternity hospital in 1975. Brochure of the annual conference of the Federated Dublin Voluntary Hospitals and St James's Hospital (1975).

Hospital and in 1987 they established one of the first joint gynaecology and urology infertility clinics in Ireland and the United Kingdom. This clinic looked at infertility as a couple's problem and not just a female one, as most people at the time regarded it. Harrison's clinics both at the Rotunda Hospital and St James's Hospital were the first to offer de-stressing techniques to couples, as research had established that emotional stress could impact on fertility. Together with Rory O'Moore from the department of clinical biochemistry, Dr Mona O'Moore from the department of education, Trinity College Dublin, and researchers from the Maudsley Hospital in London, Harrison published a paper that found that stress hormones were much higher in couples with infertility difficulties.

In 1985, seven years after Patrick Steptoe announced the world's first baby born after IVF treatment, Harrison carried out three attempts at IVF at Sir Patrick Dun's Hospital. Although unsuccessful, the attempts were leaked to the press, provoking such a controversy that a voluntary moratorium was introduced. Subsequently, the subject was debated at a contentious conference at Maynooth. After due consideration by the Institute of Obstetrics and Gynaecology of the RCPI and by the Medical Council, the use of the technique was approved. Sir Patrick Dun's Hospital had closed in the meantime so the board of St James's Hospital gave permission to Harrison to start Ireland's first assisted human reproductive service at the hospital in January 1986. The service was based at St James's Hospital until 1989, when Harrison was appointed professor of obstetrics and gynaecology in the RCSI and the clinic transferred to the Rotunda Hospital.[32]

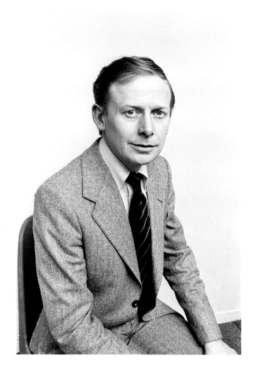

13.32   Robert Harrison, associate professor of obstetrics and gynaecology. Photograph: Bobby Studio.

Medical physics and bioengineering

The hospital's department of medical physics and bioengineering was formed in 1984. It was an amalgamation of the medical physics activities, which had been structured informally at St James's Hospital since 1976, and the medical engineering section, which had been established in Baggot Street Hospital in 1966. The department was based in Garden Hill, which had been converted in 1975 by the Eastern Health Board for the use of the department of psychiatry of University College Dublin. The building was acquired by St James's Hospital from the Eastern Health Board in 1981. Over subsequent years, under the leadership of Jim Malone, the bioengineering department developed very strongly in both the service and academic areas and also reached out to form strong collaborative research links with other departments. The department assumed de facto national responsibility for education in medical physics and bioengineering in Ireland. Malone was appointed Robert Boyle professor of medical physics in 1997.

The closure and transfer of Mercer's Hospital

On 19 October 1981, the chairman of the board of governors of Mercer's Hospital, Dr William (Bill) Watts, who was also provost of Trinity College Dublin, addressed the medical board of Mercer's about the future of the hospital. He placed emphasis on Comhairle na nOspidéal's ruling that any development at St James's Hospital necessitated a parallel reduction of activities in the federation. He explained that when the proposed medical professorial unit opened in St James's Hospital there would be a corresponding closure in either Mercer's Hospital or Sir Patrick Dun's Hospital. As Mercer's was the smaller and had a falling bed occupancy, it seemed logical that it would be the first of the Federated Hospitals to close.[33]

Intensive negotiations on the closure of the hospital and the transfer of the patients and staff to St James's began in 1982. Mercer's Hospital closed at the end of May 1983, and a total of 141 posts – including medical, nursing, paramedical, catering, clerical, administrative, portering and other services – were transferred to St James's Hospital. Forty student nurses moved to St James's to complete their training. Poignantly, one of the senior surgeons of the hospital, Richard Brenan, was the last patient to be nursed in Mercer's. He was not transferred to St James's Hospital with the other patients and he died in the hospital on 28 May.[34]

Research on the effects of winter smog

Much of the space and water heating in Dublin was effected by means of oil until the Middle East crisis in the 1970s. The oil crisis resulted in an official policy to encourage the use of bituminous coal for home heating. Consequently, there was a steep rise in the levels of winter air pollution in Dublin in the 1980s. In January 1982, a particularly severe period of pollution resulted in the doubling of the death rate of patients admitted to St James's Hospital in that month. The phenomenon was first noticed and attributed to smog by the respiratory physician Luke Clancy, who had joined the staff of the hospital in 1978.

The smog was clearly visible and although there were approximately sixteen monitoring stations, the information from this activity was not released to the public. The data for exposure to pollution and the mortality figures from the whole county of Dublin became available in 1984 and revealed that there had been a doubling of mortality in all of the Dublin hospitals. These findings led to calls for the control of pollution in Dublin, and Clancy was in the vanguard of this campaign. Success was achieved in September 1990 when a Dublin-wide ban on the sale, marketing and distribution of bituminous coal was introduced by the minister for the environment, Mary Harney. This resulted in an immediate and dramatic drop of around 70 per cent in air pollution. In a paper published in *The Lancet* in 2002, Clancy and his co-authors calculated that the introduction of the ban resulted in a reduction in respiratory and cardiovascular mortality equivalent to some 4,000 people over a ten-year period.[35] These findings led to the revision of the standards for air quality by the WHO and other international regulatory bodies, as they demonstrated the importance of reducing air pollution.

New board structure

In 1984, the minister for health and social welfare, Barry Desmond, amended the original establishment order to provide a new board structure for St James's Hospital. The representation of the Eastern Health Board and the Federated Hospitals on the board was reduced to introduce nominees of the university, the medical board, the nursing staff and the unions. This development signalled the growing significance of the hospital in relation to its 'parent' bodies, the Eastern Health Board and the Federated Hospitals, and it encouraged a sense of cohesiveness and belonging among the staff of the hospital.

There was another encouraging development in 1984 when the long-awaited construction of the clinical facilities of the new hospital, phase 1C, began in June. G & T Crampton Ltd was appointed as the main contractor. It was hoped that this phase would be completed by 1987 and that immediate progress would be made with the second phase of the hospital development, which would be completed by 1990. The central concourse of the hospital was to be built during phase 2, together with the administration facilities, supplies department, restaurant, pharmacy, rehabilitation and other ancillary facilities. However, the whole process was to take much longer and was to develop in a way that was not anticipated.

Sudden closure of designated hospitals and transfer of specialties

The year 1982 witnessed the beginning of a severe economic recession in Ireland. The financial situation placed St James's Hospital in unprecedented difficulties. The board of the hospital was informed early in 1982 by the Department of Health that there would be an abatement of £600,000 from its financial allocation. However, the annual funding was not allocated until August, when a further cut of £718,000 was imposed. This meant that the allocation for the year was cut by a total of £1,318,000 or 6.2 per cent. The board of the hospital rushed through a range of measures that included a reduction in non-pay allocation to departments, a reduction in drug stocks, elimination of non-rostered overtime, an embargo on employment of locums and the designation of some beds as semi-private to generate income.[36] The financial crisis continued throughout the 1980s and, as the decade progressed, the hospital faced deeper cuts in its annual allocations from the Department of Health.

In 1986, the first step was taken by the Department of Health to reduce the number of acute beds in south Dublin by accelerating the planned closure of the designated voluntary hospitals. It had been anticipated that these closures would commence in 1989, when the main phase of the new St James's Hospital was due to be completed. At that stage, the services provided by Sir Patrick Dun's Hospital and the Royal City of Dublin Hospital, Baggot Street, and some of the services of Dr Steevens' Hospital, were to transfer to St James's. However, in 1986, the funding given to Sir Patrick Dun's by the Department of Health meant that the hospital could only stay open to the end of August. As a consequence, St James's Hospital was placed under enormous pressure to accommodate the clinical services from Sir Patrick Dun's Hospital within its existing facilities. Sir Patrick Dun's closed on 1 September 1986 and sixty-one student nurses transferred to St James's to complete their training. Staff moved to St James's Hospital, to one of the other Federated Hospitals or accepted redundancy packages.

St James's Hospital indicated that it would need an allocation of £36.5 million from the Department of Health for 1987. However, the allocation to the hospital was £30.5 million and it was estimated that if the hospital continued delivering the same service there would be a £3.2 million overdraft by the end of June and an overdraft of £7.2 million at the end of the year. A special meeting of the board was held on 16 April, and board members reluctantly agreed to sweeping cuts and new income-generating measures.[37] Two public wards were converted into private and semi-private wards in order to generate income, the hospital's participation in the Dublin A & E rota was reduced, there was a 10 per cent reduction in outpatients and day care patients, the midwifery school was closed and there were substantial redundancies throughout the hospital. The board could not rely on bank overdrafts to tide the hospital over, as the banks had been instructed not to provide overdraft facilities beyond the limits then in place, which in St James's case was £1.25 million.

Economic pressures also brought about the precipitous closure of Baggot Street Hospital and Dr Steevens' Hospital in December 1987. With considerable regret, the decision was made to move the maternity unit from Hospital 5 in St James's Hospital to the Coombe Hospital in order to accommodate specialties from the hospitals destined to close. Gynaecology was to remain in St James's Hospital. After the closure of the obstetrics unit in September 1987, immediate preparations were made for the transfer of services from Baggot Street Hospital and Dr Steevens' Hospital. The work carried out in Hospital 5 to accommodate those services included a twin-theatre suite, a burns unit, a six-suite outpatients department, a maxillofacial plastics laboratory, a four-bed intensive care facility and a six-bed day surgical unit to facilitate the transfer of the plastic surgery and maxillofacial departments, and two theatres for ENT, thoracic surgery and gynaecology. The work was completed quickly and the services transferred from Baggot Street Hospital at the beginning of December 1987. The accident and emergency services transferred from Dr Steevens' Hospital to the Meath Hospital in June 1987 and plastic surgery and maxillofacial surgery transferred to James Connolly Memorial Hospital in October pending the completion of the structural work at St James's Hospital.[38] Dr Steevens' was scheduled to close on the 30 September but a reprieve was granted for three months. The services remaining in the hospital moved to St James's at the end of December and the hospital closed. Seventy-two nursing students transferred to the school of nursing at St James's on the closure of Baggot Street Hospital and the student nurses at Dr Steevens' Hospital went to the Meath Hospital. Ninety-six staff moved to St James's Hospital from Baggot Street Hospital, as did seventy-six staff from Dr Steevens' Hospital. The trauma and orthopaedic services of Dr Steevens' Hospital were relocated to the Adelaide Hospital and the burns unit moved to St James's Hospital.

The whole process was very difficult for many people. It was facilitated to some extent by the early retirement and voluntary redundancy scheme introduced by the Department of Health. Many of the staff of the voluntary hospitals and St James's Hospital availed of this scheme. The cutbacks meant that St James's Hospital had to provide the services of a major acute teaching hospital from a very limited number of beds, situated in old and inadequate buildings scattered over a large site. The hospital was fortunate in having a very able chief executive officer, Liam Dunbar, who gave leadership during this difficult time.

The chairman of the hospital board, Ian Howie, writing soon after these events, stressed the enormity of the task faced by the hospital, its officers and staff:

> This is probably the largest and swiftest closure and transfer of acute hospital services which has occurred either in Ireland or Britain in the history of the voluntary hospital movement and since the emergence of the major public hospitals ... The conversion of space to accommodate, often sophisticated services, in a matter of a few weeks in the latter half of 1987 was a heroic task. Simultaneously solutions had to be found to the innumerable personnel problems inevitably involved in hospital closures and the transfer of services.[39]

Those who transferred from the old voluntary hospitals integrated fully and shared the vision of developing St James's Hospital into a first-class institution of which all could be justly proud. It would have been very easy for staff to become despondent during the recession, with a resultant general malaise and loss of morale. This did not happen and despite the cutbacks inflicted to remedy the financial situation, all the staff responded well to the challenges. Wards were closed and the budget for the laboratory services was reduced significantly. Vacancies were not filled and only minimal essential locum cover was sanctioned. However, this period of managed chaos in the early years of the new hospital led to one very desirable outcome:

> Almost unnoticed against the background of corporate and individual trauma induced by the forced closures of the designated hospitals was the fact that the original aspiration of the Federated Hospitals to 'own' the new hospital had in effect been abandoned. In hindsight the reasons are plain. There was at the crucial

time no new hospital to 'own' and, more fundamentally, since it was established St James's had acquired its own corporate identity as a unique combination of municipal and voluntary hospital but belonging neither to the Health Board nor the Federation. The issue of separate managements was never discussed.[40]

The loss of the maternity service

The transfer of the maternity department to the Coombe Hospital during this process was a very significant loss to St James's Hospital. This was the only maternity unit within an acute hospital in Dublin and as a consequence it was in an ideal situation to care for women in pregnancy with medical and surgical complications requiring specialist intervention. It was staffed by highly skilled midwives and it had an associated school of midwifery. The perinatal mortality of the unit was among the lowest in Ireland and at a level that had not been achieved at that time by any of the Dublin maternity hospitals. This was remarkable as the unit served a low-income catchment area. When the maternity unit moved to the Coombe Hospital on 30 September 1987, the service within St James's Hospital was reconfigured as a division of gynaecology. The gynaecological service at Baggot Street Hospital, which was largely delivered by consultant obstetrician and gynaecologist Eamon McGuinness, was incorporated into this new development. Fourteen midwives transferred to the Coombe and Rotunda hospitals and the remaining midwives and attendants were reassigned to other areas of the hospital. The teaching staff and students of the midwifery school at St James's Hospital transferred to the Coombe Hospital.

New roles for the designated hospitals

The three designated hospitals, Mercer's Hospital, Sir Patrick Dun's Hospital and the Royal City of Dublin Hospital, had now ceased to function as acute hospitals. All the buildings were eventually used for new roles in healthcare involving service provision, education and administration. Mercer's Hospital was acquired by the RCSI and was developed as a medical library, a primary care practice for teaching and research, and student accommodation. Sir Patrick Dun's Hospital was initially acquired by the Institute of Clinical Pharmacology, a company involved in pharmaceutical research, which was led by Professor Austin Darragh. The company subsequently ran into financial difficulties and Sir Patrick Dun's was then bought by the Eastern Health Board and developed as a community hospital. The Royal City of Dublin Hospital was acquired by the Eastern Health Board, on a lease from the board of governors, to provide community health facilities. Dr Steevens' Hospital was also acquired by the Eastern Health Board and became, after extensive refurbishment, their headquarters.

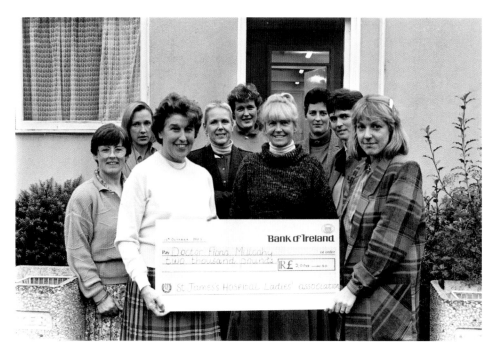

13.33   Joyce Temperley presents a cheque for clinical equipment to Dr Fiona Mulcahy on behalf of the St James's Hospital Ladies' Association in 1987. Front row, left to right: Temperley, Bella Scott and Dr Fiona Mulcahy, consultant in genitourinary medicine. Back row, left to right: Aileen Walsh, Dr Emer Keeling, Jill Casey, Linda Stephens, Mary Coakley and Angie O'Briain. Photograph: Bobby Studio.

Emergence of the HIV/AIDS pandemic

The condition that would ultimately be described as AIDS was recognized for the first time in 1981 among five homosexual men in three different hospitals in Los Angeles. Over the next two years more cases were found in homosexuals but also in individuals who acquired AIDS through heterosexual contacts and in those who had been transfused with contaminated blood products. During the 1980s, AIDS emerged as a deadly disease, killing millions worldwide. The first AIDS cases in Ireland were identified in the Mater Hospital in 1982, affecting two gay men.[41] The first death from AIDS in the country occurred a year later. The trickle of cases in the early 1980s had turned into a steady stream by the end of the decade.[42] Some of the earliest cases of AIDS in Ireland were among individuals who had received contaminated blood transfusions or blood products. As a consequence, much of the care of patients with HIV/AIDS fell on St James's Hospital.

Fiona Mulcahy was appointed as the country's first consultant in genitourinary and HIV medicine in 1987. A Trinity graduate, Mulcahy received her specialist training at Leeds General Infirmary. As soon as she returned to St James's Hospital, Mulcahy assumed a leadership role in the treatment and prevention of HIV infection in Ireland. She contributed greatly to public education by her regular appearances in the media, which alleviated fears and promoted a more informed and tolerant approach to AIDS in Irish society.

By 1987, AIDS constituted a major part of the workload of the genitourinary medical service, in terms of both medical time and counselling. There was a threefold to fourfold increase in activity on the previous year, with 135 HIV-positive patients attending, of whom 14 had AIDS. Mulcahy gradually established a skilled multidisciplinary team. Initially the service was based in cramped conditions in Hospital 7, but within a few years more extensive space was made available for the rapidly expanding clinics.[43] Although the hospital provided a specialist unit to deal with the acute problems of patients admitted with AIDS, the complexities of their care affected virtually all the disciplines throughout the hospital. The number of patients with the condition increased dramatically within a short period of time. A total of 621 HIV/AIDS patients attended the outpatient clinics in 1990 and of these 556 were intravenous drug abusers. In that year 180 HIV/AIDS patients were admitted to hospital and 23 per cent of these patients were newly diagnosed. There were 45 HIV-related deaths during the same year. Patients with AIDS presented with increasingly complex medical problems, and the death rate was rising. In the first two decades of the AIDS epidemic in Ireland, over 40 per cent of cases occurred in intravenous drug abusers. HIV/AIDS in this group was virtually confined to inner-city Dublin, with devastating consequences for families and communities. A generation of parents was lost and grandparents raised grandchildren whose parents had died. Fear gripped many communities because of false perceptions about how AIDS was transmitted. Some infected individuals were ostracized by their local community and their children were shunned at school.[44] The fear of contagion from HIV experienced by medical and nursing staff in hospitals throughout the country was addressed by a course established by St James's School of Nursing in 1992 on the care and management of HIV/AIDS.

Encouraging results of a new approach to therapy were reported in 1996 at the World AIDS Conference in Vancouver. The outlook became more optimistic, with the possibility of reducing mortality and morbidity rates by using a triple-drug regimen to manage HIV infection. Ultimately this is what happened and HIV infection became, as a result, a chronic illness. St James's Hospital remains the largest centre in the country for the provision of services for HIV medicine and sexual health.

New hospital opens

The first clinical areas of the new hospital were opened in 1987. These included the psychiatric unit and the Robert Mayne Day Hospital for older patients, which was named after one of the physicians who worked in the South Dublin Union during the

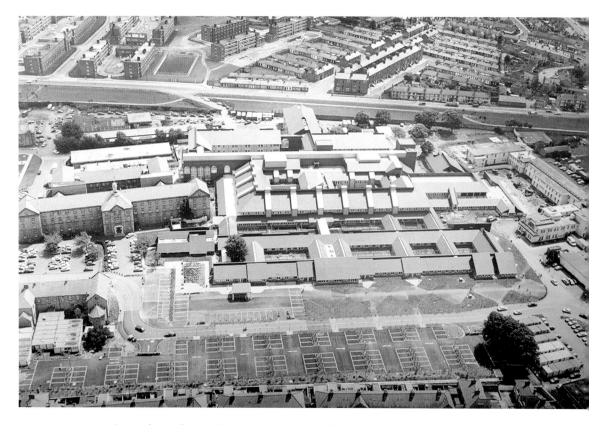

13.34 The new hospital situated between Hospital 3 (left) and Hospital 7 (right) in 1988. Courtesy of St James's Hospital.

Great Famine period. The psychiatric unit was the first inpatient unit of the new hospital and was designed with a distinctive central courtyard to make it a pleasant living and working department. It was named the Jonathan Swift Clinic because of Swift's interest in disorders of the mind and his connection with St Patrick's Hospital, the City Workhouse and the Foundling Hospital. One of the wards was named the Peter Beckett Ward to acknowledge the contribution made by Beckett as the first professor of psychiatry in the hospital and medical school.

On 30 June 1988, following three and a half years of construction work, the contractors, G & T Crampton, formally handed over the completed phase 1C to the hospital board. The new development was the biggest construction on the site since the building of the City Workhouse in the early years of the eighteenth century. The new hospital contained 279 inpatient acute beds, 11 operating theatres, an outpatient department, an A & E department, a 20-bed burns unit complete with its own operating theatres, a 22-bed intensive care unit, a coronary care unit, a department of diagnostic imaging, offices for a department of anaesthesia, a central sterile supply department and a temporary concourse.

In the design of the new hospital there was a deliberate attempt to build on a human scale and to avoid the forbidding institutional appearance of many hospitals, both old and new. The front elevation, which faces the main internal road of the hospital, presents as a single storey, behind which there are two- and three-storey ward and theatre sections. The external walls are clad with silver power-coated profiled steel sheeting. Several attractively landscaped courtyards were included in the development and as many mature trees as possible were retained during construction. The intention was that patients would derive a therapeutic effect from their proximity to pleasant and restful external surroundings.

Work began on commissioning the department of diagnostic imaging. A CT scanner and equipment for modern angiography and interventional radiology were installed. The scanner was the first in either St James's Hospital or the Federated Hospitals. The department became operational in October 1988 and was officially opened by the minister for health, Dr Rory O'Hanlon, in January 1989. It was the first fully computerized department of diagnostic imaging in the country. At the opening a plaque was unveiled in memory of Dr Edward Malone. The new A & E department was opened, together with the outpatient department, in 1990.

The opening of the ward areas and other parts of the new building, including the burns unit, the coronary care unit and the intensive care unit, together with the theatre suites, was delayed until 1992 because of financial stringencies. The minister for health, Mary O'Rourke, formally opened the hospital on 17 January 1992. The development, which cost £60 million, transformed the hospital into the largest acute general hospital in the country, equipped with the most advanced technology available. The names of the wards of the hospital and of several clinical departments reflect the history of medicine and nursing in the Federated Hospitals, St Kevin's Hospital and the school of medicine of Trinity College Dublin.

Art in St James's Hospital

A hospital committee was formed to advise on works of art, and the selected art works were incorporated into the design of the building.[45] For many years the hospital had emphasized the importance of art for patients, visitors and staff as a means of providing a milieu conducive to healing and supporting health and well-being.[46] This approach was overseen by a hospital arts committee involving staff, members of the arts community and representatives of the Irish Museum of Modern Art and the National College of Art and Design, both situated in the immediate neighbourhood of the hospital. More recently, multimedia arts projects have been used in an imaginative way to provide a virtual window on the worlds of art and nature for patients.[47]

Mercer's Institute for Research on Ageing

The Department of Health took a strong stand on the issue of the disposal of assets accruing from the sale of the designated hospitals. It claimed that it should receive the money from the sale of Mercer's Hospital as it had been funding most of its activities for several years.[48] The department also argued that the assets should be used to clear deficits that had accumulated during the difficult years before closure, and that the balance should be used as a contribution to the cost of the new facilities. This approach was strenuously resisted by Dr William Watts, provost of Trinity College, chairman of the council of the Federated Hospitals and chairman of the board of governors of Mercer's Hospital. He argued that the assets should be used to support projects that reflected the original intentions of the founders of the hospitals. Ultimately Watts' view prevailed. This had very positive outcomes,

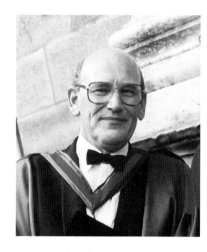

13.35   Prof. William Watts, provost of Trinity College and last chairman of the board of governors of Mercer's Hospital. Private collection.

not only in relation to the sale of Mercer's Hospital, but also in relation to the sale of several other voluntary hospitals in subsequent years, allowing their boards to fund novel developments in service, research and education, largely in St James's and in the new hospital in Tallaght. These benefactions played a pivotal role in the development of St James's Hospital.

Following the sale of Mercer's Hospital, the board of the hospital applied to the Commissioners for Charitable Donations and Bequests and to the courts for a cy-pres scheme, which would allow it to establish a new charity through which 'the funds of the hospital will be applied to the health needs of the citizens of Dublin'.[49] The cy-pres scheme was approved in 1987 and the board of the hospital was reconstituted as the Mercer's Hospital Foundation, whose function was to manage the funds that accrued from the sale. The Mercer's Hospital Foundation proposed three areas as beneficiaries of the new trust: a centre of excellence for ageing at St James's Hospital, the department of general practice in the Royal College of Surgeons and the department of general practice in Trinity College. The development of a centre of excellence for ageing, a proposal submitted by Davis Coakley and Jim Malone, was identified as their primary beneficiary. This led to the foundation of the Mercer's Institute for Research on Ageing (MIRA) in 1988. St James's Hospital made space available for the new development. The institute was awarded a major grant in 1991 by the Health Research Board (HRB) to fund research into Alzheimer's disease and to establish the first memory clinic in Ireland. The institute was very successful and made significant contributions in the field of ageing in three areas – service development, research and training. It achieved an international reputation because of the quality of the presentations made to learned societies on both sides of the Atlantic and the number of publications by staff in international peer-reviewed journals. As a consequence of this expertise, the hospital was chosen by the Department of Health in 1998 as the location for the National Dementia Services and Information Development Centre, with the remit to foster best practice in dementia care among professionals and caregivers throughout the country.

Activity levels soar

Following the closure of the designated hospitals, activity within St James's increased significantly. In 1989, outpatient attendances exceeded 100,000 per annum for the first time. Work in the hospital began to concentrate largely on medical and surgical emergencies admitted through the A & E department and from outpatients. These emergency admissions were responsible for about 70 per cent of the total admissions in 1988. During the 1980s, day care activity in medicine and surgery increased from virtually zero in 1980 to about 20,000 per annum at the end of the decade. This surge in day care activity was largely driven by the loss of acute hospital beds, which made the admission of patients for non-emergency investigations and treatment very difficult.

Until well into the 1980s it was possible for general practitioners to get their patients admitted to hospital without too much difficulty. They could ring the admissions department of the hospital and request a bed or they could ring the consultant or registrar of the specialty most appropriate for their patient and request an admission. However, in the late 1980s, because of declining bed numbers, general practitioners found themselves wasting more and more time ringing hospital after hospital seeking admission for their patients, often without success. Understandably, they became very frustrated by this and had no choice but to order an ambulance and send their patients directly to the A & E departments. Soon the A & E departments became the main route of admission of patients to hospital and they began to deal with more and more acutely ill medical patients rather than accidents. The A & E departments could not cope with the pressure of admissions, medical patients overflowed into the day care and surgical wards and, as a consequence, day care patient procedures and appointments for elective surgery were cancelled. This resulted in great frustration for patients and for their consultants. The closure of wards in the summer of 1989 to meet financial targets caused further disruption and increased use of the specialist day wards for treatment of emergency patients. The workers' union, SIPTU, described the ward closures as 'the last straw' and the nursing union threatened strike action.

In 1988 Patrick Plunkett was appointed as full-time consultant in A & E medicine in St James's Hospital and in the same year the first A & E registrar took up his post. The A & E department in the new hospital opened in December 1989. There was no

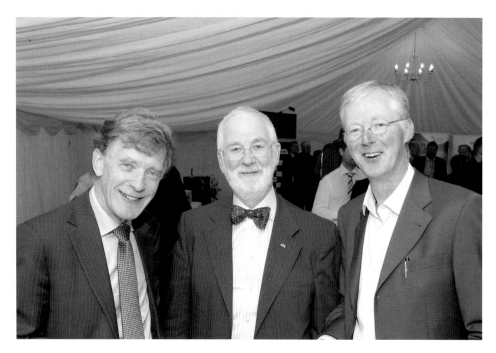

13.36   Prof. Bernard Walsh, consultant physician in geriatric medicine (left), Prof. Patrick Plunkett, consultant in emergency medicine (centre) and Prof. Joseph Keane, consultant in respiratory medicine (right). Photograph: Anthony Edwards.

honeymoon period for the new department. It came under growing pressure in its early months because of the closure of the A & E departments of Sir Patrick Dun's, Dr Steevens' and Baggot Street Hospitals and the situation was aggravated by an influenza epidemic. As a result, the A & E department was very busy from the start and has remained so ever since. Admissions to the hospital were also soaring, and between 1986 and 1989 the activity level doubled. Yet during the same period there was no increase in nursing numbers because of an embargo on recruitment. Plunkett was a very capable director of the emergency department, coping with major pressures as the numbers presenting to the department continued to increase significantly, year after year. He became a national leader in the field, and made regular appearances on radio and television news programmes. St James's Hospital was changing rapidly from an elective to an emergency hospital.[50] The hospital piloted the introduction of an emergency nurse practitioner in the A & E department in 1996. It was hoped that the initiative would reduce lengthy waiting times for patients presenting with conditions that could be treated by the emergency nurse, such as lacerations, sprains, foreign body in the eye, ear or nose and soft-tissue injuries. The initiative was a success and emergency nurse practitioners were appointed to other A & E departments throughout the country.

New levels of sophistication

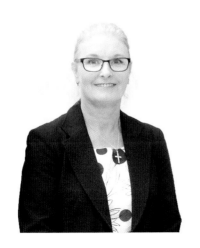

13.37   Nurse Valerie Small, first advanced nurse practitioner in St James's Hospital. Photograph: Anthony Edwards.

The 1980s was a decade that saw not only a major increase in activity but also the development of new levels of sophistication, complexity and variety throughout the hospital. At the beginning of the decade, St James's Hospital was a large institution of nearly a thousand beds, concentrating primarily on general medicine and surgery. There was a small A & E department, no intensive care unit, few specialist units and a very limited pathology service. By the end of the decade, the hospital had a wide range of highly specialized units and national referral centres. It housed the core clinical departments of the medical school of Trinity College Dublin. It had the largest A & E department in the city and the largest centralized pathology laboratory. Over the decade the number of beds within St James's fell from 1,000 to 800, primarily due to the transfer of long-stay patients to units outside St James's in order to facilitate the demolition of Hospital 3, which had been built originally as the infirmary (Hospitals 2–3) of the South Dublin Union. Its demolition was necessary to clear the site for the development of the next phase of the hospital, phase 1H. Increasing numbers of inpatient admissions were made possible by better utilization of beds. The mean patient stay throughout the hospital was reduced progressively during the decade. The development of day care in areas such as endoscopy, surgery and cancer chemotherapy represented a major change from traditional medical practice, with corresponding benefits for patient care. A diabetic day care centre was opened in 1989 to provide a five-day multidisciplinary clinical service to diabetic patients and to promote education and preventive care. The introduction of a digitalized system in the department of diagnostic imaging enabled immediate reporting. This was a very significant advance not only for the department but for all the clinical units.

Undergraduate teaching became an increasingly important activity within the hospital. Students from many disciplines were now receiving practical instruction on the wards. In addition to medicine and nursing, these disciplines included physiotherapy, occupational therapy, speech and language therapy, sociology and dietetics. By 1992, the first phase of the new hospital development was fully operational, but there remained pressing issues largely due to the fact that more than 50 per cent of patients were still housed in old and inadequate buildings throughout the campus.

14

The largest teaching hospital in Ireland

As provost of Trinity College between 1991 and 2001 I had the opportunity, through the Faculty of Health Sciences connection, to become more closely acquainted with St James's Hospital. I was always impressed by the amazing story of St James's – it is a story of drive and ambition and extraordinary commitment to public service from an extraordinary group of individuals.[1]

The board of the hospital decided to proceed with the development of the next phase of the capital programme, 1H, in 1992. This would bring the number of public beds in new accommodation to 500, providing more intensive care, burns, A & E and haematology/oncology beds, a private ward block of 90 beds, new facilities for day care and the main hospital concourse. As soon as the plans received approval from the Department of Health, construction began. The first phase of the new development was handed over to the hospital in 1995 and included the new haematology/oncology unit, incorporating the National Bone Marrow Transplant Centre and two standard wards. The National Bone Marrow for Leukaemia Trust contributed £5 million for equipment. The haematology/oncology ward was named after the famous Trinity medical graduate, Denis Burkitt. Working as a surgeon in Africa, Burkitt discovered a highly malignant lymphoma common in children in certain parts of Africa and he subsequently found that it responded well to treatment with chemotherapy.

Pioneering a new system of hospital management

With the development of computerized information systems it became possible to move the management and decision-making closer to the clinical activity to improve patient care, efficiency and cost-effectiveness. The clinical directorate system, pioneered in Johns Hopkins Hospital, was selected as the form best suited to St James's

Hospital. The system involved dividing the clinical specialties in a hospital into groups, called clinical directorates, with a number of specialties forming each directorate. Each group was led by a clinical director, elected by the consultants, and by a nurse manager and a business manager. The Department of Health supported the development of the directorate system and agreed to fund two departments in St James's Hospital as pilot directorates in 1993. These were CResT (cardiology, respiratory medicine and thoracic surgery), with Luke Clancy as director and MedEL (medicine for the elderly), with J. Bernard Walsh as director. The whole process was overseen by John O'Brien, deputy CEO and operations manager. The two pilot directorates were very successful: the financial and activity performances surpassed those in the previous year and also the outcomes that had been forecast. The board of the hospital concluded that the clinical directorate model was the way forward and decided to implement it hospital-wide.[2] By 1999 there were nine clinical directorates in the hospital. The clinical directors together with senior corporate staff formed the executive management group. This group functioned as the 'cabinet' of the hospital. The Department of Health and Children was impressed by the success of the model and established it in other hospitals throughout the country.[3]

A major teaching hospital

St James's Hospital provided a wide range of diagnostic and treatment services, many with a regional or national remit, and consolidated its position as a major teaching hospital in Ireland during the 1990s. During this period, the quality of its services and its commitment to education and research were increasingly acknowledged. The composition of the hospital board was altered in 1998 but it continued to reflect the unique mix of municipal and voluntary representation that had characterized St James's from the beginning.

The hospital was eager to establish its credentials and a core group of its consultants was academically focused. They had returned from prestigious teaching hospitals in North America, the United Kingdom and Australia and were anxious to maintain their research and teaching interests as well as to develop their clinical departments. These consultants were given part-time academic appointments in the Faculty of Health Sciences of Trinity College Dublin. A number of them went on to develop major academic teaching and research units. The medical school, although very old and bearing a venerable reputation, was small and perceived itself as vulnerable, so it welcomed the hospital consultants and encouraged them to pursue academic interests, and the university opened its academic promotional system to them. The initiative was led by Professor John Bonnar, who was the dean of the Faculty of Health Sciences at the time. This synergistic relationship was one of the key factors that led to what can only be described as the phenomenal development of the hospital in such a short period of time.

Michael Cullen was one of the first of this group to be appointed to St James's Hospital. He was a graduate of University College Dublin and did his postgraduate training in Boston. When he returned to Dublin he worked with Peter Gatenby at the Meath Hospital and was appointed as consultant endocrinologist to St James's Hospital in 1978. He was committed to teaching and research and he published in international journals. Cullen also made a significant contribution to the development of the hospital by establishing the consultant appointments committee. This changed the appointment of new consultants from an ad hoc system, which was sometimes dictated by the influence of those promoting new posts, to a methodical system where the need for consultants in a particular specialty was identified, together with the resources necessary to create and sustain the new posts.[4]

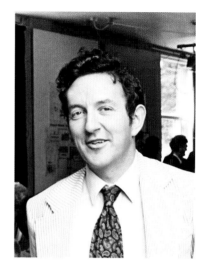

14.1   Prof. Michael Cullen, consultant endocrinologist. Photograph: Bobby Studio.

The Trinity Centre for Health Sciences

It had been a key objective of the hospital and university to erect a clinical sciences complex and dental hospital at St James's Hospital on the site formerly occupied by the buildings of the old City Workhouse and the Foundling Hospital. Medical and dental education, together with the Dental Hospital, came under the remit of the Department of Education. In 1980, John Wilson, minister for education, wrote to the board of St James's Hospital confirming that the Department of Education would be responsible for funding both the Clinical Sciences Centre and the Dental Hospital.[5] A project team was formed to draw up a brief, and work on the new proposal was expected to begin in 1987. However, as a consequence of the recession in the 1980s, government funding was not forthcoming to finance the project. Subsequently, the sale of the designated voluntary hospitals presented an alternative source of capital, albeit on a more modest scale.

Following the closure of Sir Patrick Dun's Hospital, the governors obtained approval for a cy-pres scheme under which the assets of the hospital were to be divided between Trinity College and the RCPI. The funding the university received was designated for a new Trinity Centre for Health Sciences at St James's Hospital. The board of Dr Steevens' Hospital also contributed towards the Trinity Centre through their cy-pres scheme. This funding, together with donations received from graduates, a grant from the Department of Health for nursing education and the

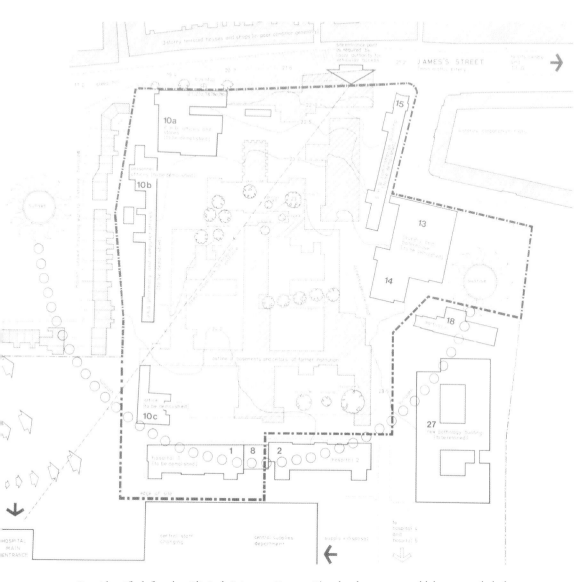

14.2   Site identified for the Clinical Sciences Centre. The development would have entailed the demolition of the old stone buildings and Hospital 1. Reproduced from 'Brief for the Clinical Sciences Centre', St James's Hospital.

Chester Beatty Fund (a gift the university had received for medical education from the Chester Beatty Trust), provided the capital to build the first phase of the Trinity Centre for Health Sciences. The new centre included space for the clinical professorial departments, lecture theatres, seminar rooms, a library, the nursing school, and teaching and research laboratories. The clinical departments of the medical school began to move into the completed centre in 1993. The nursing school transferred

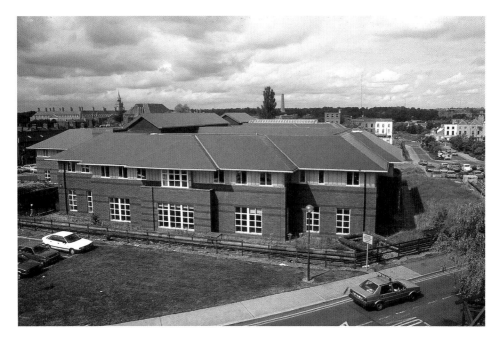

14.3   Phase 1 of the Trinity Centre for Health Sciences. Photograph: David Smyth.

from the old convent to purpose-built accommodation in the new development in November 1993.

There was an aspiration to move the existing William Stokes Postgraduate Centre, which was based at the Rialto end of the hospital, into the new academic centre. The existing accommodation was based in a temporary structure that was not big enough to host large clinical meetings, and it was generally agreed that the centre should be situated in a more central location. Funding from the Royal City of Dublin Hospital Trust, together with funding raised by the director of postgraduate medical education, Con Feighery, from the hospital consultants, the Eastern Health Board, the National Lottery and the pharmaceutical companies, was used to build a new postgraduate centre as part of the Trinity Centre. St James's Hospital acquired the existing postgraduate facility from its steering committee and it was subsequently used as a social and recreational amenity in the hospital. The new two-storey postgraduate centre contained a lecture theatre, conference and teaching rooms and, because of its location, it had direct access to the 250-seat tiered lecture theatre in the Trinity Centre.

The development of the Trinity Centre for Health Sciences strengthened the relationship between the hospital and Trinity College and created a first-class facility for the education of students. There were two days of celebrations on 26 and 27 September 1994 to mark the opening of the new Trinity Centre. These included an academic ceremony in the public theatre on the university campus when the lord mayor, John Gormley, spoke of the link between the foundation of the college and the origins of medical education in the city of Dublin. The ceremony was preceded by an academic procession comprising members of the college and senior academic representatives from the medical schools of Yale, Leiden, Prague, Oxford and Tours. Sir Peter Froggatt, vice chancellor of Queen's University Belfast and a Trinity medical graduate, launched *The School of Physic, Trinity College Dublin: a retrospective view* by Peter Gatenby on the evening of the first day. The book traced the history of the medical school since its bicentenary in 1911. The following day, Donald Weir chaired a symposium in the new building entitled 'The importance of research for clinical practice'. In a keynote address, he emphasized the

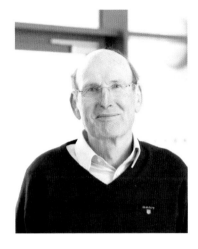

14.4   Prof. Conleth Feighery, consultant immunologist. Photograph: Anthony Edwards.

range, number and standard of the academic publications in international journals produced by the staff of the department of clinical medicine over the previous five years. He stressed that this research was largely funded by grants from international research funding bodies such as the Wellcome Trust, the National Institutes of Health in Bethesda, Maryland and the European Union. Weir concluded:

> Research in Ireland is a growth industry which is employing our medical and science graduates who would otherwise emigrate to America or Europe – the modern equivalent of the Irish Wild Geese. These graduates are now bringing credit to Ireland instead of to other countries. The government has failed to realize that 'seed money' for clinical research is essential if we are to build on this success story.[6]

Nursing education

The nursing school at St James's Hospital had thrived since its foundation in 1967, with an average of 250 students undertaking the general nursing programme at any one time. These numbers were augmented when student nurses from the nursing schools associated with the designated hospitals transferred to St James's.[7] Peta Taaffe, who was appointed director of nursing in 1989, made a major contribution to nurse education at St James's Hospital by facilitating the development of post-registration education for nurses. In 1989, the first course was established in burns, plastics and oromaxillofacial nursing. It was quickly followed by others including courses in intensive/coronary care (1989), theatre nursing (1990), gerontological nursing (1991) and accident and emergency nursing (1993). All of these programmes were subsequently developed into postgraduate diplomas and master's degrees with Trinity College. In 1997, four nurses from St James's Hospital were awarded a master's in gerontological nursing, becoming the first nurses to graduate from the university with a degree in nursing. In the short period since its foundation, the school of nursing had grown to become the school with the largest intake of pre-registration student nurses and with the highest number of post-registration nurse education programmes in the country.

Traditionally, pre-registration nurse education in Ireland was firmly based in the hospital service, with student nurses being an integral part of the nursing workforce. Pre-registration nurse education was a certificate programme in Ireland until 1996. During the 1990s, nursing education began to form affiliations with universities and, in

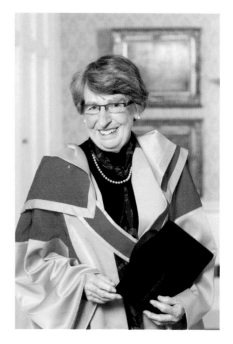

14.5   Dr Peta Taaffe when she received the honorary degree of LLD from the University of Dublin. Photograph: Trinity College Dublin.

line with these developments, the school of nursing began to plan an undergraduate nursing course with Trinity College. Initially this took the form of a diploma course and in 1996 the programme commenced with the first intake of seventy student nurses at St James's Hospital in conjunction with the newly established school of nursing and midwifery studies in Trinity College. These student nurses undertook supernumerary placements on hospital wards as opposed to being part of the nursing workforce. The move to a pre-registration diploma in nursing led to the establishment of the Nursing Practice Development Unit in St James's to support and guide students while on clinical placement on the wards. The registration and diploma programme was an interim phase while preparations went ahead to move nursing education to a degree-based programme, fully integrated within the higher education system. The new degree course in nursing commenced nationwide in 2002, the nursing students at St James's becoming undergraduate students at Trinity College. Initially based at St James's Hospital, the school of nursing and midwifery moved to a new location in D'Olier Street in 2002. The clinical base for nursing education at St James's Hospital is still housed in the Trinity Centre for Health Sciences. The changes in nursing education resulted in an overall reduction in the numbers of nurses qualified in Ireland. The resultant short-

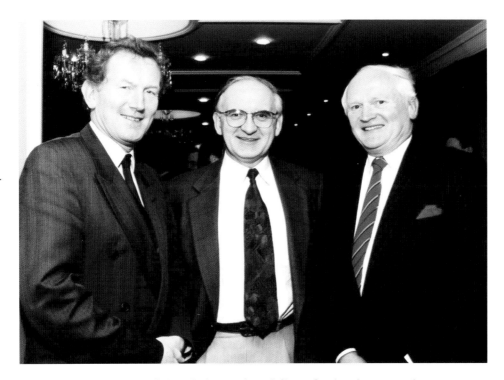

14.6   John Feely, professor of clinical pharmacology (left), Prof. Luke Clancy, consultant respiratory physician (centre) and Prof. Michael Walsh, consultant cardiologist (right). Private collection.

age of nurses in St James's Hospital peaked in 2000 and this led to a radical review of nurse recruitment and retention. The review recommended the international recruitment of nurses to meet service needs, an increase in the number of places available on pre-registration degree programmes and active encouragement of nurses who had left the health service to return to practice. Retention of nurses became a major goal and emphasis was placed on continuing professional development.

The development of new national centres

It was a sign of the growing significance of St James's Hospital that the Department of Health supported the establishment of a number of national medical centres on its campus. The National Medicines Information Centre (NMIC) was established in 1994, led by John Feely, professor of pharmacology and therapeutics and Kamal Sabra, chief pharmacist at St James's, to provide independent information about medicines to members of the healthcare professions, including general practitioners, community pharmacists, hospital doctors, pharmacists, nurses, dentists and professions allied to medicine. The National Centre for Pharmacoeconomics, with a remit to advance the discipline of health economics in relation to drug therapy in Ireland, was established by Feely in 1997. The centre undertakes research on the cost-effectiveness of different therapies for a range of conditions, and it monitors the comparative cost of medicines in European countries. Michael Barry was appointed as its first director. The success of these two developments made St James's Hospital the natural home for another innovative centre in 2001, which was also led by Feely. This was the Centre for Advanced Clinical Therapeutics, a non-profit organization with a remit to enable healthcare professionals and the pharmaceutical industry to keep abreast of advances in pharmaceutical medicine.

John Feely was appointed professor of pharmacology and therapeutics at Trinity College and physician to St James's Hospital in 1984. Feely studied medicine at University College Dublin and graduated in 1971. He undertook his general professional training in the Mater Hospital and subsequently did his specialist training in the medical school of the University of Dundee and in the department of clinical pharmacology in Vanderbilt University, Nashville. He built up a strong department of clinical pharmacology and therapeutics at St James's Hospital and Trinity College. He was particularly interested in the cause and treatment of high blood pressure and he developed a very successful hypertension clinic in the hospital. He published over 300 research papers, many of which appeared in international journals of high repute. He was also an inspirational registrar of the RCPI for many years. John Feely died at the age of 61 in 2009.

Health informatics

The latter half of the twentieth century saw an increasing awareness of the power of modern technology to improve communication systems in healthcare. Rory O'Moore, associate professor of clinical biochemistry at St James's Hospital and Trinity College, played a key role in the development of health informatics. This is a multidisciplinary field in which clinicians collaborate with other healthcare and information technology professionals. O'Moore was one of the pioneers of health informatics in Europe and led the development of the field in Ireland. In 1982, he organized the first major international conference on the subject to be held in Dublin. O'Moore was quick to realize the potential benefits that information and communications technology could offer to improve

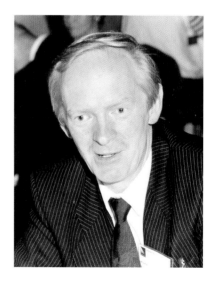

14.7   Rory O'Moore, professor of clinical biochemistry. Courtesy of Prof. Mona O'Moore.

the efficiency and effectiveness of laboratory medicine. He brought together a group of researchers in the department of computer science at Trinity College and in the department of electrical engineering at the Dublin Institute of Technology, as well as leading researchers in the health IT industry in hospitals and universities across Europe.

O'Moore led a highly innovative project, OpenLabs, funded by the European Commission between 1992 and 1995. OpenLabs focused on improving the efficiency and effectiveness of clinical laboratory services by integrating clinical decision support systems with laboratory information systems and equipment. This was a ground-breaking project that developed intelligent solutions to assist physicians in requesting laboratory tests and interpreting the results. OpenLabs was able to demonstrate that the adoption of these solutions could result in a significant reduction in unnecessary tests, thereby not only saving money but also ensuring that patients received the appropriate treatment as soon as possible. In 1991, O'Moore, in collaboration with Professor Jane Grimson of the department of computer science, established the Centre for Health Informatics in Trinity College Dublin.

Developments in cardiology and cardiac surgery

Michael Walsh, consultant cardiologist, submitted a proposal to the Royal City of Dublin Hospital (RCDH) Trust in 1994 requesting support to develop an institute for research and education in the specialities of cardiology, respiratory medicine and cardiothoracic surgery. The trust agreed to support this development, which became known as the RCDH Research and Education Institute. Based in Hospital 7, it was officially opened in 1996 by Dr Thomas (Tom) Mitchell, provost of Trinity College Dublin. Numerous peer-reviewed publications, master's and doctoral theses have been produced by researchers in the institute, and it has supported significant national and international collaborations in research. In 2004, the success of the RCDH Research and Education Institute led to the development of the Institute of Cardiovascular Science.

In 1996, at the request of the Department of Health, the hospital developed and submitted a competitive bid to establish a cardiac surgery unit in St James's, which would undertake 500 open-heart surgery cases annually. The department accepted the proposals from St James's Hospital, and a cardiac surgery unit, which cost £6 million, was opened in 2000. It was named in honour of Keith Shaw, who had introduced cardiac surgery to the Royal City of Dublin Hospital, Baggot Street, and who played a key role in the establishment of a national cardiac unit in the Mater Hospital. The new unit at St James's Hospital, which was led by Eilis McGovern, consultant cardiothoracic surgeon, dramatically reduced the waiting time for cardiac surgery in Ireland.

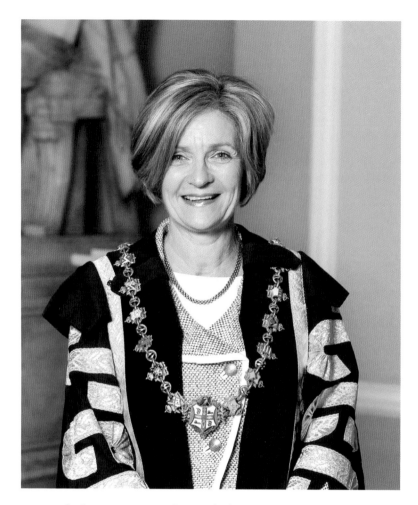

14.8   Prof. Eilis McGovern, consultant cardiothoracic surgeon, who became the first woman to be elected president of the Royal College of Surgeons in Ireland. Courtesy of the Royal College of Surgeons in Ireland.

Twenty-fifth anniversary celebrations

At the end of 1996, the first of a series of events took place to celebrate the twenty-fifth anniversary of the establishment of St James's Hospital. To symbolize the partnership that had successfully overseen the development of St James's as a major acute teaching hospital, three trees were planted, one by Jerry O'Dwyer, secretary of the Department of Health, representing the Department of Health, a second by Davis Coakley, dean of health sciences, representing Trinity College Dublin and a third by Ian Howie on behalf of the board of the hospital. Following the ceremony, O'Dwyer addressed the hospital board and his remarks are summarized in the minutes of the board:

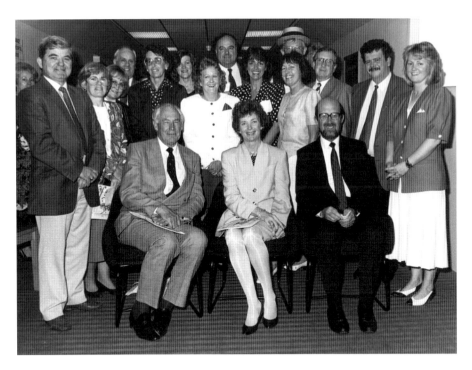

14.9   Visit of the president of Ireland, Mary Robinson, to St James's Hospital in 1997. Front row, left to right: Ian Howie, chairman of the board of St James's Hospital; the president; and John Scott, professor of biochemistry and experimental nutrition. Middle row: Jack Kelly, Aileen Walsh, name unknown, Peta Taaffe, Margaret Kelleher, Ita Cadwell, name unknown, name unknown, Jimmy Cullen and Mary Dooley. Back row: Jean Cullen, John Malone, Philomena Flood, John Fitzpatrick and Bob Fogarty. Courtesy of St James's Hospital.

He said that he was very pleased to be asked to participate in the ceremony as the Department of Health was very proud of St James's and its association with the hospital. He described St James's as a hospital with ambition and said it had realised all the goals it had set itself. He referred to the integration of other hospitals into St James's during the 1980s and the difficulties encountered during that period. He mentioned the remarkable series of firsts achieved at the hospital, e.g. in relation to haematology/oncology/bone marrow transplantation, HIV/AIDS, and management initiatives ... Mr O'Dwyer also referred to the developments in teaching, particularly post-graduate teaching. He mentioned the relationships fostered with other hospitals and the community, particularly with GPs in the area, which he said were remarkable.[8]

A number of celebrations took place throughout 1997, with the major event occurring in early September. This was inaugurated by President Mary Robinson in her last week in office as president of Ireland. A variety of activities took place over a three-day

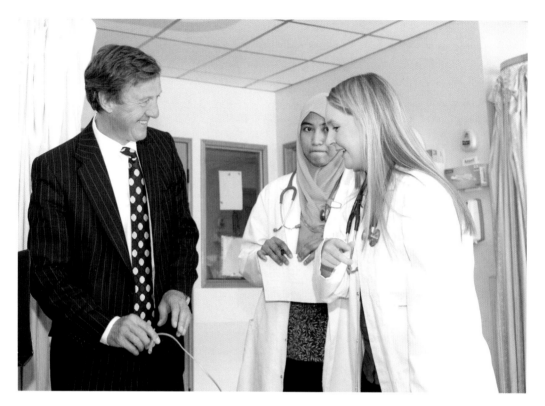

14.10 Dermot Moore, consultant vascular surgeon, teaching students. Photograph: Anthony Edwards.

period that were designed to highlight the hospital's achievements over the previous twenty-five years and to strengthen its links with the local community. Many of these events took place in an anniversary marquee that was erected in the grounds. One afternoon was devoted to a 'community showcase', when young people from the local area presented their talent through a range of performances, arts and craftwork. A number of public lectures on health issues were delivered in the Trinity Centre for Health Sciences. On the final day there was a series of academic and clinical lectures in the Trinity Centre that concentrated on recent medical research within the hospital.

The formal launch of the St James's Hospital Foundation was hosted by the Bank of Ireland in the house of lords on College Green, in 1997, with the taoiseach, Bertie Ahern, and the tánaiste, Mary Harney, as guests of honour. The foundation was established to raise additional funding for the hospital from private sources. During the launch, the chairman of St James's, Ian Howie, recalled the long tradition of private support for Dublin hospitals and went on to say: 'I believe the voluntary commitment that sustained the hospitals that preceded St James's still exists, especially as much of the care we provide is for the less-privileged sections of the community.'[9] Dermot Moore, a consultant vascular surgeon, was the first chairman of the foundation.

The year 1997 also marked the thirtieth anniversary of the establishment of the school of nursing, and to celebrate the occasion, the 1997 Nursing Awards ceremony was held in the marquee. Ninety student nurses were presented with their badges, certificates and prizes and the Anne Young Memorial Lecture was delivered by Cecily Begley, professor of nursing and midwifery and founding director of the school of nursing and midwifery studies at Trinity College. The celebrations concluded with a gala reception in the state apartments in Dublin Castle, hosted by the minister for health, Brian Cowen.

Ian Howie was awarded an honorary degree by the University of Dublin in 1998 to mark his major contribution to the development of St James's Hospital. The oration during the ceremony was read in Latin by Trinity's public orator, Professor John Luce. Having described Howie's major contributions to the university as a professor of zoology, registrar of the college and vice provost, Luce went on to say:

> But if you ask for an even loftier monument to his endeavours, you must contemplate the extended hospital complex at St James's. You see before you the chief architect of this most ample structure. From the start of the project (over 25 years ago) there has scarcely been a year when he has not been chairman of the St James's Hospital Board. It was his sweat, and his tears, that won most of the victories.[10]

Blood Transfusion Service Board moves to St James's

As a result of the adverse publicity surrounding the treatment of patients with infected blood products, there was a loss of public confidence in the Blood Transfusion Service Board (BTSB). In order to restore the institution's reputation, the minister and the Department of Health sought to improve the quality of both the management and the scientific laboratories of the BTSB. With these goals in mind they asked the board of St James's Hospital to second the hospital's CEO, Liam Dunbar, to act as CEO of the Blood Transfusion Service and Shaun McCann, consultant haematologist and director of the bone marrow transplant service, to act as medical director. It was a big request but, in the final analysis, the board accepted that the needs of the health service as a whole should be given priority and agreed to the secondments. John O'Brien took over as acting CEO of the hospital and the transition occurred smoothly. Dunbar was offered and accepted the permanent post of CEO of the Blood Transfusion Service in 1996 and O'Brien succeeded him as CEO of the hospital.

The Department of Health decided that the National Blood Centre, the new headquarters of the Blood Transfusion Service, should be located on an acute hospital campus. St James's Hospital was selected in 1997 and work began on a new building for the National Blood Centre a year later. On the grounds of St James's Hospital, the centre has its own independent board and management systems. The Blood Transfusion Service Board's name was changed to the Irish Blood Transfusion Service (IBTS) in 2000.

National Blood Centre

Micheál Martin, minister for health and children, officially opened the new pur-pose-built National Blood Centre in 2000. Apart from its core work of providing safe blood for transfusion, the new build-ing houses a number of related national centres including the National Blood Group Reference Laboratory under the auspices of the WHO, the National Tissue Typing Reference Laboratory and Ser-vices, the National Heart Valve Bank, the National Eye Bank and the Irish Unre-lated Bone Marrow Donor Registry.[11] The

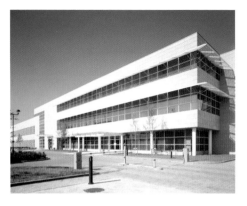

14.11   The National Blood Centre. Courtesy of the National Blood Centre.

presence of the IBTS on the St James's campus facilitates cooperation between the staff of the two institutions in haematological and molecular medicine. The IBTS possesses a well-equipped facility for the manufacture of molecular and cell-based therapies, which has led to joint collaborative research with several departments in the medical school and hospital. Emer Lawlor and Joan O'Riordan, both consultant haematologists to the IBTS, were allocated sessions in St James's Hospital. Lawlor took responsibility for blood transfusion and O'Riordan for the matched unrelated bone marrow trans-plant programme and long-term follow-up of patients in St James's. All these advances supported the management of patients with complex and challenging malignancies and bleeding disorders.

Scott Tallon Walker were the architects of the National Blood Centre. The shape of the building was dictated by the long, narrow nature of the site in the south-east-ern corner of the hospital, which is curved at its southern end by the Luas light-rail system. The building, clad in Wicklow granite, takes up this curve and creates a dynamic atrium space, which floods the centre with light.[12]

Creation of an academic square

The decision to locate the National Blood Centre in St James's Hospital yielded another significant benefit. The Trinity school of physiotherapy was on the site chosen for the new centre. The Eastern Health Board and the Department of Health offered the old Queen Mary building (former offices of the EHB), which was on the eastern side of the Trinity Centre for Health Sciences, to facilitate the decanting of the school of physiotherapy. The dean of health sciences, Davis Coakley, was aware that the 'Queen Mary' building was scheduled for demolition in the longer term, so he suggested that the Foundling Hospital buildings on the western side of the Trinity Centre would be more suitable. These buildings included the Georgian house used as the headquarters of the 4th Battalion of the Irish Volunteers during the Easter Rising. This option was agreed in negotiations between Trinity College, the Eastern Health Board, St James's Hospital and the Department of Health. The buildings were sensitively restored by the architects Maloney O'Beirne and Partners, to provide accommodation for the school of physiotherapy until phase 2 of the Trinity Centre for Health Sciences was completed. A two-storey concourse running the entire length along the back of the long, low building provides an attractive mingling space for staff and students. It is envisaged that these buildings will form the western range of an academic square, which will mirror the old squares on the Trinity College campus.

The recognition of hepatitis C and its consequences

It was known from the mid 1970s that some patients treated with blood products subsequently developed jaundice. Unlike infections with hepatitis A and hepatitis B, the virus causing the jaundice could not be identified with a serological test and was known as non-A, non-B hepatitis. When this form of hepatitis first presented, doctors thought that it generally followed a benign course, but in the 1980s it became apparent that in some patients, this form of hepatitis could lead to chronic liver disease, liver failure and liver cancer. In 1987, the virus causing non-A, non-B hepatitis was identified and it became known as hepatitis C. In 1991, a blood test became available that could be used as a screening test and this revealed that a significant number of patients who had been treated with blood products had been infected with the virus. Patients who were treated with infected blood concentrates, women who were given anti-D immunoglobulin during pregnancy and patients with haemophilia, had a high incidence of hepatitis C.

Consultants Donald Weir and Nap Keeling in the department of gastroenterology developed a special expertise in dealing with the condition and patients were offered treatment with recombinant interferon.[13] In 1994, Dermot Kelleher established a hepatology centre in Hospital 5, which formed part of the national response to the emergence of cases of hepatitis C. It provided integrated services for the treatment of all forms of liver disease and became a focus for research on viral diseases, such as hepatitis C, as well as other liver diseases.

Another significant development took place at this time. Owen Smith, consultant haematologist, who became director of the National Haemophilia Centre in 1995 following the retirement of Ian Temperley, organized the funding required to build a haemophilia centre. The centre was renamed the National Centre for Hereditary Coagulation Disorders. Apart from treating patients with haemophilia, the centre undertakes advanced research on coagulation deficiency syndromes. The hepatology centre and the coagulation centre moved, in 1998 and 2000 respectively, into a new building located near the Rialto entrance to the hospital.

The end of a long association

The long relationship between the Carmelite order and the chaplaincy in St James's Hospital came to an end in 2001 after 140 years. The departure was marked by a number of ceremonies and presentations and the hospital authorities expressed their enormous gratitude for the contribution and dedication of the Carmelite priests over many years. The Carmelites withdrew because of the problems caused by diminishing new vocations, together with the increasing number of elderly priests in need of care. In a commemorative booklet describing the history of the Carmelites in St James's Hospital, Revd Paddy Smyth, one of the chaplains, wrote:

> I wish to say thank you, not only on behalf of generations of chaplains, but also on behalf of the Carmelite order itself for the precious resource that the Union and St Kevin's especially, and in latter years St James's Hospital has been for our Irish Province.
>
> For many years we used the Union and St Kevin's as a pastoral training ground for most of our newly ordained priests. In the days when there were no such courses as clinical pastoral education, when there were no lectures available on listening skills, on grief counselling and on various other psychological aids that are available today, this campus was our private university. This is where most of our young priests spent 6 or 9 months learning the basics of pastoral care under the tutelage of older and wiser men like Fr John Coffey just to recall one name.
>
> Here they picked up those counselling and listening skills, not in the classroom or the lecture hall, but at the bedsides of the sick and the old and the dying and the poor. This too is where they learned the art of sharing the pain of the bereaved.[14]

Comprehensive capital developments

There were significant capital developments in the hospital in the opening years of the twenty-first century. A new chest pain assessment unit, designed to provide rapid assessment of chest pain in patients attending the emergency department, was completed in 2001. The hospital was experiencing great pressure to find beds for acutely ill patients presenting to the emergency department. This led to an excessive number of patients waiting for admission to a hospital bed. Patients on trolleys overflowed into areas of the hospital such as the day care unit and, as a consequence, people with appointments waiting for procedures to be carried out in the day care unit frequently had their appointments postponed, as did those waiting at home to be admitted for elective procedures. The government responded by making recurrent and capital funding available to the acute hospitals. As a result of this initiative, seventy-four additional beds were provided at St James's Hospital in 2003.

The main concourse of the new hospital was opened in 2004. Designed by Moloney O'Beirne, the spacious concourse includes six retail and restaurant units in a glazed

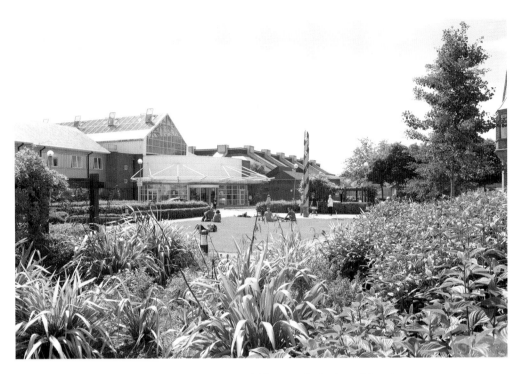

14.12 The new main entrance to St James's Hospital. Photograph: Anthony Edwards.

14.13 The new concourse of the hospital. Photograph: Anthony Edwards.

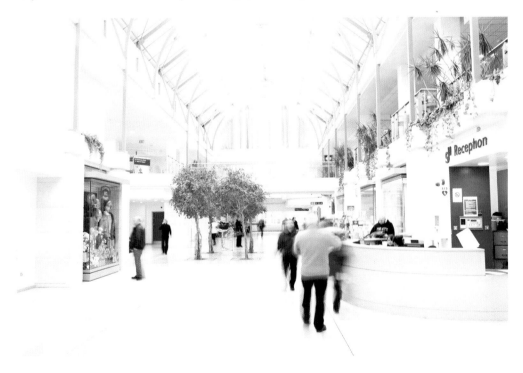

two-tier mall. This marked a commercial departure from the traditional Irish hospital, which typically had a small shop and canteen. Apart from being bright and spacious, the new concourse, with its shops and restaurants, provides a stream of income for the hospital. The number of patients, visitors and staff walking through make it resemble a 'busy shopping street'.[15] An underground car park with 375 spaces formed part of the development. This phase of the capital development also included the construction of a comprehensive range of day care facilities for endoscopy, haematology/oncology and surgery, three theatres, an outpatients department and an additional ward. The new facilities trebled day surgery capacity and doubled the capacity for the other specialties.

Ian Howie retires

Ian Howie retired as chairman of the board on 31 March 2002 and was succeeded by Dr Thomas Mitchell, former provost of Trinity College Dublin. Mitchell paid the following tribute to his predecessor:

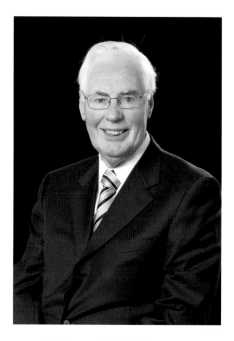

> For more than thirty years Professor Howie was at the centre of the remarkable redevelopment of the St James's site, helping shape the vision and providing continuity, drive, experience and wisdom. His tireless work for the hospital in a voluntary capacity is an inspiring example of a generous civic spirit and of the importance of voluntarism to the effective working of our public services. The hospital and the country are in his debt.[16]

The capital redevelopment programmes that Ian Howie had led over his thirty years of association with the hospital had changed the environment of St James's Hospital beyond recognition.

14.14   Dr Thomas Mitchell, chairman of the board of St James's Hospital. Photograph: Anthony Edwards.

Tom Mitchell graduated in classics from University College Galway and subsequently studied at Cornell University in New York. He was appointed professor of classics at Swarthmore College in Pennsylvania, and in 1979 was appointed professor of Latin at Trinity College Dublin. He served as provost of Trinity between 1991 and 2001. Mitchell identified the Faculty of Health Sciences as one of his priority areas for development, and this resulted in a very productive relationship between the teaching hospitals and Trinity College during his provostship.

Significant expansion of the Trinity Centre

A further phase of development of the Trinity Centre took place between 1999 and 2002, which included a substantial extension to provide accommodation for the schools of physiotherapy, occupational therapy, radiation therapy, the academic unit of oncology, and the department of pharmacology and clinical therapeutics. Two major research developments, the Institute of Molecular Medicine and the John Durkan Leukaemia Research Laboratories, were added to this phase. This involved a significant expansion and permission was granted by Dublin Corporation to add an extra floor to the Trinity Centre, converting it from a two-storey to a three-storey building. The vaults of the original City Workhouse, which were constructed in 1703, lay under the site of the development. When made aware of these vaults, the Dublin City Council planning department decided they should be retained. As a result, the architects had to redesign the whole of the proposed building.

The scene was now set for the hospital's objective to create centres of international standing. This strategy was outlined by the chairman of the board, Tom Mitchell, in 2003:

> The hospital is already moving energetically and creatively to develop even stronger centres of international quality in areas such as cancer care, ageing, haematology and cardiovascular diseases and continues to explore possibilities for partnership that would facilitate the creation of a world-class academic health centre with the facilities and critical mass of expert clinicians and researchers capable of providing advanced services of the highest international standard. As the government proceeds to create a knowledge society, its strategy should give a central place to medical science, where Ireland's human resources and research potential are second to none. A major centre of international stature, such as that envisaged by St James's, would then become a necessity.[17]

The Institute of Molecular Medicine

An Institute of Molecular Medicine was established under the auspices of the department of medicine in 1995. The purpose of the institute was to promote the use of genetics in the management of cancer, degenerative diseases and birth defects. An MSc in molecular medicine was introduced in 1997, which was the first of its kind in Europe. Dermot Kelleher, consultant gastroenterologist, obtained a grant from the Higher Education Authority (HEA) to provide accommodation for the Institute of Molecular Medicine, and this grant was used to add 4,000 square metres of research space as part of the second phase of construction of the Trinity Centre for Health Sciences.

It was opened in November 2003 by the minister for education, Noel Dempsey, and John Scott, professor of experimental nutrition, delivered the first Institute of Molecular Medicine lecture. The proximity of the Institute of Molecular Medicine

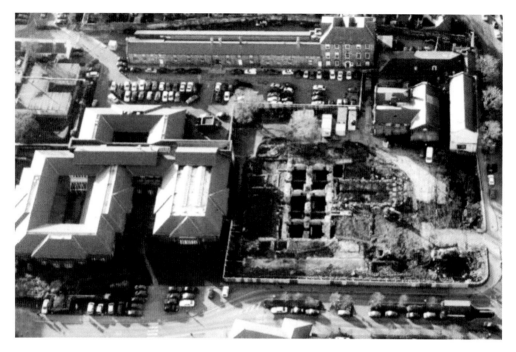

14.15 Aerial view of the construction of Phase 2 of the Trinity Centre for Health Sciences, showing the vaults of the dining hall of the Foundling Hospital and the foundations of the Victorian Church of Ireland chapel attached to the front. Private collection.

14.16 Phase 2 of the Trinity Centre for Health Sciences. Photograph: Anthony Edwards.

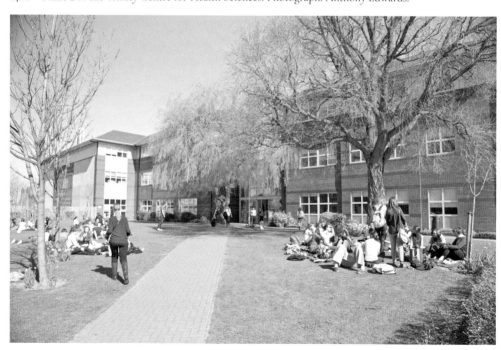

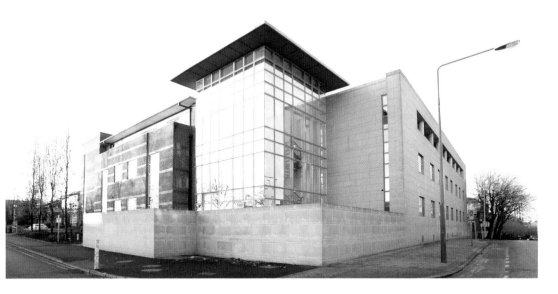

14.17　The Institute of Molecular Medicine and the Trinity Centre for Health Sciences, which stand on the right of the main entrance to the hospital on James's Street. Photograph: Anthony Edwards.

to the hospital wards provided a close link between research and healthcare delivery. The institute became a fulcrum for interdisciplinary research, where scientists and clinicians work side by side.[18] It attracts international researchers to the school of medicine, and research in the institute concentrates on areas such as cancer, inflammatory disease, immunity, neuropsychiatric disorders and the genetics of common conditions. It provides a range of postgraduate research programmes and a four-year PhD programme in molecular medicine.[19]

In 2016, the Institute of Molecular Medicine was merged with the Sir Patrick Dun's Laboratory to form a new entity, the Trinity Institute of Translational Medicine. This institute brings together over 40 principal investigators and 150 scientists. Translational research brings advances made in the laboratory to patients in the wards and forms a key aspect of cancer research at the hospital.

The John Durkan Leukaemia Research Laboratories

The John Durkan Leukaemia Research Laboratories in the Institute of Molecular Medicine were funded by a donation of €2.5 million from the John Durkan Leukaemia Trust and by support from the Bone Marrow for Leukaemia Trust. John Durkan was a very successful Irish jockey and trainer who died in St James's Hospital at the age of 31 from leukaemia. Research in the laboratories is focused on leukaemia and other haematological malignancies. This purpose-built facility has allowed researchers at St James's Hospital to undertake significant research programmes with a number of international partners. The development, which was led by Shaun McCann, included a lecture theatre, also named after John Durkan. The laboratories and lecture theatre were opened in 2003.

Major refurbishment of the Burkitt Ward was necessary at this time to make it more suitable for the management of severely immuno-compromised patients. The alterations provided twenty-one air-conditioned en-suite rooms for the treatment of leukaemia and related diseases, and six new beds were added. These changes greatly facilitated the development of the National Blood and Bone Marrow Transplant Programme.

St Luke's Radiation Oncology Centre

In 2000, the minister for health, Micheál Martin, appointed an expert working group on the future configuration of Irish radiation oncology services. The group was chaired by Donal Hollywood, Marie Curie professor of clinical oncology. In 2003 the group published its report, which proposed that radiation services should be situated either in an existing multidisciplinary hospital or as part of a comprehensive cancer centre.[20] This recommendation led to a decision to base two major radiotherapy centres in Dublin, one in Cork and one in Galway.[21] Mary Harney, the minister for health and children, established an international committee, chaired by the chief medical officer, Dr Jim Kiely, to advise on the location of the radiation oncology centres in Dublin. All the Dublin hospitals were invited to submit proposals to the committee. The St James's proposal was coordinated by Hollywood and it was chosen as the centre for south Dublin.

St Luke's Radiation Oncology Centre in St James's Hospital provides a comprehensive service encompassing clinical care, education and research. It was a major step forward in the hospital's strategy to develop an excellent multidisciplinary cancer treatment service spanning all areas of cancer care. The radiation centre building forms the eastern limb of the central hospital square and was designed by O'Connell Mahon Architects in partnership with Murray O'Laoire Architects. It is a three-storey structure over basement with an atrium at the core of the building, which provides natural light. The treatment, examination and research facilities, together with inpatient beds, form the perimeter of the building. The facility contains four linear accelerators and it was formally opened by the minister for health and children, Dr James Reilly, in 2011. It greatly improved the service to patients as well as creating an ideal environment for world-class research.

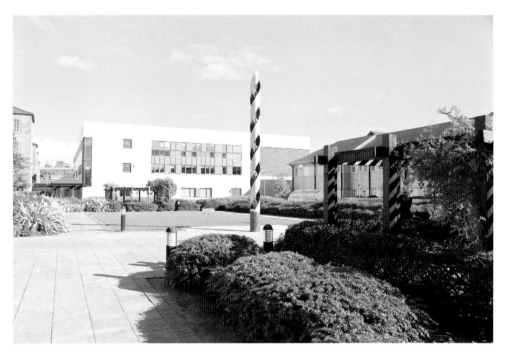

14.18   St Luke's Radiation Oncology Centre. Photograph: Anthony Edwards.

14.19   The central square of the hospital. Courtesy of St James's Hospital.

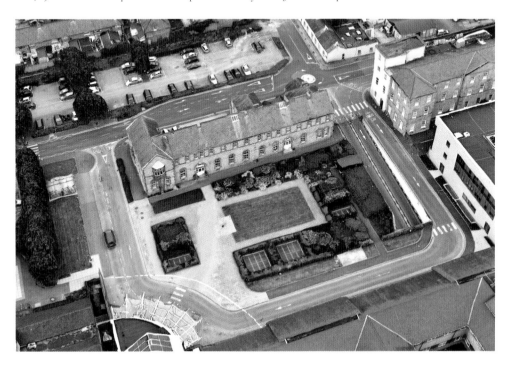

An outstanding oncologist

Donal Hollywood established the multidisciplinary Academic Unit of Clinical and Molecular Oncology (AUCMO), the first academic oncology department in Ireland. The centre linked up with the National Institutes of Health (NIH) Telesynergy system, creating a unique association between American, European and Irish centres of excellence in cancer treatment. This system enables scientists and clinicians at multiple laboratories to participate in teleconferences to discuss the optimum treatment for patients with complex and rare tumours. It also promotes national and international expertise in cancer research and treatment. The school of radiation therapy relocated to the Trinity Centre for Health Sciences in St James's Hospital from St Luke's Hospital in 2010. All these developments represented a major step forward for cancer treatment, research and education in Ireland.[22]

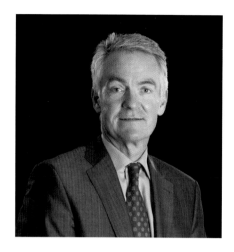

14.20   Donal Hollywood, Marie Curie professor of clinical oncology. Photograph: Anthony Edwards.

Hollywood, who had become a household name for over a decade in Ireland for the role he played in devising a plan for the roll-out of radiotherapy services across the state, died from cancer in May 2013 at the age of 53.[23] He had studied medicine at University College Dublin, graduating in 1983. After general professional training in Dublin he worked at the Hammersmith Hospital (London), the Imperial Cancer Research Fund (London) and Baylor College of Medicine (USA), where he developed his expertise in clinical and molecular oncology. His main research interest was the development of biologically optimized radiation therapy using novel targeted agents and precision radiation. He was president-elect of the European Society of Radiotherapy and Oncology at the time of his death.

Irish National Cancer Control Programme

To achieve best outcomes from cancer treatment, patients need multidisciplinary care at specialized cancer centres. Over the years, cancer surgery was divided into a number of subspecialties and the role of multidisciplinary team conferences in decision-making became increasingly important in line with best international practice. Key elements of the current cancer programme at St James's Hospital have been led by John Reynolds, professor of surgery at St James's Hospital and Trinity College. Reynolds held fellowships at the University of Pennsylvania and Wistar Institute in

Philadelphia and at the Memorial Sloan Kettering Cancer Center in New York before his return to Dublin in 1996, where he developed an international reputation for his clinical and research activities in oesophageal and stomach cancer.

As part of the Good Friday Agreement, signed in Belfast in 1998, there was a specific mention of cancer services on the island of Ireland and the need to improve the quality and range of these services. In 1999, the National Cancer Institute (NCI) in Bethesda, Maryland, embarked on an international partnership with the developing programmes on the island of Ireland. The All Ireland–NCI Cancer Consortium was established to improve cancer treatment, educa-

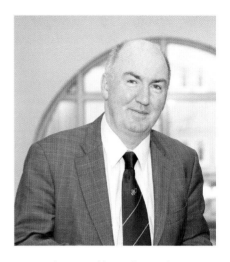

14.21　John Reynolds, professor of surgery. Photograph: Anthony Edwards.

tion and research across the island. The consortium was an important milestone in the development of cancer services in Ireland as it placed pressure on the governments, north and south, to deliver resources. Peter Daly represented the oncology community in the Republic of Ireland on the consortium.

In 2002 a consortium of hospitals, which included Our Lady's Children's Hospital, the Coombe Women's Hospital and the Midland Health Board, under the leadership of St James's Hospital, applied successfully for funding from the HRB to strengthen infrastructure for cancer clinical trials within the participating institutions. John Kennedy, consultant medical oncologist, was appointed as the clinical director and John Reynolds as the scientific director. The Cancer Clinical Trials Office (CCTO) was opened at St James's Hospital in 2003. Recruitment to clinical trials increased dramatically after the establishment of the CCTO.

The National Cancer Forum was established in 2000 as the national advisory body on cancer policy to the minister for health and children. In 2006, a report by the National Cancer Forum recommended that all cancer care should be provided through a national system of four major cancer control networks and eight cancer centres. St James's Hospital was designated as one of the major centres.[24] The hospital has emerged as the largest single provider of cancer treatment in Ireland with national and supra-regional centres for bone marrow transplantation, leukaemia and lymphoma, oesophageal and gastric cancer, early upper gastrointestinal neoplasia and skin, lung, prostate, breast, gynaecological, head and neck, and maxillofacial cancers. Rapid-access clinics have been developed in all of the cancer programmes.

A psycho-oncology service was established by consultant psychiatrist Anne Marie O'Dwyer in 2003 with the purpose of supporting the psychological well-being of patients with cancer. This service was the first of its kind in Ireland and filled a significant shortcoming in the holistic approach to the care of patients. The hospital has also developed a dedicated specialist cancer genetics service. The centre provides risk assessment, counselling and genetic testing for individuals and families at increased risk of cancer. David Gallagher was appointed as a consultant medical oncologist with a special interest in cancer genetics in 2011. It is anticipated that targeted treatment based on genetic information for individuals with cancer will become much more common in the years ahead. Cancer treatment at St James's is facilitated by the quality and scale of the diagnostic services on site, which include molecular diagnostics, PET and CT scanning and MRI. International evidence demonstrates that patients with cancer who are treated in academic-led and research-orientated hospitals have a better prognosis.

Building on these strengths, there was a proposal, led by John Kennedy, John Reynolds, Paul Browne and John O'Leary, to develop a Trinity Cancer Institute at St James's Hospital. In October 2016, the chairman of St James's Hospital, Paul Donnelly, and the provost of Trinity College, Dr Patrick Prendergast, signed an agreement to establish a cancer institute. One of the principal objectives of the new institute is to build up a core of international cancer experts to attract major clinical trials in oncology. Speaking of the new development the provost said:

> We will be educating the next generation of cancer clinicians, health professionals and scientists. Both Trinity and St James's Hospital share a long history together training medical doctors, nurses and health professionals who have treated the people of Dublin and Ireland with expertise and dedication. With this new institute we intend to lead the way in innovative new cancer treatment.[25]

Paul Browne, head of the medical school and professor of haematology, pointed out that, whereas the majority of children suffering from cancer enter clinical trials, the rate for adults in Ireland in 2016 was between 5 and 10 per cent. Browne is director of the National Adult Stem Cell Transplant Programme at St James's Hospital. He trained in Dublin and in the University of Minnesota, and since returning to Ireland in 1997 he has led the development of therapeutic programmes for leukaemia and myeloma.

Centre for Advanced Medical Imaging

The Health Research Board (HRB) awarded a major grant (€3.5 million) in 2006 for the development of the Centre for Advanced Medical Imaging on the St James's campus. The centre evolved out of a collaborative endeavour between the department of diagnostic imaging and the departments of cardiology and oncology. The Centre for Advanced Medical Imaging explores concepts that have the potential to lead to clinical benefit using advanced imaging equipment. The development, led by James (Jim) Meaney, consultant radiologist, opened in 2008.

The first PET-CT scanner was installed in 2008 on the ground floor of Hospital 1, one of the surviving Foundling Hospital buildings, which was designed by the architect Francis Johnston in 1801. This highly sensitive scanner is of great value to patients with a variety of conditions, as it is capable of identifying small lesions with great precision and is a most important tool in the staging of various malignancies.

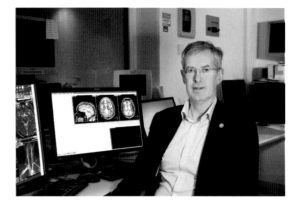

14.22   Prof. James Meaney, consultant radiologist. Photograph: Anthony Edwards.

Departure of CEO

John O'Brien, the CEO, left the hospital in 2006 on a five-year secondment to the Health Services Executive (HSE). O'Brien made a very significant contribution to the development of the hospital. According to the chairman, Tom Mitchell, he brought:

> an unusually wide range of experience and skill to the post, and during the last ten years he has presided over a remarkable era of development at the hospital, which has brought an array of new facilities, major organisational changes, and the development of a range of specialties that has elevated St James's to a leading position as a national provider of tertiary and fourth level services.[26]

O'Brien was succeeded by the deputy CEO, Ian Carter, and Eilish Hardiman, the director of nursing, was appointed deputy CEO.

Mercer's Institute for Successful Ageing

The development of the Mercer's Institute for Research on Ageing, which was established in 1988, was a significant milestone in the development of a centre of excellence for older people in St James's Hospital. However, new capital was needed to provide modern clinical and rehabilitation facilities together with accommodation for teaching and research. The construction of a new purpose-built centre became a major goal for Davis Coakley, Bernard Walsh and Conal Cunningham, consultant physicians in geriatric medicine, and for Brian Lawlor, consultant in old age psychiatry. A draft brief was submitted to the Department of Health and to the design team of the hospital in 1986, and the development control plan of the hospital was

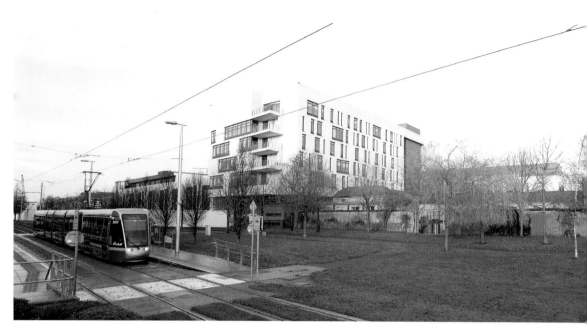

14.23   Mercer's Institute for Successful Ageing (MISA). Photograph: Anthony Edwards.

revised to ensure that the proposed centre would fit on the campus and relate to the diagnostic and service departments of the new hospital. The construction of the centre did not go ahead at that time because Ireland was in the midst of the severe economic depression of the 1980s and capital funding was not available.

A greatly revised and updated proposal for a centre of excellence was submitted to the Eastern Regional Health Authority (ERHA) in 2002. The chances of seeing the centre built increased significantly when Atlantic Philanthropies, an American charity established by Chuck Feeney, decided to shift its investment programme in Ireland from third-level education to ageing. The charity decided to support the centre initially by co-funding with the Department of Health and Children a full-time chair and a senior lecturer in geriatric medicine together with support staff. Rose Anne Kenny, who has an international reputation in falls and syncope, was appointed to the chair in 2005 and Joseph Harbison, who has a special interest in stroke, was appointed senior lecturer in 2006.

St James's Hospital received a grant of almost $17.1 million from Atlantic Philanthropies towards the construction costs of the centre in 2006. The grant was conditional on the Department of Health and Children and the HSE providing the balance needed to build the centre, which was to cost in the region of €50 million. Not long after the American funding was approved, the country found itself in the biggest financial crisis since the foundation of the state. During this critical period, the chair-

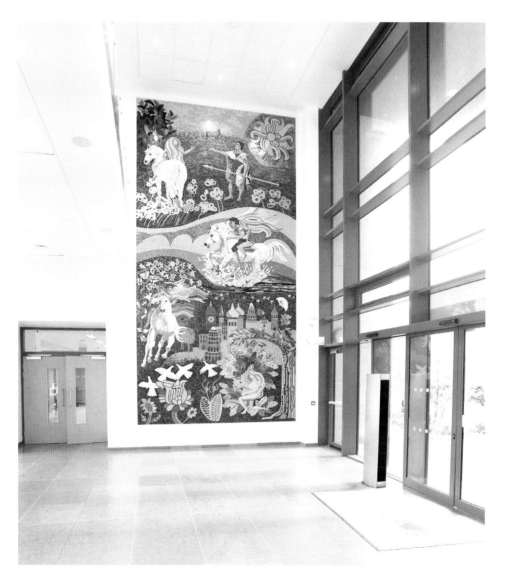

14.24   Tír na nÓg mosaic by Desmond Kinney in the entrance foyer of the Mercer's Institute for Successful Ageing (MISA) building. Photograph: Anthony Edwards.

man of the board, Tom Mitchell, continued to give the project his full support. Mary Harney, the minister for health and children, was also very supportive of the development and in 2009, the minister and the HSE made the commitment to provide the necessary funding.

Moloney O'Beirne Architects was appointed as the design team, and BAM Building Ltd secured the construction contract. The completed building was handed over to the hospital in April 2016. The building is seven storeys high and contains a large

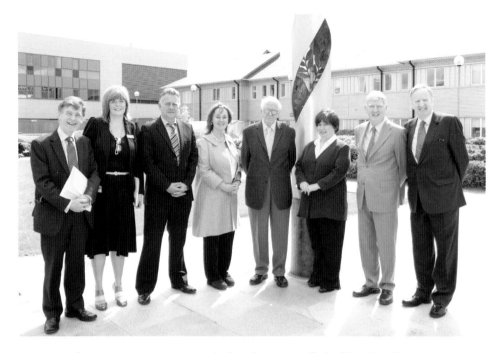

14.25   At a function in St James's Hospital when the minister for health and children, Mary Harney, announced the funding for Mercer's Institute for Successful Ageing (MISA). Left to right: Prof. Bernard Walsh (MISA steering group); Carol Murphy (steering group); Ian Carter (CEO of St James's Hospital and steering group); Prof. Rose Anne Kenny (steering group); the late former taoiseach Garret FitzGerald (steering group); Harney; Colin McCrea (senior vice president, Atlantic Philanthropies); and Prof. Davis Coakley (steering group). Courtesy of St James's Hospital.

ambulatory care facility with specialist clinical areas for falls and blackouts, bone disorders, stroke prevention and memory disorders together with extensive rehabilitation facilities. The Martha Whiteway Day Hospital, which provides day care for older people with all types of mental health problems, was moved from St Patrick's University Hospital to the ground floor of the new institute.

The institute has 116 beds with acute, general rehabilitation and stroke rehabilitation wards. There are extensive research laboratories in a four-storey wing off the main building. The institute also has a specially designed creative life centre to explore the role of art, music and other cultural activities in enriching the ageing experience. There are extensive education and training facilities to help up-skill professionals and carers and to encourage positive attitudes to ageing among healthcare workers and students. The Mercer's Institute for Successful Ageing (MISA) was opened by the president of Ireland, Michael D. Higgins, in December 2016. The MISA building won the Royal Institute of the Architects of Ireland (RIAI) award for 'best health building' in 2017.

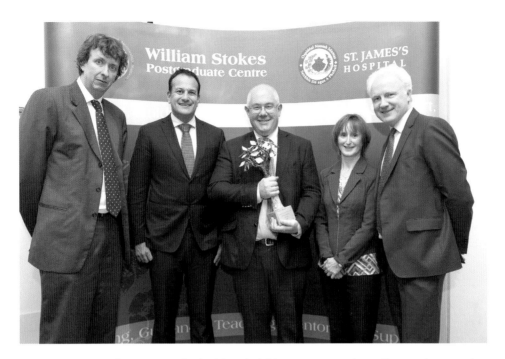

14.26   Dr Leo Varadkar, minister for health and children, presenting the William Stokes Award to Professor Joseph Harbison. Left to right: Paul Donnelly, chairman of the board of St James's Hospital; Varadkar; Harbison; Prof. Gaye Cunnane, director of postgraduate education; and Lorcan Birthistle, CEO. The William Stokes Postgraduate Award was established in St James's Hospital to recognize consultants who have made innovative clinical contributions and important research discoveries, with a particular emphasis on the benefits to patient care and well-being. Photograph: Anthony Edwards.

Leadership and commitment

Tom Mitchell stepped down as chairman of the board in 2011 after holding the office for nine years. Speaking of Mitchell's achievements, John Scott told the board of the hospital that St James's had become a great teaching hospital and that much of this could be attributed to Mitchell's leadership and commitment. The hospital had the widest range of services in the country and the highest throughput of patients. It was also the most successful research hospital, and its consultants were being increasingly recognized for their contributions to Irish medicine.[27] There was a seamless transition between Mitchell and the next chairman of the board, Diarmuid (Derry) Shanley. Shanley was professor of oral health in Trinity College and had considerable administrative experience. He was dean of dental affairs for many years and subsequently dean of the Faculty of Health Sciences. He played a major role in international dental affairs and he was the main driver behind the construction of a new dental hospital and school of dentistry in Lincoln Place.

Financial crisis

The moratorium imposed on recruitment during the difficult years following the 2008 financial crisis had a major impact on services and staff. By 2011, costs were rising and the hospital was facing more cutbacks. The staff struggled to maintain services to patients, and despite the cutbacks there was a significant increase in inpatient, day care and outpatient activity. In 2011, there was a cut of €21 million in the annual hospital budget, and this was followed by a further cut of €25 million in 2012. This called for measures such as the restructuring of staff replacements and staff overtime, a plan to increase the income from private patients and the renegotiation of contracts with vendors. Major efforts were made by all the staff to protect the clinical services. In 2012, the hospital, despite

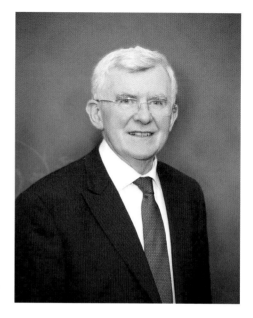

14.27 Prof. Diarmuid Shanley, chairman of the board of St James's Hospital, 2011–14. Photograph: Anthony Edwards.

suffering the sixth successive reduction in its allocation, delivered a further increase in patient services, providing treatment for 25,406 inpatients, 95,047 day care patients and 223,650 outpatients. Commenting on this phenomenon, the chairman of the board wrote:

> The essential role played by all our staff in the care of patients including security, catering, administrative, maintenance, executive colleagues, with clinical and consultant staff, is to their credit. Much appreciation is due to all of them for the palpable spirit of collegiality they generate. Each day and night they do everything in their power to provide the highest standard of care to promote the comfort, health and dignity of our patients despite resource challenges.[28]

In 2013, the budget reduction was less severe, with a cut of €9 million. The hospital was instructed by the HSE to reduce staffing by 140. The reduction in hospital staffing occurred at the same time as resources for social support in the community were being cut, making it difficult to discharge many of the more dependent patients. The hospital faced major challenges in the emergency department as a consequence of delayed discharges and this in turn led to the postponement of the admission of patients for elective surgical and medical procedures. The situation was further aggravated as a result of the significant reduction in consultant salaries, which was introduced in 2012.

This led to predictable difficulties in the filling of both new and replacement posts with high-calibre candidates.

During this period of great financial uncertainty the hospital had a strong, highly competent and lateral-thinking senior management. This team, which included CEO Ian Carter, deputy CEO Eilish Hardiman and director of finance Brian Fitzgerald, worked closely with the clinicians to ensure that services to patients were protected as much as possible under very difficult circumstances.

Clinical Research Facility

Despite the cutbacks, the infrastructure of the hospital continued to develop. In 2006, a team led by Dermot Kelleher received a grant from the Wellcome Trust and the HRB to build a clinical research facility at St James's Hospital that would be linked to a wider network of clinical research teams in Dublin. Kelleher had graduated from Trinity College in 1978 and completed his specialist training in gastroenterology in Sir Patrick Dun's Hospital under Donald Weir. He subsequently received a Fogarty scholarship for a research fellowship in the University of California, San Diego, where he carried out research in immunology and coeliac disease. On his return to Ireland, he was appointed Wellcome senior fellow in clinical sciences at Trinity College and consultant gastroenterologist at St James's Hospital. He succeeded Weir as professor of clinical medi-

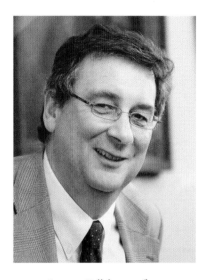

14.28   Dermot Kelleher, professor of medicine and head of the medical school. Photograph: University of British Colombia.

cine in 2001 and in 2006 he was elected head of the school of medicine and vice provost for medical affairs. The Clinical Research Facility (CRF) provides a means for clinicians, the healthcare industry and other partners to explore and test innovative therapies and technologies in areas such as infectious diseases, cardiovascular disease, haematology and hepatology. It also reduces the time it takes to introduce new research advances into everyday clinical practice.

The CRF has high-technology features to enable cutting-edge experimental medical research. These include a research pharmacy capable of safely compounding cancer drugs and handling novel gene therapies and vaccines. It contains inpatient isolation rooms in which to nurse patients with infections or compromised immune systems, a neuropsychology suite for high-quality assessment of brain activity, and a sample processing laboratory for rapid preparation and storage of biolog-

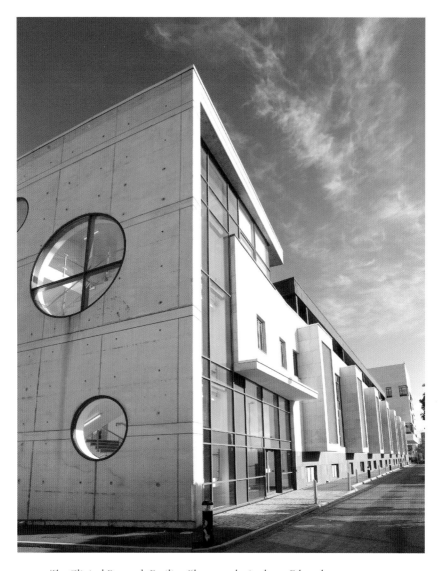

14.29   The Clinical Research Facility. Photograph: Anthony Edwards.

ical samples. The new centre was opened in May 2013 by the taoiseach, Enda Kenny. The chairman of the hospital described it 'as a landmark development that means Irish clinical science is being recognized internationally as world-class'.[29] The three-storey building also houses the Institute of Cardiovascular Science and an inpatient facility for haemophilia and hepatology.

Kelleher resigned as professor of medicine and head of the school of medicine in 2012, when he was appointed principal of the Faculty of Medicine in Imperial College London.

The Institute of Cardiovascular Science

The Institute of Cardiovascular Science, which was established in 2004, was funded by the Royal City of Dublin Hospital Trust. It was a partnership between the university and its two main teaching hospitals, St James's Hospital and the Adelaide and Meath Hospital incorporating the National Children's Hospital (AMNCH) in Tallaght. The institute facilitates all cardiac and cardiovascular research on the campus. The aims of the institute are to increase the understanding of cardiovascular disease in order to improve and develop prevention, diagnosis, treatment and rehabilitation strategies. The main focus of the institute is on research, but it is also engaged in the development and delivery of education and in coordinated service development.

The institute's multidisciplinary research programme comprises four main themes: cardiac imaging; cardiovascular risk estimation and health; inflammation and vascular biology; and invasive cardiology. There is a focus on cardiovascular imaging and the institute works closely with the Centre for Advanced Medical Imaging on the St James's campus. The development of the institute was led by Michael Walsh, associate professor of cardiology. Walsh graduated from UCD in 1965 and, after filling a number of senior house officer positions, he decided to specialize in cardiology. He was a registrar in cardiology in the Ulster Hospital, Belfast, and in the Mater Hospital, Dublin, before moving to Canada in 1975, where he was chief resident in cardiology at the University of Alberta Hospital in Edmonton. He was appointed consultant cardiologist in Craigavon Hospital in 1977 and two years later he joined the staff of St James's hospital. He became a founding fellow of the European Society of Cardiology in 1988. Michael Walsh, who died in 2016, was highly respected as a cardiologist and teacher of both undergraduate and postgraduate students.

Drug-resistant tuberculosis

Over the last twenty years tuberculosis has presented a new challenge to the health services due to the increase in multidrug-resistant tuberculosis (MDR TB). Most cases emanate from countries of high prevalence, where local public health is poor. MDR TB occurs when patients fail to take their anti-tuberculosis treatment properly. The treatment required for MDR TB is rigorous and takes at least two years, including the use of injections for the first six months. The breakdown in public health services in Eastern Europe, caused by the collapse of the Soviet Union, resulted in the emergence of MDR TB which was then carried to other countries by migrants. There were also cases of MDR TB in Irish patients, many of them due to substance abuse, but in more recent years, patients with MDR TB have been largely from Eastern Europe and Africa. St James's Hospital was seen as being in a strong position to confront this new challenge, as the TB service had access to the excellent facilities in the National Mycobacteria Reference Laboratory, which was established in the microbiology department in 2001.

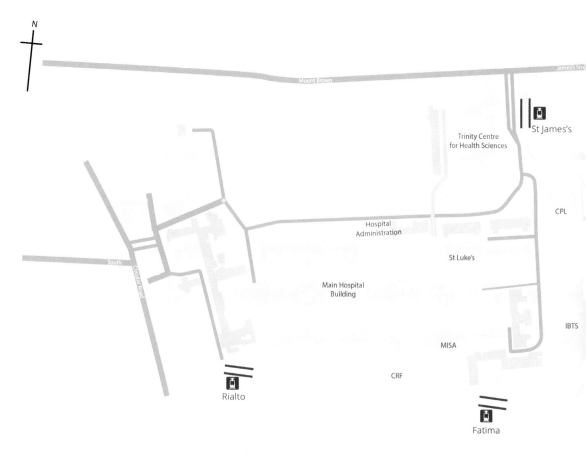

14.30   St James's campus in 2015, with new developments in grey and older buildings in blue. Image:
Anthony Edwards.

The TB service transferred from Peamount Hospital to St James's Hospital in
2005. As part of the transfer, the HSE agreed to fund the development of a dedicated
building for the management of TB. This would include modern inpatient and outpatient facilities for patients with complicated TB, including MDR TB. A temporary
facility was developed in Hospital 5, which included the construction of three negative pressure rooms to nurse patients with TB. In 2006, the HSE gave the go-ahead
to proceed with the development of a fit-for-purpose supra-regional TB unit with a
target opening date in 2009. However, the funding of the unit was one of the casualties of the economic collapse and the stringent cutbacks that resulted from it. Joseph
(Joe) Keane, the director of the service, continued to develop the TB programme in
very inadequate facilities. He now leads a world-class translational TB programme in
liaison with Trinity College and the Institute of Molecular Medicine, with funding
from the HRB, Science Foundation Ireland and the Royal City of Dublin Hospi-

tal Trust. The team has an active and highly successful research programme. Their work has greatly improved the understanding of the immune response to TB, and this knowledge is helping the search for a better and more effective vaccine.

Proposal for a private hospital

In 2005, the minister for health, Mary Harney, received government approval to locate private hospitals on the grounds of eight public hospitals throughout the country. The minister hoped to move private patients out of public beds to the new private hospitals and in the process free up approximately a thousand beds for public patients. A consortium named Synchrony Healthcare signed an agreement with the HSE and St James's Hospital to build an eight-storey private hospital near the Rialto entrance, which would provide 195 inpatient beds, 72 day care beds and eight operating theatres. There was considerable local opposition to the plan, as it entailed demolishing the early twentieth-century chapel.

The overall scheme was affected by the economic downturn, and the HSE service plan for 2009 stated that the plan to build private hospitals on public hospital sites would only proceed to the construction phase 'subject to satisfactory banking arrangements'. The promoters of the private hospitals had to deal with a rapidly changing funding climate. As the recession progressed, it became increasingly difficult to get support from the banks. Moreover, there was a fall in the number of Irish people who were able to afford private health insurance. In 2011, Synchrony Healthcare received full planning permission to proceed with the construction of the private hospital at St James's. At this stage, it was obvious that the deepening financial crisis was proving to be an insurmountable obstacle to the private hospital strategy. As a consequence, the HSE made no mention of co-located hospitals in its service plan for 2011. Strategies were now being put in place to bring about a seismic contraction in the number of hospital beds rather than an expansion. In this environment, Synchrony Healthcare failed to get banking support and the plan to build a private hospital at St James's was not realized. Just a few years later, the land identified for the private hospital would become part of the site for new national children's hospital.

The new children's hospital

Hospital care for children in Dublin has been divided between three hospitals since 1956: Our Lady's Children's Hospital, Crumlin; the National Children's Hospital, Tallaght; and Temple Street Children's University Hospital. Of these, Our Lady's Children's Hospital, Crumlin, which was founded in 1956, is the largest, with 227 beds and cots, including 38 day-case beds. It is a national centre for a range of specialties, including childhood cancers and blood disorders, cardiac diseases, burns, cystic fibrosis and clinical genetics. It is a teaching hospital for students from University

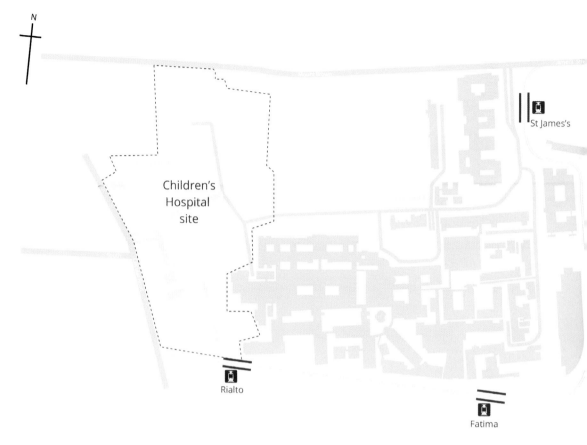

14.31 St James's Hospital in 2018, with the site of the new children's hospital. Image: Anthony Edwards.

College Dublin, Trinity College Dublin and the Royal College of Surgeons in Ireland. The National Children's Hospital was founded in 1821 and was the first hospital in Ireland and Great Britain to be established specifically for the care and treatment of children. In 1965, the first paediatric haematology service in Ireland was established in the hospital. The National Children's Hospital moved from Harcourt Street to Tallaght in 1998 to form part of the new Adelaide and Meath Hospital incorporating the National Children's Hospital. Temple Street Hospital, which was founded in 1872, has a number of national centres including the National Centre for Paediatric Ophthalmology, the National Craniofacial Centre, the National Airways Management Centre, the National Meningococcal Laboratory and the National Centre for Inherited Metabolic Disorders.

The Faculty of Paediatrics of the RCPI advocated a single tertiary children's hospital in 1993. The minister for health, Mary Harney, initiated a review of tertiary paediatric hospital services in 2005. In 2006, the resultant report (McKinsey Report)

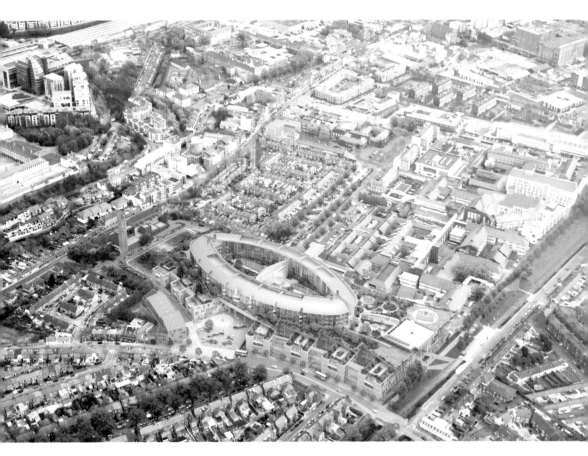

14.32   Architect's impression of the new children's hospital. Reproduced with permission of the National Paediatric Hospital Board.

recommended a single national children's hospital, and subsequently a task force, established by the HSE, chose the Mater Misericordiae University Hospital as the site for the development. In 2007, Harney established the National Paediatric Hospital Development Board. A planning application was submitted to An Bord Pleanála in 2011 for a fourteen-storey building on the Mater Hospital site. After due consideration, An Bord Pleanála refused planning permission in February 2012. The minister for health, Dr James Reilly, established a review group that proposed St James's Hospital as the new site in November 2012. The project brief for the new hospital at St James's Hospital was approved by the HSE two years later and planning permission was granted for the new development by An Bord Pleanála in April 2016. Two months later work on clearing the site for the hospital began.

The children's hospital is a first step in a national model for paediatric care that will combine the specialties of maternity, paediatric and adult hospitals in a tri-located facility.[30] With this goal in mind, the Government Capital Investment Plan 2016–21 has

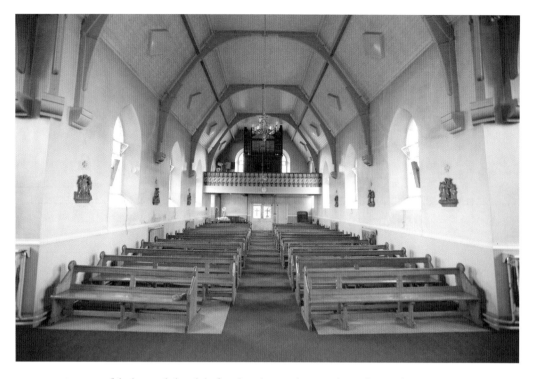

14.33   Interior of the hospital church before demolition. Photograph: Anthony Edwards.

allowed for the transfer of the Coombe Women and Infants University Hospital to the St James's Hospital campus.

The new children's hospital will be seven storeys high, with 380 single inpatient rooms, 42 critical care beds, 22 operating theatres, 122 consulting rooms and a neonatal critical care unit with a capacity of 18. It will have a rooftop therapeutic garden designed for children. There will be two satellite centres, one in Connolly Hospital and the other in Tallaght Hospital. The planning decision also included approval for the development of a Children's Research and Innovation Centre on the St James's campus. The location identified for this centre lies on the site occupied by the eighteenth-century Foundling Hospital. Speaking of the development, Owen Smith, special adviser to the children's hospital group and consultant paediatric haematologist at Our Lady's Children's Hospital, Crumlin, said:

> this centre will be at the heart of innovation and research helping to find cures to diseases that currently pose a serious threat to children and young people. Our ability to partner in research with colleagues on the St James's campus will fundamentally change the approach to research and will be a major catalyst for driving breakthrough results and outputs.[31]

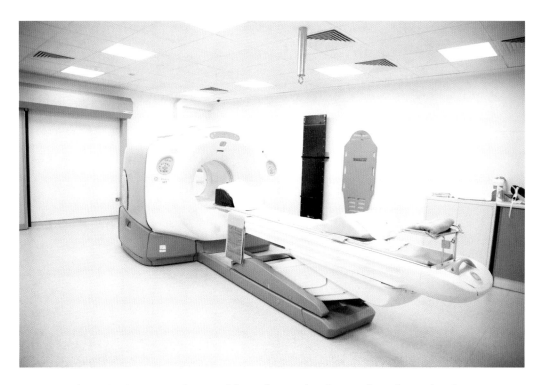

14.34   The PET-CT scanner in the ground floor of Hospital 1. Photograph: Anthony Edwards.

Costing in the region of €1 billion, the new hospital has been described in the Government's Capital Investment Plan 2016–21 as the largest health-infrastructure project ever undertaken in Ireland.[32]

Implications for St James's Hospital

The project has had major implications for St James's Hospital, as it has involved the demolition of around twenty-three buildings and the relocation of over thirty clinical, administrative and outpatient departments in order to clear the site for the children's hospital. Two of the remaining workhouse buildings, Hospitals 2 and 4, have been extensively refurbished to provide accommodation for several specialties and services. The ground floor of Hospital 1 had already been refurbished to accommodate the hospital's PET-CT scanner, which in recent years has revolutionized medical diagnosis and treatment.

The buildings demolished include Garden Hill and the early twentieth-century church near the Rialto gate. The church has been replaced by a new interdenominational place of worship, the Camino Rest, which opens onto the main concourse of the hospital. Some modern buildings, including the National Centre for Hereditary

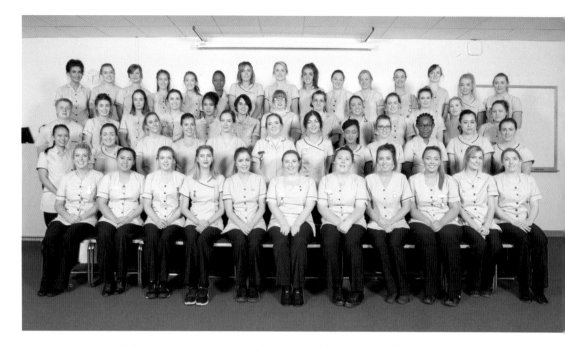

14.35   St James's Hospital B.Sc. in nursing graduates, 2016. Photograph: Anthony Edwards

Coagulation Disorders, have also been demolished. The pressures on the staff and infrastructure of St James's Hospital are reminiscent of the mid 1980s, when the designated hospitals were closed precipitously and their staff and services were accommodated by St James's, which was already functioning as a busy general hospital. This period proved subsequently to have been a major catalyst in the development of the hospital.

A shared vision

Since the foundation of St James's Hospital in 1971, there have been key shifts in the hospital's patient base and in the types of illness and injury that present. The increasing proportion of older people in the catchment area has had a major impact on the hospital's facilities and resources. Despite the demands of complex national clinical specialties, the hospital has maintained its focus on the provision of a wide range of medical and surgical services to the local population.

The rapid rise in international diversity in Ireland has not only changed the patient profile, but also the profile of the staff, which is now made up of employees of many nationalities. National and international students from several different disciplines including medicine, clinical speech and language studies, nursing, physiother-

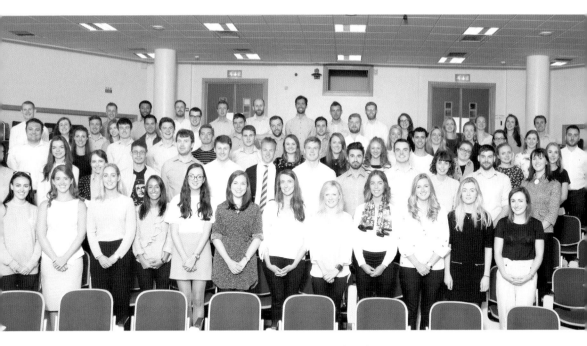

14.36   St James's Hospital interns, 2017. Photograph: Anthony Edwards.

apy, occupational therapy, social work, human nutrition and dietetics, receive clinical training in the hospital.

St James's Hospital was created by the shared vision of the Department of Health, the Federated Dublin Voluntary Hospitals, the Dublin Area Health Authority and Trinity College Dublin, to deliver comprehensive, state-of-the-art healthcare to the local catchment area. The hospital has been transformed into the largest and busiest university hospital in Ireland. It is home to many national and regional specialties, academic disciplines and professorial units. Research is deeply embedded in its culture, and there are several institutes of international standing on its campus. The development of the hospital has been driven from the start by criteria of excellence, continuous improvement and innovation, and its services focus on clinical care and bringing the most recent advances in diagnosis and treatment to the bedside of the patient.

Chronology of St James's Hospital, 1971–2016

Major events and senior appointments

Events	Appointments	Retirements and resignations
1971		
The minister for health, **Erskine Childers**, made an order establishing St James's Hospital board as a statutory body (June 1971).	The following full-time and visiting medical staff of St Kevin's Hospital transferred to St James's Hospital:	
The first meeting of the board of St James's Hospital took place on 2 July.	**K.M. Aboud** – medical officer	
The old convent was upgraded to provide accommodation for the school of nursing.	**P.G. Beckett** – psychiatrist	
	G.T. Berney – dental surgeon	
First discussions held between National Children's Hospital (NCH) and St James's Hospital on a proposal from the NCH to move the Children's Hospital to the St James's campus.	**P.J. Blaney** – physician	
	M. Buckley – physician	
	V. Coffey – paediatrician	
	J.P. Conroy – anaesthetist	
New maternity unit opened.	**W. Cremin** – physician	
New geriatric day hospital opened by the minister for health, Erskine Childers. This was the first geriatric day hospital in the country and was the initiative of **J.J. (Jack) Flanagan**, consultant physician in geriatric medicine.	**M. Fenton** – ophthalmologist	
	J.J. Flanagan – geriatrician	
	E.S.T. Foley-Taylor – radiologist	
	J. Gately – radiologist	
	T.D. Hanratty – obstetrician and gynaecologist	
	V. Lane – urologist	
	H. MacCarthy – surgeon	

Events	Appointments	Retirements and resignations
1971 (cont.)		
	W.T.E. McCaughey – pathologist	
	M.G. Magan – radiologist	
	J.R. Mahon – physician	
	E.W. Malone – radiologist	
	P. Moore – biochemist	
	P.J. Mullaney – pathologist	
	D. O'Brien – obstetrician and gynaecologist	
	G.T. O'Brien – respiratory physician	
	M. O'Connor – ENT surgeon	
	J. St L. O'Dea – medical administrator	
	J.D. O'Flynn – urologist	
	B. O'Neill – thoracic surgeon	
	T.D. O'Reilly – rheumatologist	
	P.M. O'Toole – anaesthetist	
	R.W. Ryder – haematologist	
	E. Tempany – paediatrician	
	F.J. Timoney – physician	
	F. Ward – surgeon	
1972		
The first outpatient department was opened in Hospital 7. The minister for health, **Erskine Childers**, formally renamed the hospital St James's Hospital and installed the new autonomous hospital board (November 1972).	**Kibon Aboud** as deputy medical administrator. **Victoria Beckett** as the first director of postgraduate medical education. **Ronald Draper** as consultant psychiatrist.	**William O. Cremin**, who served in the South Dublin Union, St Kevin's Hospital and St James's Hospital as visiting physician. **Anne Young** as matron.

Events	Appointments	Retirements and resignations
1972 (cont.)		
A teaching agreement was signed by representatives of Trinity College Dublin and St James's Hospital. A combined scheme of nurse training commenced with Our Lady's Hospital for Sick Children, Crumlin. It was a new experimental course leading to dual qualification in general and paediatric nursing in four years. Temporary huts were transferred from Trinity College to St James's Hospital to house the medical school. Senior house officer (SHO) rotation was established involving the Federated Hospitals and St James's Hospital.	**Lorcan Hogan** as hospital administrator. **Fergus Lawler** as accountant/assistant secretary. **John Stockton** as principal of the school of physiotherapy.	
1973		
A new premature-infants unit was built in Hospital 5, and the radiology department was relocated to Hospital 7. The school of physiotherapy was officially opened by the minister for health, **Erskine Childers**. The first medical students from Trinity College Dublin took up residence in the hospital.	**Padraig Dalton** as technical superintendent. **Peter B. Gatenby**, professor of medicine, as honorary consultant to St James's Hospital. He was given 50 long-stay beds on the top floor of Hospital 4. **Dermot Hourihane** as professor of histopathology and morbid anatomy. **Nora McCarthy** as matron. **James McCormick**, professor of social medicine, as honorary physician. **Pamela Woods** as superintendent physiotherapist.	**W.T.E. (Elliott) McCaughey** as professor of pathology.

Events	Appointments	Retirements and resignations
1974		
Death of **Peter Beckett**, dean of medicine and professor of psychiatry. Establishment of the first postgraduate centre. A child psychiatric outpatient unit was opened on the site by the Eastern Health Board (EHB) and the director of the child psychiatric service, **Paul McCarthy**, was appointed honorary consultant to St James's Hospital. **James McCormick**, professor of social medicine, was elected dean of the Faculty of Medicine and Dentistry. **James McCormick** took over the care of 50 patients on top floor of Hospital 4 following the departure of Peter Gatenby to take up a position in the United Nations. Letter sent to National Children's Hospital supporting the development of a substantial children's hospital in St James's Hospital.	**Michael Butler** as consultant urologist. **Eoin Casey** as consultant rheumatologist. **John Dinn** as consultant neuropathologist. **James Gardiner** as consultant anaesthetist. **Marjorie Young** as consultant dermatologist.	**Peter Gatenby** as professor of medicine.
1975		
Staff of the central council of the Federated Dublin Voluntary Hospitals moved into temporary accommodation on the St James's Hospital site. A project team was established to prepare a brief for the new St James's Hospital.	**John Bonnar** as professor of obstetrics and gynaecology. **Thomas Hennessy** as Regius professor of surgery. **Graham Neale** as professor of medicine. **Robert Quill** as senior lecturer/ consultant in surgery. **Hector Warnes** as professor of psychiatry.	

Events	Appointments	Retirements and resignations
1976		
Death of **Elizabeth Foley-Taylor**, consultant radiologist. The medical professorial unit transferred from the Meath Hospital to St James's Hospital, occupying the top floor of Hospital 1. Work began on a centralized facility for physiotherapy on the ground floor of Hospital 3. Architects **Moloney O'Beirne Guy**, and **Hutchinson Locke and Monk**, were appointed as design team for the new hospital.	**John Goodbody** as consultant anaesthetist. **Robert Harrison** as senior lecturer/consultant in obstetrics and gynaecology. **James Malone** as medical physicist. **Eamon Sweeney** as senior lecturer/consultant in histopathology.	**Victoria Beckett** as director of postgraduate medical education. **Victoria Coffey** as consultant paediatrician. **James Gardiner** as consultant anaesthetist. **Patrick J. Mullaney** as chief pathologist. **Thomas J. O'Reilly** as consultant rheumatologist.
1977		
Clinical haematology was transferred to St James's Hospital from the Meath Hospital. Department of vascular surgery was established by **Gregor Shanik**, who went on to develop the first vascular laboratory and the first endovascular operating suite in Ireland. A temporary building was erected to house the ambulance control centre of the EHB. Children's unit closed. Work began on the following developments in Hospital 7: 1) a third operating theatre and recovery room; 2) an accident and emergency unit; 3) a surgical professorial unit; 4) an outpatients department; and 5) paramedical accommodation.	**Conor Keane** as associate professor of clinical microbiology. **Brendan Lawless** as consultant anaesthetist. **Peter O'Connor** as director of postgraduate medical education. **John Prichard** as senior lecturer/consultant in medicine. **Gregor Shanik** as consultant vascular surgeon. **Ian Temperley** as consultant haematologist. **Marcus Webb** as professor of psychiatry.	**Maurice Fenton** as consultant ophthalmologist. **Edward Tempany** as consultant paediatrician. **Bridín Tierney**, principal nurse tutor, as head of the school of nursing. She had been director of the school from its opening in January 1967. She was succeeded by **Ita Leydon**. **Hector Warnes** as professor of psychiatry.

Events	Appointments	Retirements and resignations
1978		
Ultrasound facilities were installed in the radiology department. The minister for health, **Charles J. Haughey**, announced his approval of the development control plan for the new St James's Hospital at a ceremony in the staff restaurant.	**Luke Clancy** as consultant in respiratory medicine. **Michael Cullen** as consultant endocrinologist. **Doreen Dowd** as consultant in respiratory medicine. **Matthew McHugh** as consultant in plastic surgery. **Michael Walsh** as consultant cardiologist. **Frank Ward**, consultant surgeon, as director of the accident and emergency service.	**Peter O'Connor** as director of postgraduate medical education. **Joseph Timoney** as consultant physician.
1979		
A new central pathology laboratory to serve St James's and the Federated Hospitals was completed. **Dermot Hourihane**, professor of histopathology and morbid anatomy, was elected dean of the Faculty of Medicine and Dentistry. A medical intensive care and coronary care unit was opened in Hospital 2. The hospital was designated for the reception of accident victims. First outpatient fibreoptic bronchoscopy service in Ireland established by **Luke Clancy**. **Ronald Draper** was appointed as postgraduate coordinator.	**Davis Coakley** as consultant physician in geriatric medicine. **Peter A. Daly** as consultant physician with an interest in malignant disease. **Bernard Fallon** as consultant urologist. **Patrick Freyne** as consultant radiologist with special interest in nuclear medicine. **Aidan Kennedy** as consultant anaesthetist. **Ron Kirkham** as consultant anaesthetist. **Fiona O'Higgins** as consultant anaesthetist.	**James Mahon** as consultant physician. **James St L. O'Dea** as medical administrator (his services were retained in a consultancy capacity to work on the new hospital).

Events	Appointments	Retirements and resignations
1979 (cont.)		
Luke Clancy was appointed as director of postgraduate medical education. The social work building, formerly a children's unit, was demolished.		
1980		
The new central pathology laboratory was handed over to the hospital. Immunology and histopathology were transferred to the laboratory. It was formally opened in 1981. The chief technologists in the new central pathology laboratory were: **Sean Collins** – haematology; **Derek Cullen** – histopathology; **Liam English** – microbiology; **Liam Field** – biochemistry; **Paul Lynam** – blood transfusion; **Alex Whelan** – immunology; and **Noel White** – overall responsibility. The board proposed closing wards in order to stay within a restricted budget.	**Kibon Aboud** as medical administrator. **Michael Brady** as supplies officer. **Barry Breslin** as consultant in radiotherapy and clinical oncology. **Paul Byrne** as catering superintendent. **Liam Duffy** as Grade VII officer. **Mary Ennis** as consultant radiologist with special interest in ultrasound. **Niall Gallagher** as consultant histopathologist. **George McDonald** as senior lecturer in histopathology. **Jane Mahon** as theatre sister. **George Mullett** as consultant psychiatrist. **Martin Molloy** as consultant radiologist with special interest in vascular radiology. **Donal Sean O'Briain** as consultant histopathologist. **John O'Brien** as Grade VI officer. **Michael O'Hagan** as Grade VI officer. **Rory O'Moore** as consultant pathologist (clinical biochemist).	**Graham Neale** as professor of medicine.

Events	Appointments	Retirements and resignations
1980 (cont.)		
	Gerard Sheahan as consultant histopathologist.	
	Richard Stephens as consultant general surgeon.	
	Paul Wagstaff as head of the school of physiotherapy following the retirement of John Stockton.	
1981		
Long-stay ward closures in Hospital 3 to stay within budget.	Hugh Cassidy as consultant ophthalmologist.	Bernard Fallon as consultant urologist.
A new common contract for consultants was introduced nationally.	Liam Dunbar as group nursing administrator.	Ronald Draper on transfer of his sessions to St Patrick's Hospital.
	Conleth Feighery as consultant immunologist.	
	John Fitzpatrick as consultant urologist.	
	Stanley Miller as consultant radiologist.	
	Eric Mulvihill as consultant microbiologist.	
	Ernst Robinson as chief executive officer.	
1982		
The murder of Nurse Bridie Gargan in the Phoenix Park.	Garry Fenelon as consultant orthopaedic surgeon.	Patrick Blaney as consultant physician.
Phase 1A – the communications centre and the new entrance at Rialto – was completed.	Clayton Love as senior lecturer in clinical biochemistry.	
Vascular laboratory established.	Donald Weir as professor of medicine.	
Member of the board, Councillor Dan Browne, was elected lord mayor of Dublin.		

Events	Appointments	Retirements and resignations
1983		
Closure of Mercer's Hospital and transfer of services to St James's Hospital. This resulted in the establishment of a joint department of clinical haematology and oncology, located in Hospital 1, top floor, the first such department in Ireland.	**John Feely** as professor of pharmacology and therapeutics.	**Jack Flanagan** as consultant physician in geriatric medicine.
	Philomena Flood as senior dietician.	**Nora McCarthy** as matron.
	Michael Gibney as lecturer in the department of nutrition, which was linked to the department of medicine.	
The total staff complement following the transfer of the staff from Mercer's Hospital was 1,815.		
	Napoleon Keeling as senior lecturer/consultant gastroenterologist.	
John Bonnar, professor of obstetrics and gynaecology, was elected dean of the Faculty of Medicine and Dentistry.	**Shaun McCann** as consultant haematologist.	
	James McKeever as head of security.	
A new healthcare centre, which included a day ward and endoscopy facilities, opened in Hospital 5.	**Ann McNeill** as deputy matron.	
	Noel O'Connell as consultant radiologist.	
Bronchoscopy service moved from Hospital 1 to the new Health Care Centre.	**Thomas Wilson** as consultant otolaryngologist.	
	Alfred Wood as cardiothoracic surgeon.	
Gastroenterology unit transferred from Sir Patrick Dun's Hospital.		
Opening of Sir Patrick Dun's Research Laboratory.		
Martin Molloy, consultant radiologist, introduced an angioplasty service. This new technique permitted dilatation of narrowed arterial segments by means of a balloon catheter. Streptokinase infusion to dissolve recent obstructing clot formation was also employed.		
A new ambulance control centre was erected for the EHB.		
The department of medical physics and bioengineering was established under the leadership of **Jim Malone**.		

Events	Appointments	Retirements and resignations
1983 (cont.)		
Development of a respiratory-function laboratory under the direction of **Doreen Dowd**, consultant in respiratory medicine. There were 2,422 deliveries in the maternity unit. Apart from its commitment to staff and inpatients, the hospital's catering department had a major commitment to outside bodies, and each year prepared meals for community services. For instance, it supplied 15,500 meals to Meals on Wheels, 12,400 meals to the day centre in Whitefriar Street and 36,590 meals to a night shelter in Back Lane in 1983.		
1984		
The first bone marrow transplant was carried out in Hospital 1, top floor, by **Shaun McCann**, consultant haematologist. **Davis Coakley** appointed as director of postgraduate medical education. Work began on phase 1C of the new hospital. **G.T. Crampton** were the contractors. The main energy centre for the new hospital was completed. A revision of the statutory order of establishment of St James's Hospital gave Trinity College direct representation on the hospital board. A comprehensive teaching agreement was signed with Trinity College Dublin.	**Erc Kealy** as energy services officer. **James Liston** as security officer. **Francis Powell** as consultant dermatologist. **J. Bernard Walsh** as consultant physician in geriatric medicine.	**Thomas Hanratty** as consultant obstetrician. **Gerard Sheahan** as consultant histopathologist.

Events	Appointments	Retirements and resignations
1985		
The academic department of obstetrics and gynaecology moved to St James's Hospital from the Rotunda Hospital. The staff managed the maternity unit in St James's and based their research activities in the Sir Patrick Dun's laboratory.	Liam Dunbar as acting CEO.	Noel O'Connell as consultant radiologist.
In vitro fertilisation service introduced.	Lesley Fox as consultant anaesthetist.	Francis Powell as consultant dermatologist.
Laser therapy was introduced in the department of gastroenterology.	Eoin Gaffney as consultant histopathologist.	
CEO Ernst Robinson granted leave of absence for two years.	Peter Gray as consultant neonatologist.	
The hospital introduced its own drug formulary.	Lorcan Hogan as director of research and development. He relinquished his post as hospital administrator.	
The postgraduate centre published its first book, *Emergencies in clinical practice*, which was based on lectures given at the centre. It was edited by **Michael Buckley**.	Eamon McGuinness as consultant obstetrician and gynaecologist.	
Summer ward closures as a cutback measure.	James Milliken as consultant vascular surgeon.	
Smoking ban implemented in patient areas.	Dermot Moore as consultant vascular surgeon.	
	Hugh Smyth as consultant orthopaedic surgeon.	
	Michael Walsh as consultant otolaryngologist.	
1986		
Death of **Edward Malone**, consultant radiologist.	Mary Dooley as financial controller.	John Fitzpatrick as consultant urologist.
Patrick Freyne succeeded Malone as director of radiology.	Edwina Dunne as head of occupational therapy.	
Closure of Sir Patrick Dun's Hospital on 1 September and transfer of services to St James's Hospital.	John Kirker as consultant physician with an interest in neurology, on the closure of Sir Patrick Dun's Hospital.	

Events	Appointments	Retirements and resignations
1986 (cont.)		
The postgraduate centre was extended and refurbished. The centre was named the William Stokes Postgraduate Centre and formally opened by **Dr Barbara Stokes**, a member of the family.	**Fergus Lawler** as head of internal audit.	
	Martin O'Connor as consultant ophthalmologist.	
A major refurbishment of Hospital 4 on receipt of funding from the Department of Health for the geriatric services.	**Gina O'Donoghue** as senior speech therapist.	
	Francis O'Loughran as consultant otolaryngologist.	
The transfer of the sexually transmitted diseases unit to St James's Hospital from Dr Steevens' Hospital.	**Patrick Scanlon** as consultant anaesthetist.	
The Friends of St James's Hospital was established to raise funds for the provision of additional facilities and equipment for the patients of the hospital.	**David Shanley** as consultant general adult psychiatrist.	
	Celine Traynor as consultant anaesthetist.	
Chemotherapy day care unit moved to Hospital 5, Health Care Centre, transferring from Hospital 1.		
Oesophageal investigation unit was established.		
St James's Hospital Ladies' Association was established to answer a widely felt need to create opportunities to bring staff together on an informal basis. Several events were organized each year, including the annual carol service in the hospital chapel.		
1987		
Closure of the Royal City of Dublin Hospital (RCDH), Baggot Street, on 7 December, and transfer of its services to St James's Hospital.	**Louise Barnes** as consultant dermatologist.	**John Gately** as consultant radiologist.

Events	Appointments	Retirements and resignations
1987 (cont.)		
Closure of Dr Steevens' Hospital on 31 December and transfer of its services to St James's Hospital.

Robert Mayne Day Hospital for older patients opened in April. This was the first clinical facility of the new hospital to open.

Ian Temperley, professor of haematology, elected dean of the Faculty of Health Sciences.

Clayton Love, consultant clinical biochemist, was awarded the 1987 Wellcome Prize by the Association of Clinical Biochemists in recognition of his outstanding contribution to the practice of clinical biochemistry.

Transfer of obstetrics service to the Coombe Hospital.

The Jonathan Swift Clinic for psychiatry opened in December with accommodation for fifty-six beds and fifty day places.

Stress echocardiography introduced.

Comprehensive pulmonary function laboratory including a sleep laboratory established by **Luke Clancy**, consultant in respiratory medicine.

The angiography unit transferred to Hospital 1, ground floor.

The closure of Hospital 3, which housed long-stay older patients, to make way for the next phase of the new hospital. The patients were moved to Bru Chaoimhin in Cork Street and to Leopardstown Park Hospital. | **Hugh Barry** as consultant oral surgeon, on the closure of Dr Steevens' Hospital.

Frank Brady as consultant maxillofacial surgeon, on the closure of Dr Steevens' Hospital.

Peter Crean as consultant cardiologist.

Ted Dinan as senior lecturer/consultant psychiatrist.

Liam Dunbar as CEO.

Gerald Edwards as consultant plastic surgeon, on the closure of Dr Steevens' Hospital.

Edward Fitzgerald as consultant radiologist.

Gerard Gearty as consultant cardiologist, on the closure of Baggot Street Hospital.

David Hogan as consultant anaesthetist, on the closure of Baggot Street Hospital.

Stanley Jagoe as general physician, on the closure of Baggot Street Hospital.

Brigid P. Kelly as director of nursing.

Gerard King as chief cardiac technician.

Geoff Kronn as consultant dental surgeon, on the closure of Dr Steevens' Hospital.

Denis Lawlor as consultant plastic surgeon, on the closure of Dr Steevens' Hospital. | **Peter Gray** as consultant neonatologist.

Robert Harrison as associate professor of obstetrics and gynaecology.

Anne McNeill as deputy director of nursing.

James Milliken as consultant vascular surgeon.

Patrick E. Moore as head of biochemistry.

Maureen Prendergast as acting director of nursing.

Ernst Robinson as CEO. |

Events	Appointments	Retirements and resignations
1987 (cont.)		
The occupational health department was established, with **Christopher Dick** as occupational health physician and **Joan McNamara** as sister-in-charge. A new entrance on James's Street.	**David Luke** as consultant cardiothoracic surgeon, on the closure of Baggot Street Hospital. **Myles McEvilly** as consultant anaesthetist. **Eilis McGovern** as consultant cardiothoracic surgeon. **James McNulty** as consultant radiologist. **Vincent Morris** as consultant orthodontist, on the closure of Dr Steevens' Hospital. **Fiona Mulcahy** as consultant physician in genitourinary medicine.	
1988		
Handover of the new main hospital building. The postgraduate centre was replaced by a new building on the same site and was officially opened by **Dr Maeve Hillery**. The new diagnostic imaging department opened. A new diabetic care centre was established in August. This development was led by **Michael Cullen**, consultant endocrinologist. Transfer of the Mercer's Institute for Research on Ageing to the refurbished old day hospital. Introduction of flexible cystoscopy in the urology department.	**Ronald Grainger** as consultant urologist. **T.E.D. McDermott** as consultant urologist. **Patrick Plunkett** as consultant in emergency medicine.	**Brigid P. Kelly** as director of nursing. **Frank Ward** as consultant surgeon and director of the accident and emergency department.

Events	Appointments	Retirements and resignations
1989		
Death of **Paul Wagstaff**, director of the school of physiotherapy. Opening of new accident and emergency department, which included an observation ward. Opening of new coronary care unit. Installation of two cardiac catheterization laboratories. Intraluminal vascular stents introduced in vascular surgery. The department of speech therapy in collaboration with **Patrick Freyne**, consultant radiologist, established a video fluoroscopy service to assess patients with swallowing problems. The management of the psychiatric unit (Jonathan Swift Clinic) transferred from St Patrick's Hospital to St James's Hospital.	**Betty Coyle** as director of human resources. **Noirin Noonan** as occupational health physician. **Kamal Sabra** as chief pharmacist. **Peta Taaffe** as director of nursing services. **Peter Vaughan** as consultant anaesthetist. **Graham Wilson** as consultant radiologist.	**Edward Fitzgerald** as consultant radiologist. **Therese MacDonogh** as catering superintendent.
1990		
Death of **John Dinn**, consultant neuropathologist. A portrait of **Anne Young** by **Thomas Ryan** was unveiled in the nursing school. Opening of the new outpatient department. **Conleth Feighery** appointed as director of postgraduate medical education. The Mercer's Institute for Research on Ageing (MIRA) was launched by the provost, **Dr William Watts**, in the Royal College of Physicians of Ireland.	**Bernadette Moran** as superintendent of diagnostic imaging department. **Seamus O'Riain** as consultant plastic surgeon. **Mary Toner** as consultant histopathologist.	**Aidan Kennedy** as consultant anaesthetist. **Margaret McMahon** as superintendent of diagnostic imaging department.

Events	Appointments	Retirements and resignations
1990 (cont.)		
Introduction of the use of percutaneous gastrostomy tubes by the department of gastroenterology. A five-day investigation ward was opened in the new hospital.		
1991		
An honorary degree of ScD was conferred on **Gerard Gearty**, consultant cardiologist, by the University of Dublin. Establishment of the memory clinic. Establishment of old age psychiatry service by **Brian Lawlor**. Closure of hospital laundry.	**James Clinch** as consultant gynaecologist. **Edward Fleming** as financial controller. **Brian Lawlor** as consultant in old age psychiatry. **Raymond Murphy** as consultant neurologist. **Rosemarie Watson** as consultant dermatologist.	**Mary Dooley** as financial controller.
1992		
New ward accommodation (291 beds) opened, along with the National Burns Unit, the coronary care unit, the intensive care unit and eleven operating theatres. Commissioning phase of new hospital, which was overseen by **Michael Brady** as commissioning officer, was completed in January. Insertion of an implantable defibrillator for the first time in a patient in the Republic.	**Martin Buckley** as manager of information and management services. **Jeanne Moriarty** as consultant in anaesthesia and critical care medicine. **John O'Brien** as deputy CEO. **Desmond O'Neill** as consultant physician in geriatric medicine. **Janice Redmond** as consultant neurologist.	**Barry Breslin** as consultant in radiotherapy and clinical oncology. **Betty Coyle** as director of human resources. **Ted Dinan** as senior lecturer/ consultant psychiatrist.

Events	Appointments	Retirements and resignations
1992 (cont.)		
Introduction of functional endoscopic sinus surgery in the treatment of sinusitis and nasal polyposis. Introduction of a new acute hepatitis B diagnostic service for staff who have had an accidental needle-stick injury.	**Thomas Schnittger** as consultant anaesthetist. **Mary White** as consultant anaesthetist.	
1993		
Death of **Nurse Valerie Place** on voluntary work in Somalia. She had trained in St James's and had worked in the hospital as a staff nurse. Introduction of continuous renal replacement therapy in intensive care. The school of nursing moved from the old convent to the new Trinity Centre for Health Sciences. **Davis Coakley** elected dean of the Faculty of Health Sciences. The department of cardiology introduced an MSc course in diagnostic and interventional cardiology, which was led by **Michael Walsh**. The catering department introduced new cook-chill kitchens.	**Francesca Brett** as consultant neuropathologist. **Niall Hughes** as consultant anaesthetist. **Gillian Lacey** as director of human resources. **Conrad Timon** as consultant otolaryngologist.	
1994		
The Trinity Centre for Health Sciences was officially opened by the minister for health, **Brendan Howlin**. **Thomas Hennessy**, Regius professor of surgery, elected president of the Royal College of Surgeons in Ireland. Opening of the high-dependency unit.	**Patricia Eadie** as consultant in plastic and reconstructive surgery. **Michael Gill** as senior lecturer/consultant in psychiatry. **Marie Guidon** as superintendent physiotherapist.	

Events	Appointments	Retirements and resignations
1994 (cont.)		
Opening of the neurophysiology laboratory.	**Donal Hollywood** as consultant radiotherapist.	
The National Medicines Information Centre, established at St James's Hospital under the direction of John Feely and Kamal Sabra, was opened by the minister for health, **Brendan Howlin**.	**Eamonn McKiernan** as consultant orthodontist.	
	Liam O'Siorain as consultant in palliative medicine.	
Desmond O'Neill appointed as director of postgraduate medical education.		
A laser unit was established in the department of plastic surgery following the donation of laser equipment by **Norma Smurfit**. It was opened by the minister for health, **Brendan Howlin**, and was the first such laser unit in the country.		
1995		
Specialist palliative care service established.	**Cliff Beirne** as consultant oral surgeon.	**Liam Dunbar** as CEO
Shaun McCann appointed as George Gabriel Stokes professor of haematology.	**Sean Connolly** as consultant neurophysiologist.	**Niall Gallagher** as consultant histopathologist.
The new William Stokes Postgraduate Centre was officially opened by the minister of state at the Department of Health, **Austin Curry**.	**Brendan Foley** as consultant cardiologist.	**Gerard Gearty** as consultant cardiologist.
	Mairead Griffin as consultant histopathologist.	**Lorcan Hogan**, former hospital secretary.
	Dermot Kelleher as consultant gastroenterologist.	**Donal O'Brien** as consultant gynaecologist.
	Emer Lawlor as consultant haematologist.	**Ian Temperley** as professor of haematology.
	George Mellotte as consultant nephrologist.	
	Joan O'Riordan as consultant haematologist.	

Events	Appointments	Retirements and resignations
1995 (cont.)		
	Owen Smith as consultant haematologist and director of the National Haemophilia Centre.	
1996		
Death of **John Prichard**, associate professor of medicine and consultant physician.	**Patrick Byrne** as chief technician in the gastrointestinal functional laboratory.	
The new haematology /oncology unit, incorporating the National Adult Bone Marrow Transplant Unit, was opened and named the Denis Burkitt Ward.	**Ian Carter** as deputy CEO. **Noreen Gleeson** as consultant gynaecologist. **John Nolan** as consultant endocrinologist.	
Private wing of 90 beds and two new standard wards completed.	**John O'Brien** as CEO.	
Board approved development of private clinic.	**Finbarr O'Connell** as consultant in respiratory medicine.	
Refurbishment of the Victorian nursing school and former convent to house the boardroom and offices of the CEO and his team, the nursing administration and a consultants' common room.	**Michael O'Hagan** as director of human resources. **John Reynolds** as consultant surgeon.	
Launch of St James's Hospital Foundation. The foundation was set up to raise additional funding for the hospital from private sources.		
Twenty-fifth anniversary celebrations of the hospital.		
Formal opening of the RCDH Research and Education Institute by **Dr Thomas Mitchell**, provost of Trinity College Dublin.		
Davis Coakley appointed professor of medical gerontology.		

Events	Appointments	Retirements and resignations
1996 (cont.)		
Launch of the hospital's website. Board approves Luas (light rail) plans in relation to their impact on St James's Hospital. This transport system would link Trinity College, St James's Hospital and Tallaght Hospital.		
1997		
National Centre for Pharmacoeconomics was established by **John Feely**, professor of pharmacology and therapeutics. Launch of St James's Hospital Foundation with **Dermot Moore**, consultant vascular surgeon, as first chairman. Signing of collaborative agreement between St James's and AMNCH (Tallaght). **Peta Taaffe**, director of nursing services, appointed as chief nursing officer in the Department of Health and Children. Appointment of **John Reynolds**, consultant surgeon, as director of cancer services for the south-west area of the Eastern Health Region (EHR). **Jim Malone** appointed as Robert Boyle professor of medical physics. The John Prichard postgraduate education room in the RCDH Research and Education Centre was opened.	**Michael Barry** as senior lecturer/consultant in pharmacology and therapeutics and medical director of the National Centre of Pharmacoeconomics. **Paul Browne** as consultant haematologist. **Eamonn Keenan** as consultant psychiatrist. **Niall McEniff** as consultant radiologist. **Hugh O'Connor** as consultant gynaecologist. **John O'Leary** as consultant histopathologist. **Thomas Ryan** as consultant anaesthetist.	**Hugh Barry** as consultant oral surgeon. **James Clinch** as consultant gynaecologist. **Gillian Lacey** as director of human resources. **R.W. (Kim) Ryder** as consultant haematologist.

Events	Appointments	Retirements and resignations
1997 (cont.)		
A multidisciplinary specialized breast clinic was established as part of the cancer service at St James's Hospital. Patients receive triple evaluation consisting of clinical examination and counselling, diagnostic imaging investigations and pathology evaluation in a single visit.		
The first four students to be awarded the MSc in gerontological nursing qualified. The course was based at St James's Hospital and it was the first nursing degree conferred by Trinity College Dublin.		
New consultant private clinic established. The clinic incorporated ten consulting rooms together with ECG, radiology, pathology facilities and a reception area.		
Establishment of Eastern Regional Health Authority (ERHA).		
1998		
Death of **Derek Cullen**, chief technologist of histopathology and cytology.	**David Borton** as consultant orthopaedic surgeon.	**Thomas Hennessy** as Regius professor of surgery.
In 1997–8 the department of genitourinary medicine transferred to the renovated section of Hospital 5. The facilities included a dedicated ward for HIV/infectious diseases patients.	**John Kennedy** as consultant medical oncologist.	**Dermot Hourihane** as professor of histopathology and morbid anatomy.
Department of accident and emergency was renamed department of emergency medicine by the hospital board. Triage system introduced in the department.	**Margaret O'Donnell** as consultant in plastic and reconstructive surgery. **David Orr** as consultant in plastic and reconstructive surgery. **Rosemary Ryan** as director of nursing services.	**Desmond O'Neill**, consultant physician in geriatric medicine, on transfer of his sessions to the new AMNCH (Tallaght).

Events	Appointments	Retirements and resignations
1998 (cont.)		
An acute haemodialysis unit opened in St Kevin's ward.		
Department of microbiology recognized as the Centre for European Antimicrobial Resistance Surveillance System (EARSS). **Conor Keane**, professor of clinical microbiology, appointed to the EU central committee.		
First treatment of liver cancer with chemoembolization performed in the department of diagnostic imaging.		
The minister for health, **Brian Cowen**, announced the development of cardiac surgery service.		
Introduction of narrowband UVB phototherapy in the dermatology day centre.		
Collaboration between vascular surgery and radiology led to the introduction of stent grafts for the management of aortic aneurysms.		
'Dubdoc', an out-of-hours general practitioner centre, was established in St James's Hospital by twenty-five general practitioners. The purpose of the centre was to provide a rapid assessment, diagnosis and treatment centre for local patients.		
Opening of new hepatology unit for the treatment of all forms of liver disease by minister for health, **Brian Cowen**.		
The department of social work celebrated the 50th anniversary of its foundation.		

Events	Appointments	Retirements and resignations
1998 (cont.)		
The Haughton Institute was launched at a special ceremony in Trinity College Dublin. An independent corporate body wholly owned by its three members, Trinity College, St James's Hospital and AMNCH, Tallaght, it was founded to facilitate and develop the common interests of its three constituent members in research, postgraduate education and training. **Jim Malone** was appointed as its first executive director.		
Establishment of the National Dementia Services and Information Centre. The aims of the centre included promoting an awareness of dementia, improving and expanding services for persons with dementia and providing education and training to practitioners working in the field.		
The closure of the Meath and Adelaide Hospitals and their transfer to the new hospital at Tallaght had a significant impact on St James's Hospital and its catchment area. The city-centre population, which now dominated the catchment area, had a significantly higher age profile than the population served previously.		
1999		
Establishment of a Molecular Medicine Diagnostic Laboratory for leukaemia and related disorders, which would work closely with the National Genetics Centre at Our Lady's Children's Hospital, Crumlin.	**Mark Abrahams** as consultant anaesthetist. **Colm Bergin** as consultant in infectious diseases.	**John Bonnar** as professor of obstetrics and gynaecology. **Micheal Buckley** as consultant general physician.

Events	Appointments	Retirements and resignations
1999 (cont.)		
A rheumatology day centre was established. The Arthritis Foundation contributed to this development, which was led by **Eoin Casey**, consultant rheumatologist. Agreement on the establishment of a supra-regional vascular surgery unit to serve the population of the South West Area and Midland Health Boards was concluded. Services will be distributed over four sites at St James's Hospital, AMNCH, Naas and Tullamore. **Jim Malone**, Robert Boyle professor of medical physics, was elected dean of the Faculty of Health Sciences. **Barry O'Connell** appointed as director of postgraduate medical education. **Brian Lawlor** appointed as Conolly Norman professor of old age psychiatry. Opening of Conolly Norman unit in the Jonathan Swift Clinic. Temporary relocation of the school of physiotherapy to the refurbished old stone buildings adjacent to the Trinity Centre.	**Conal Cunningham** as consultant physician in geriatric medicine. **Thomas D'Arcy** as consultant gynaecologist. **Noreen Dowd** as consultant cardiothoracic anaesthetist. **Mark Lawler** as chief molecular geneticist. **Fionnuala Lyons** as consultant cardiothoracic anaesthetist. **Geraldine McMahon** as consultant in emergency medicine. **Linus Offiah** as associate emergency physician. **Noreen O'Shea** as physiotherapy manager. **Ellen O'Sullivan** as consultant anaesthetist. **Michael Tolan** as consultant cardiothoracic surgeon. **Vincent Young** as consultant cardiothoracic surgeon. Six cancer care coordinators appointed.	**Fergus Lawler** as head of internal audit. **Clayton Love** as senior lecturer in clinical biochemistry. **David Luke** as cardiothoracic surgeon, on transfer of his sessions to St Vincent's University Hospital. **John McSweeney** as principal biochemist. **Donald Weir** as Regius professor of physic and professor of medicine.
2000		
Death of **George Mullett**, consultant psychiatrist. St James's Hospital became the first Irish hospital to start a new insulin pump programme (continuous subcutaneous insulin infusion, CSH) for patients with diabetes.	**Grainne Courtney** as associate specialist in genitourinary medicine. **Aongus Curran** as consultant otolaryngologist. **Brian Graham** as chief technologist, transfusion laboratory.	**Kibon Aboud** as medical administrator. **Mary Ennis** as consultant radiologist. **David Hogan** as consultant anaesthetist.

Events	Appointments	Retirements and resignations
2000 (cont.)		
The Metabolic Research Unit was opened in the department of endocrinology, with a focus on clinical research in type 2 diabetes.	**Eilish Hardiman** as director of nursing.	**Stanley Jagoe** as consultant general physician.
The first Irish cases of carotid angioplasty with cerebral protection were performed.	**Martin Healy** as principal biochemist.	**Paul Lynam** as chief technologist, transfusion laboratory.
Establishment of a liaison psychiatry service by consultant psychiatrist **Anne Marie O'Dwyer**.	**Dermot Kelleher** as professor of medicine.	**Niamh O'Sullivan** as consultant microbiologist.
National Centre for Hereditary Coagulation Disorders opened. The centre's main focus is on haemophilia.	**Prakash Madhavan** as consultant vascular surgeon.	**Rosemary Ryan** as director of nursing.
The Keith Shaw Cardiac Surgery Unit opened. The unit consisted of 6 intensive care beds, 12 ward beds and 2 dedicated cardiothoracic theatres.	**Joseph Murphy** as consultant radiologist.	**Marjorie Young** as consultant dermatologist.
	Siobhan Nicholson as consultant histopathologist.	
Endovascular suite opened. This facility enhanced the care of patients with vascular disease by the use of less invasive methods of treatment.	**Emily O'Connor** as associate emergency physician.	
The installation of a pneumatic tube transport system to link the laboratory with the wards and units to speed up the transport of samples to the laboratory.	**Ann Marie O'Dwyer** as consultant liaison psychiatrist.	
Formation of new management unit called SCOPe, which embraced speech and language therapy, social work, clinical nutrition and occupational therapy. **Bernie McNally**, occupational therapy service manager, was appointed as the first manager of SCOPe.		
A patient advocacy committee was established as a subcommittee of the board.		
Opening of the new National Blood Centre.		

Events	Appointments	Retirements and resignations
2001		
The Carmelite order left St James's Hospital. The order had provided chaplaincy services to the hospital for 140 years.	**David Aberdeen** as director of human resources.	**Gerard T. Berney** as consultant oral surgeon.
Magnetic resonance imaging (MRI) suite opened in the diagnostic imaging department.	**Gerard Boyle** as principal physicist.	**Edward Fleming** as financial controller.
Centre for Advanced Clinical Therapeutics was established by **John Feely**.	**Terence Boyle** as consultant in general surgery.	**Mary Flynn** as assistant director of nursing.
A chest pain assessment unit was established within the emergency department.	**Eibhlin Conneally** as consultant haematologist.	**Mary Harte** as deputy director of nursing.
Extended care wards in Hospital 4 were refurbished on a 'home from home' principle.	**Vincent Doherty** as financial controller.	**Dermot O'Brien** as principal biochemist.
Opening of new endovascular suite.	**Carl Fagan** as consultant in anaesthesia and critical care medicine.	**Michael O'Hagan** as director of human resources.
Breast cancer service received additional staff and the diagnostic facilities were improved.	**Stephen Froese** as consultant anaesthetist.	**Owen Smith** as director of the National Centre for Hereditary Coagulation Disorders.
The reconstruction of the Burkitt Ward to make it suitable for care of highly immunocompromised patients was completed and the Walter Stevenson Ward was opened for haematology and oncology services.	**Declan Gasparro** as principal biochemist.	**Marcus Webb** as professor of psychiatry.
The National TB Reference Laboratory was established in the department of clinical mircrobiology.	**Nicholas Kennedy** as senior lecturer in clinical medicine (nutrition).	**Mary White** as consultant anaesthetist.
Opening of new interventional radiology suite.	**Deirdre McCoy** as consultant anaesthetist.	
Brief for the new centre of excellence for older patients submitted to ERHA.	**Connail McCrory** as consultant in anaesthesia and pain medicine.	
Rheumatology day centre officially opened by the minister for health and children, **Micheál Martin**.	**Mairín McMenamin** as consultant dermatopathologist.	
	James Meaney as consultant radiologist.	
	Concepta Merry as consultant in infectious diseases.	
	Beatrice Nolan as consultant haematologist.	
	Deirdre O'Riordan as consultant general physician.	
	John Reynolds as professor of surgery.	

Events	Appointments	Retirements and resignations
2001 (cont.)		
Demolition of the Eastern Health Board building (the Queen Mary) at the James's Street entrance of the hospital to facilitate the development of the Luas light-rail service.	**Paul Scully** as consultant psychiatrist. **Bernard Silke** as consultant general physician. **Elisabeth Vandenberghe** as consultant haematologist. **Barry White** as consultant haematologist and director of the National Centre for Hereditary Coagulation Disorders.	
2002		
Death of **Padraig Dalton**, project and technical services manager. He played an important role in the development of the hospital. **Derry Shanley**, professor of oral health, was elected dean of the Faculty of Health Sciences. The new National MRSA Reference Laboratory was opened by the minister for health and children, **Micheál Martin. Conor Keane** was appointed as director. Epidermolysis bullosa service was established in the department of dermatology by **Rosemarie Watson**. The respiratory assessment unit was opened. It concentrates on the management of patients with acute exacerbations of chronic obstructive pulmonary disease to facilitate their early discharge from hospital. A haemachromatosis centre was established in the Hepatology Centre. Student nursing degree course commenced in Trinity and the nursing school moved to D'Olier Street.	**Miriam Casey** as consultant physician in geriatric medicine. **Brendan Conlon** as consultant otolaryngologist. **Gaye Cunnane** as consultant rheumatologist. **Una Geary** as consultant in emergency medicine. **Alan Irvine** as consultant dermatologist. **Joseph Keane** as consultant respiratory and general physician. **Mary Keogan** as consultant radiologist. **Thomas Lynch** as consultant urologist. **Ronan McDermott** as consultant radiologist. **Susan McKiernan** as consultant gastroenterologist. **Eleanor McNamara** as consultant microbiologist.	**Michael Brady** as commissioning officer. **Liam English** as chief scientist in clinical microbiology. **Conor Keane** as associate professor of clinical microbiology. **James McNulty** as consultant radiologist. **James Malone** as head of medical physics and bioengineering. **Francis O'Loughran** as consultant otolaryngologist.

Events	Appointments	Retirements and resignations
2002 (cont.)		
The school of nursing accommodation in the Trinity Centre became the location for the new Centre for Learning and Development. The purpose of the centre is to provide high-quality education and training for members of different disciplines throughout the hospital. Bone clinic established by **J. Bernard Walsh**, consultant physician in geriatric medicine. A dermatology nurse-led day care centre was established by **Louise Barnes**, consultant dermatologist. A telecardiology facility was established to enable digital angiography images and data to be transferred to St James's Hospital from regional hospitals to allow interactive teleconferencing. Opening of Cancer Molecular Diagnostics Laboratory.	**Suzanne Norris** as consultant gastroenterologist and general physician. **Brian O'Connell** as consultant microbiologist. **Aisling O'Mahony** as consultant in restorative dentistry (prosthodontics). **Owen Smith** as professor of haematology.	
2003		
Opening of the John Durkan Laboratories and Lecture Theatre. Opening of the Institute of Molecular Medicine. **Sean O'Briain**, head of the department of histopathology, was appointed dean of the Faculty of Pathology and associate professor of pathology. Funding obtained for major extension to the emergency department. A new mortuary and autopsy suite were completed.	**Mairead Condren** as consultant psychiatrist **Brendan Crowley** as consultant microbiologist. **Michelle Doran** as consultant rheumatologist. **Brian Fitzgerald** as financial controller. **Gerry Heffernan** as deputy director of human resources. **David Keane** as consultant cardiologist.	**Eoin Casey** as consultant rheumatologist. **Aongus Curran** as consultant otolaryngologist. **Vincent Doherty** as financial controller. **Geoff Kronn** as consultant dental surgeon. **Rory O'Moore** as associate professor and consultant clinical biochemist. **Alex Whelan** as chief laboratory scientist.

Events	Appointments	Retirements and resignations
2003 (cont.)		
Seventy-four new beds came on stream under the aegis of capacity-expansion initiatives introduced by the Department of Health. Fifty-nine of these were provided for the purpose of creating an acute medical admissions unit (AMAU).	**Niall Mulvihill** as consultant cardiologist.	
Establishment of a falls and blackout unit.	**Kenneth O'Byrne** as consultant medical oncologist.	
The Open Window project was initiated with funding from the British Cancer Society. Led by **Shaun McCann**, George Gabriel Stokes professor of haematology, the project was developed to provide artistic images, films and music to the rooms of patients who were undergoing stem cell transplantation.	**John O'Leary** as professor of pathology.

Fionnuala O'Loughlin as consultant general adult psychiatrist.

Catriona O'Sullivan as consultant radiation oncologist.

Leo Stassen as professor of oral and maxillofacial surgery. | |
Development of psycho-oncology service by consultant psychiatrist **Anne Marie O'Dwyer**.		
The Dementia Services Information and Development Centre organized the first national dementia care conference.		
Establishment of a prostate cancer research network between experts in St James's Hospital and the Mater Hospital. This development was funded by the Irish Cancer Society.		
Establishment of interventional cardiac electrophysiology with appointment of **David Keane**, consultant cardiologist.		
A risk management strategy was established for the hospital under the leadership of the deputy CEO, **Ian Carter**.		

Events	Appointments	Retirements and resignations
2003 (cont.)		
On the initiative of **Ian Carter**, St James's Hospital joined an international performance indicator programme. Participating hospitals included University Hospital of Wales, Guy's and St Thomas' NHS Trust, Belfast City Hospital, St Luke's Hospital Malta, University Hospital Brussels and Groningen Hospital, Netherlands. The process enables participating hospitals to learn best practice in different fields through a process of benchmarking. A vacuum tube system was piloted to deliver frozen sections of tissue to the department of histopathology from the operating theatres.		
2004		
The following services opened in phase 1H: endoscopic and day surgery centre, outpatient unit, haematology/oncology day care service centre, together with the new hospital concourse and a 31-bed inpatient ward. Department of medical physics and bioengineering twenty-first anniversary celebrations. A 'one stop shop' clinic was established for patients with haemochromatosis. Interventional pain medicine service established. The main concourse was the venue for a summer concert by the Greystones orchestra. The Luas transport system was completed and trams began running in October.	**Eamon Beausang** as consultant in plastic and reconstructive surgery. **Vivion Crowley** as consultant chemical pathologist. **Barbara Dunne** as consultant histopathologist. **John Kinsella** as consultant otolaryngologist. **Peter Lawlor** as consultant in palliative medicine. **Cian Muldoon** as consultant histopathologist. **Muireann O'Briain** as legal manager. **David O'Donovan** as consultant in plastic and reconstructive surgery. **Catherine O'Malley** as consultant anaesthetist.	**David Aberdeen** as director of human resources. **Eamonn Keenan** as consultant psychiatrist. **Matthew McHugh** as consultant plastic surgeon. **Martin Molloy** as consultant radiologist. **Eamon Sweeney** as associate professor of histopathology.

Events	Appointments	Retirements and resignations
2004 (cont.)		
	J. **Mark Ryan** as consultant in interventional radiology.	
2005		
An international design team appointed to provide an outline development control plan for the future development of the hospital campus. The HSE replaced the existing health board structure on 1 January. Departure of CEO, **John O'Brien**, on a five-year secondment to the HSE. **Gerard King**, chief cardiac technician, was conferred with Ireland's first clinical science PhD in echocardiography. A new falls and syncope unit, led by **Rose Anne Kenny**, professor of geriatric medicine, was officially opened by **Mary Harney**, tánaiste and minister for health and children. Watts clinical research fellowship was established in the Mercer's Institute for Research on Ageing (MIRA). It was named in honour of **Dr William Watts** who was the first chairman of the Mercer's Hospital Foundation. A diabetic retinal screening clinic was established in a collaborative venture between endocrinology (led by **John Nolan**) and ophthalmology (led by **Susan Mullaney**). Development of an interim tuberculosis (TB) facility in Hospital 5 as a result of the transfer of TB services from Peamount Hospital to St James's Hospital.	**Colette Adida** as consultant histopathologist. **Susan Clarke** as consultant in infectious diseases. **Elizabeth Connolly** as consultant in anaesthesia and intensive care medicine. **John M. Cooney** as consultant liaison psychiatrist. **Colin Doherty** as consultant neurologist. **Aoife Doyle** as consultant ophthalmologist. **Ruairi Fahy** as consultant respiratory physician. **Michael Gill** as professor of psychiatry. **Rose Anne Kenny** as professor of geriatric medicine. **James O'Donnell** as consultant haematologist. **Dearbhaile O'Donnell** as consultant medical oncologist. **Rory A. O'Donnell** as consultant respiratory and general physician. **Patrick Ormond** as consultant dermatologist. **Jenny Porter** as consultant anaesthetist.	**Hugh Cassidy** as consultant ophthalmologist. **Lesley Fox** as consultant anaesthetist. **Ron Kirkham** as consultant anaesthetist. **Brendan Lawless** as consultant anaesthetist. **Myles McEvilly** as consultant anaesthetist. **Jane Mahon** as assistant director of nursing. **David Shanley** as consultant psychiatrist.

Events	Appointments	Retirements and resignations
2005 (cont.)		
The hospital was designated the Dublin centre for a supra-regional tuberculosis service. This unit will act as the hub of a comprehensive service extending into the community. Development of a new breast clinic.		
2006		
A comprehensive physician-directed transoesophageal echocardiographic service was established in the day surgery centre by cardiologists **Ross Murphy** and **Angie Browne**. The third annual live intervention course took place with live images from the cardiac catheterization laboratory being transmitted to an audience in the Trinity medical school building. The hospital's supra-regional role in the management of lung cancer continued to develop. A new endobronchial ultrasound (EBUS) service commenced. The hospital received approval to proceed with the development of a supra-regional TB unit and a project team was established. The launch of a major Irish longitudinal study on ageing (TILDA Study) under the direction of **Rose Anne Kenny**. Introduction of laparoscopic colorectal surgery. Official launch of the rapid access breast care department by the taoiseach, **Bertie Ahern**.	**Mary Anglim** as consultant gynaecologist. **Breida Boyle** as consultant microbiologist. **Michael Carey** as consultant anaesthetist. **Ian Carter** as CEO. **Daniel Collins** as consultant in anaesthesia and intensive care medicine. **Aidan Corvin** as senior lecturer/ consultant in psychiatry. **Alison Dougall** as dental consultant. **Brian Fitzgerald** as director of finance. **Joseph Fitzgerald** as consultant in anaesthesia and pain medicine. **Paul Gallagher** as director of nursing. **Elaine Greene** as consultant in old age psychiatry. **Michael Guiney** as consultant radiologist. **Joseph Harbison** as senior lecturer/ consultant in medical gerontology.	**Tony Bates** as principal psychologist. **Luke Clancy** as associate professor and consultant in respiratory medicine. **Michael Cullen** as associate professor and consultant endocrinologist. **Aileen Egan** as assistant director of nursing. **Joanna Fitzgerald** as assistant director of nursing (formerly principal midwifery tutor until closure of maternity department in 1987). **Eilish Hardiman** as director of nursing. **David Keane** as consultant cardiologist. **Mary Kennedy** as head medical social worker. **Denis Lawlor** as consultant plastic surgeon. **Eamon McGuinness** as consultant obstetrician and gynaecologist.

Events	Appointments	Retirements and resignations
2006 (cont.)		
An unreported molecular variant of haemoglobin in an Irish patient was discovered by the haemoglobinopathy laboratory. This variant has been entered in the international database as 'Haemoglobin Dublin'.	**Eilish Hardiman** as deputy CEO. **Ken Hardy** as director of human resources. **Marie Louise Healy** as consultant endocrinologist. **Angela Keane** as head medical social worker. **Fiona Lyons** as consultant physician in genitourinary medicine. **Brian Mehigan** as consultant general surgeon. **Ross Murphy** as consultant cardiologist. **Thomas Rogers** as professor of clinical microbiology. **David Sweeney** as administrative director of the William Stokes Postgraduate Centre. **Carmel Wall** as consultant cardiothoracic anaesthetist.	**Celine Traynor** as consultant anaesthetist. **Michael Walsh** as associate professor and consultant cardiologist.
2007		
Completion of the outline development control plan which set out a template for major capital developments in the hospital. The hospital's breast unit was designated as one of the eight specialist centres for symptomatic breast disease in Ireland by the National Cancer Control programme (NCCP). **Peter Daly**, consultant medical oncologist, was awarded the cancer strategic development award for his pivotal role in establishing adult genetic cancer services in Ireland.	**Catherine Flynn** as consultant haematologist. **Martina Hennessy** as senior lecturer in clinical pharmacology and medical education/consultant clinical pharmacologist. **Niall McElwee** as project and technical services manager.	**Mary McKenna** as assistant director of nursing. **Eric Mulvihill** as consultant microbiologist.

Events	Appointments	Retirements and resignations
2007 (cont.)		
The lord mayor of Dublin, **Cllr Vincent Jackson**, presented **Patrick Plunkett**, consultant in emergency medicine, with the Lord Mayor's Award 2007.	**Nasir Mahmud** as senior lecturer/ consultant gastroenterologist.	
The respiratory assessment unit won the Irish Health Care award, 'Best Hospital Project', in recognition of the comprehensive chronic obstructive airways disease (COPD) service provided by the unit. The unit consists of a multidisciplinary team led by **Barry O'Connell**, consultant in respiratory medicine.	**Nikolay Nikolov** as consultant anaesthetist. **Veronica O'Keane** as consultant psychiatrist. **Sean O'Neill** as consultant vascular surgeon. **Dermot O'Toole** as senior lecturer/ consultant gastroenterologist. **Craig Robertson** as general support services manager.	
The tánaiste and minister for health and children, **Mary Harney**, officially launched the Mohs micrographic surgery service provided by **Patrick Ormond**, consultant dermatologist. The initiative means that patients with complicated skin cancers do not have to travel abroad for treatment.		
The rheumatology multidisciplinary team embracing occupational therapy, physiotherapy and clinical nurse specialist, won the Bernard Conor award for the RAISE project (rheumatoid arthritis informed support and education). This was an initiative to help patients with early inflammatory arthritis.		
A weekly homeless persons' clinic was initiated by the social workers in the emergency department in conjunction with the homeless persons' unit in James's Street.		

Events	Appointments	Retirements and resignations
2008		
Barry White, consultant haematologist, appointed as hospital medical director.	**Elizabeth Connolly** as senior lecturer/consultant general surgeon.	**Cliff Beirne** as consultant oral surgeon.
Eoin Gaffney, consultant histopathologist, and **Blanaid Mee**, laboratory assistant, established the St James's Hospital Cancer Biobank.	**Moya Cunningham** as consultant radiation oncologist.	**Peter Daly** as associate professor and consultant medical oncologist.
Opening of the Centre for Advanced Medical Imaging.	**Caroline Daly** as consultant cardiologist.	**Fiona O'Higgins** as consultant anaesthetist.
Donald Weir elected chairman of St James's Hospital Foundation.	**Charles Gillham** as consultant radiation oncologist.	**Gregor Shanik** as associate professor and consultant vascular surgeon.
Positron emission tomography (PET-CT) facility opened in Hospital 1.	**Niall Hogan** as consultant orthopaedic surgeon.	
A new improved treatment for dialysis patients called Online Haemodiafiltration was introduced in the renal dialysis unit.	**Gerard Kearns** as consultant oral and maxillofacial surgeon.	
The department of neurology received innovation funding in 2008 for the epilepsy management programme. The purpose of the programme is to reduce the need for admission of epileptic patients.	**Thomas McCarthy** as consultant orthopaedic surgeon.	
Clinical Skills Laboratory established.	**John McKenna** as consultant orthopaedic surgeon.	
Transcatheter aortic valve implantation (TAVI) was introduced as a new procedure for patients who are suffering from aortic stenosis and for whom surgery is not appropriate. The procedure is minimally invasive and takes place in the cardiac catheter laboratory without the need for a general anaesthetic.	**Neil O'Hare** as head of medical physics and bioengineering.	
	Deirdre O'Mahony as consultant medical oncologist.	
	Veronica Treacy as director of pharmacy.	
Gerard King, chief cardiac technician, won the cardiology award at the Irish Journal of Medical Science Doctor Awards for research on myocardial stiffness and compliance in elite athletes.		

Events	Appointments	Retirements and resignations
2008 (cont.)		
St James's Hospital obtained a licence for stem cell transplantation from the Irish Medicines Board becoming the only hospital licensed for this procedure in Ireland.		
The transfer of the management of the psychiatric service at St James's Hospital from St Patrick's Hospital to the HSE was completed and subsequently all the staff in the service were employed either by the HSE or by St James's Hospital.		
The department of anaesthesia, intensive care and pain medicine moved to a purpose-built unit comprising offices, an IT room and a seminar room to accommodate the needs of twenty-three consultants and twenty-eight trainees.		
2009		
Death of **John Feely**, professor of pharmacology and therapeutics.	**Noel Boyle** as consultant cardiologist.	**David Borton** as consultant orthopaedic surgeon.
Paul Browne, consultant haematologist, appointed as hospital medical director.	**Angela Fitzgerald** as deputy CEO in place of **Eilish Hardiman** who was seconded to the National Paediatric Development Board as CEO.	**Frank Brady** as consultant oral and maxillofacial surgeon.
Barry White, consultant haematologist, appointed as National Director for Quality and Clinical Care by the HSE. He established the National Clinical Programmes. His role was subsequently changed to National Director, National Clinical Programmes in 2010.	**Ciaran Johnston** as consultant radiologist. **Christoph Kemps** as consultant anaesthetist. **Una Kennedy** as consultant in emergency medicine.	**Garry Fenelon** as consultant orthopaedic surgeon. **Angela Keane** as social work manager. **Peter Lawlor** as consultant in palliative medicine.
Jeanne Moriarty, consultant in anaesthesia and critical care medicine, elected president of the College of Anaesthetists of Ireland.	**Yvonne Langan** as consultant clinical neurophysiologist.	**Shaun McCann** as George Gabriel Stokes professor of haematology and consultant haematologist.

Events	Appointments	Retirements and resignations
2009 (cont.)		
Gaye **Cunnane** appointed as director of postgraduate medical education. Construction commenced on radiation oncology building. FEES (fibreoptic endoscopic examination of swallow) service established by the speech and language therapy department. The first radio frequency ablation (HALO) performed in Ireland was carried out in the endoscopy unit. This is a treatment for premalignant lesions of the oesophagus and was introduced by consultant surgeon **Narayanasamy Ravi** and consultant gastroenterologist **Dermot O'Toole**. Commencement of a rapid access prostate clinic. The twenty-first anniversary of the founding of the Mercer's Institute for Research on Ageing marked by the performance of Handel's *Solomon* in St Patrick's cathedral by the Guinness choir and orchestra.	**Paul McCormick** as consultant general surgeon. **Anne-Marie McLaughlin** as consultant respiratory and general physician. **Sylvia O'Keeffe** as consultant radiologist. **Finbar O'Shea** as consultant rheumatologist. **Mark Rafferty** as consultant otolaryngologist. **Narayanasamy Ravi** as consultant gastrointestinal surgeon. **Niall Sheehy** as consultant radiologist.	**Bernadette Moran** as radiographic services manager. **Beatrice Nolan** as consultant haematologist. **Richard Stephens** as consultant general surgeon.
2010		
Eilis McGovern, consultant cardiothoracic surgeon, elected president of the Royal College of Surgeons in Ireland, the first woman to hold this office. **Louise Barnes**, consultant dermatologist, appointed as National Clinical Lead for Dermatology. **Colm Bergin**, consultant in infectious diseases, appointed as National Clinical Lead for Outpatient Parenteral Antimicrobial Therapy programme.	**Sinead Brennan** as consultant radiation oncologist. **Susan Dennan** as radiographic service manager. **Stephen Finn** as senior lecturer/ consultant in histopathology. **Mark Halligan** as consultant anaesthetist. **Patrick Hayden** as consultant haematologist.	**Noel Boyle** as consultant cardiologist. **Martin Buckley** as manager of information and management services. **Mary Foley** as assistant director of nursing. **Patrick Freyne** as consultant radiologist. **Nuala Kennedy** as assistant director of nursing.

Events	Appointments	Retirements and resignations
2010 (cont.)		
Colin Doherty, consultant neurologist, appointed as National Clinical Lead for Neurology. **Joe Harbison**, consultant in medical gerontology/stroke medicine, appointed as National Clinical Lead for Stroke. **Mary Harney**, minister for health and children, announced the development of the new Mercer's Institute for Successful Ageing at a function in the hospital boardroom. A manual and DVD for patients and their families entitled *Understanding and Managing Persistent Cancer Related Fatigue* was produced by **Ann-Marie O'Dwyer**, consultant psychiatrist, and **Sonya Collier**, clinical psychologist.	**Siobhan Hutchinson** as consultant neurologist. **Rachael Kidney** as consultant general physician. **Padraig O'Ceallaigh** as consultant maxillofacial surgeon. **Niamh O'Connell** as consultant haematologist. **Enda O'Connor** as consultant in intensive care medicine. **Paula Phillips** as assistant director of nursing. **Ronan Ryan** as consultant cardiothoracic surgeon. **Bairbre Wynne** as consultant dermatologist.	**Emer Lawlor** as consultant haematologist. **Stanley Miller** as consultant radiologist. **John Nolan** as associate professor and consultant endocrinologist. **Donal Sean O'Briain** as associate professor and consultant histopathologist. **Linus Offiah** as associate emergency physician. **Veronica O'Keane** as consultant psychiatrist. **Fionnuala O'Loughlin** as consultant general adult psychiatrist. **Paula Phillips** as assistant director of nursing. **Mark Rafferty** as consultant otolaryngologist. **Hugh Smyth** as consultant orthopaedic surgeon.
2011		
J. Bernard Walsh, consultant physician in geriatric medicine, appointed as hospital medical director. **James O'Donnell** appointed George Gabriel Stokes professor of haematology.	**Peter Beddy** as consultant radiologist. **Paul Browne** as professor of haematology. **Grainne Flynn** as consultant psychiatrist. **David Gallagher** as consultant medical oncologist/geneticist. **Grainne Govender** as consultant radiologist.	**Davis Coakley** as professor of medical gerontology and consultant physician in geriatric medicine. **Conleth Feighery** as associate professor of immunology. **Eilish Hardiman** as deputy CEO.

Events	Appointments	Retirements and resignations
2011 (cont.)		
A collaborative agreement was signed by St James's Hospital, Tallaght Hospital and Trinity College Dublin to establish Trinity Health (Ireland). The agreement allowed for the incorporation of operational activities between the school of medicine and its major teaching hospitals.	**Susannah Harte** as consultant radiologist.	**Deirdre O'Mahony** as consultant medical oncologist.
	Waseem Kamran as consultant gynaecologist.	**Liam O'Siorain** as consultant in palliative medicine.
The Trinity Biomedical Sciences Institute (TBSI) on Pearse Street was opened by the taoiseach, **Enda Kenny**, and EU commissioner, **Maire Geoghegan-Quinn**. The preclinical training of medical students is based in the institute.	**Niamh Leonard** as consultant histopathologist.	
	Zenia Martin as consultant vascular surgeon.	
	Kieran O'Shea as consultant orthopaedic surgeon.	
James Meaney elected chairman of St James's Hospital Foundation.	**David Robinson** as consultant physician in geriatric medicine.	
Radiation Oncology Cancer Care Centre opened by the minister for health and children, **Dr James Reilly**.	**Kevin Ryan** as consultant haematologist.	
	Odhran Shelley as consultant in plastic and reconstructive surgery.	
Expansion of magnetic resonance imaging (MRI) with two new scanners installed.	**Pierre Thirion** as consultant radiation oncologist.	
Intensive care unit upgrades completed with nine new beds.		
Heart failure outreach service commenced under the direction of consultant cardiologist, **Caroline Daly**.		
The inaugural lecture of the Mercer's Institute for Successful Ageing, 'Ageing and the Life of the Mind' was delivered by **Dr Thomas Mitchell** in the Dining Hall, Trinity College.		

Events	Appointments	Retirements and resignations
2012		
Patrick Plunkett was awarded honorary fellowship of the European Society for Emergency Medicine for his outstanding contribution to the development of the specialty in Europe. **Ellen O'Sullivan**, consultant anaesthetist, elected president of the College of Anaesthetists of Ireland. Submission of a proposal to have the new national children's hospital based at St James's Hospital. A respiratory palliative care pathway was developed in conjunction with Our Lady's Hospice, Harold's Cross, to provide palliative care services for patients with end-stage non-malignant respiratory diseases. Establishment of ankylosing spondylitis clinic in the rheumatology day care centre. Establishment of capital project office. Secondment of **Eilis McGovern** to the HSE as Director of National Doctors Training and Planning.	**Dhafir Alazawi** as consultant general surgeon. **Lucy Balding** as consultant in palliative medicine. **Rupert Barry** as consultant dermatologist. **Rebecca Fanning** as consultant anaesthetist. **Brian Fitzgerald** as CEO. **Richard Flavin** as consultant histopathologist. **Finbar MacCarthy** as consultant gastroenterologist and general physician. **Diarmuid Ó Donghaile** as consultant haematologist. **Neil O'Hare** as director of informatics. **Norma O'Leary** as consultant in palliative medicine. **Esther O'Regan** as consultant histopathologist. **Niamh Phelan** as consultant endocrinologist. **Darragh Shields** as consultant in emergency medicine.	**Margaret Byrne** as senior medical social worker. **Ian Carter** as CEO. **Brian Fitzgerald** as director of finance. **Philomena Flood** as manager, clinical nutrition. **Eoin Gaffney** as associate professor and consultant histopathologist. **Ronald Grainger** as consultant urologist. **Napoleon Keeling** as associate professor of gastroenterology. **Dermot Kelleher** as professor of medicine. **Kieran O'Shea** as consultant orthopaedic surgeon. **Bernard Silke** as consultant general physician.
2013		
Death of **Donal Hollywood**, Marie Curie professor of clinical oncology. Official opening of Clinical Research Facility by the taoiseach, **Enda Kenny**.	**Nadim Akasheh** as consultant in respiratory and general medicine. **Larry Bacon** as consultant haematologist.	**Angela Fitzgerald** as deputy CEO. **Christoph Kemps** as consultant anaesthetist.

Events	Appointments	Retirements and resignations
2013 (cont.)		
Paul Gallagher, director of nursing, was elected president of the Nursing and Midwifery Board. The administration of first dose of intravenous medication by nursing staff was introduced throughout the hospital. The minister for health and children, **Dr James Reilly**, launched a ten-year cancer audit report for St James's Hospital. The report, 'The Establishment of Hospital Groups as a Transition to Independent Hospitals Trusts', was launched by the minister for health and children **Dr James Reilly**. It included a proposal to incorporate St James's, Tallaght, the Coombe Women and Infants University Hospital, Naas, Tullamore and Portlaoise hospitals into a new hospital trust which will be known as the Dublin Midlands Hospital Group. The Coombe Women and Infants University Hospital joined Trinity Health (Ireland).	**David Bradley** as consultant neurologist. **David Burke** as consultant cardiologist. **Declan Byrne** as consultant in general and geriatric medicine. **Sinead Cuffe** as consultant medical oncologist. **Ann Dalton** as deputy CEO. **Nazmy ElBeltagi** as consultant radiation oncologist. **Cliona Grant** as consultant medical oncologist. **Claragh Healy** as consultant plastic and reconstructive surgeon. **Tara Kingston** as consultant general adult psychiatrist. **Kevin McCarroll** as consultant physician in geriatric medicine. **Niall McElwee** as director of capital projects. **Andrew Maree** as consultant cardiologist. **Clodagh O'Dwyer** as consultant in general and geriatric medicine. **James Paul O'Neill** as consultant otolaryngologist. **Ciaran O'Riain** as consultant histopathologist.	**Dermot Moore** as consultant vascular surgeon. **Kenneth O'Byrne** as consultant medical oncologist.
2014		
Patrick Plunkett, consultant in emergency medicine, appointed as hospital medical director.	**Catherine Bossut** as consultant orthopaedic surgeon.	**Niall Mulvihill** as consultant cardiologist.

Events	Appointments	Retirements and resignations
2014 (cont.)		
Paul Browne, professor of haematology, appointed head of the medical school. **Owen Smith** appointed Regius professor of physic. The medical oncology ward was named the Donal Hollywood ward. The National Stereotactic Radiotherapy programme was launched in the Radiation Oncology Cancer Care Centre. The directorate system was reorganized with the absorption of six longstanding clinical directorates into two new directorates, the medicine and emergency directorate (MED) and the surgery, anaesthetics and critical care directorate (SACC). A new quality and safety improvement directorate was established with **Una Geary** as director. Speech and Language Therapy moved to new accommodation on Brookfield Road. The new medical residence near the main concourse was opened. The hospital commenced development of an off-site medical records centre.	**Niall Conlon** as consultant immunologist. **Sarah Early** as consultant cardiothoracic surgeon. **David Kevans** as consultant gastroenterologist and general physician. **Rosaleen Lannon** as consultant physician in geriatric medicine. **John Larkin** as consultant surgeon. **Rustom Manecksha** as consultant urologist. **Ignacio Martin-Loeches** as consultant in intensive care medicine. **Simon Moores** as director of finance. **Adrian O'Callaghan** as consultant vascular surgeon. **Terence Tan** as consultant anaesthetist. **Emma Tuohy** as consultant haematologist.	**Martin O'Connor** as consultant ophthalmologist. **Veronica Tracey** as director of pharmacy. **J. Bernard Walsh** as clinical professor and consultant physician in geriatric medicine.
2015		
Professor **Charles Normand** appointed as acting chairman of the hospital board, January to September 2015. **Patrick Plunkett** appointed as acting CEO, February to June 2015.	**Conor Barry** as consultant oral and maxillofacial surgeon. **Lorcan Birthistle** as CEO. **Ian Brennan** as consultant radiologist. **Fiona Browne** as consultant dermatologist.	**Brian Fitzgerald** as CEO. **Mairead Griffin** as consultant histopathologist. **Clodagh O'Dwyer** as consultant physician in general and geriatric medicine.

Events	Appointments	Retirements and resignations
2015 (cont.)		
Fiona Lyons, consultant physician in genitourinary medicine, appointed as National Clinical Lead for sexual health services.	**Patricia Daly** as consultant radiation oncologist.	**Catriona O'Sullivan** as consultant radiation oncologist.
The Irish Society of Gastroenterology awarded **Donald Weir** a Lifetime Achievement Award in recognition of his research achievements on folate and vitamin B12 metabolism, coeliac disease and colon cancer.	**Niall Fanning** as consultant anaesthetist. **Jennifer Kieran** as consultant in infectious diseases and internal medicine.	**Patrick Scanlon** as consultant anaesthetist. **Rosemarie Watson** as consultant dermatologist.
A Memorandum of Understanding was signed in 2015 between St James's Hospital and the School of Pharmacy and Pharmaceutical Sciences, TCD, forging strong links and a commitment to collaborate in teaching, training and research.	**Aoife Maguire** as consultant histopathologist. **Gail Melanophy** as director of pharmacy. **Patricia O'Connor** as consultant physician in clinical pharmacology and therapeutics.	
The National Burns Unit set up an allograft skin bank at the Irish Transfusion Service.	**Christopher Theopold** as consultant plastic and reconstructive surgeon	
The Regional Oncology Programme Office (ROPO) was established. The aim of ROPO is to coordinate and consolidate oncology initiatives and to optimize resources. **John Reynolds**, professor of surgery, is the director.		
The residential unit for patients requiring extended care in Hospital 4 was transferred to the new Hollybrook Lodge Care Centre in Inchicore. This was the last extended care unit in St James's Hospital.		
Christopher Soraghan, senior medical physicist and clinical engineer, and Anthony Edwards, clinical photographer, completed the design of an app to assist patients to navigate the St James's Hospital campus.		

Events	Appointments	Retirements and resignations
2015 (cont.)		
The St James's Hospital Research and Development Hub was established to increase centralized research oversight, building on the strong research culture on the campus. It is the first hospital-based hub of its kind in the country and is a joint venture between St James's Hospital and the Clinical Research Facility.		
The Cancer Molecular Diagnostics laboratory developed the clinically accredited Next Generation Sequencing cancer profiling service.		
The Haemoglobinopathies (eg. sickle cell/thalassaemia) service for adults was initiated. This is a rapidly growing condition in the Irish setting with increasing numbers of people affected, due to migration from African, Caribbean, Asian and Mediterranean countries.		
2016		
Louise Barnes, consultant dermatologist, appointed as hospital medical director.	**Alan Broderick** as consultant anaesthetist.	**Margaret Codd** as assistant director of nursing.
Suzanne Norris, consultant gastroenterologist, appointed as National Clinical Lead for hepatitis C.	**Joseph Browne** as consultant physician in general and geriatric medicine.	**Kenneth Hardy** as director of human resources.
An honorary degree of LLD was conferred on **Peta Taaffe**, retired director of nursing, by the University of Dublin.	**John Cosgrave** as consultant cardiologist.	**T.E.D. McDermott** as consultant urologist.
Institute of Translational Medicine established.	**Brenda Griffin** as consultant nephrologist.	**Patrick Plunkett** as clinical professor and consultant in emergency medicine.
	Crothur Fergal Kelleher as consultant medical oncologist.	

Events	Appointments	Retirements and resignations
2016 (cont.)		
Mercer's Institute for Successful Ageing formally opened by the president, **Michael D. Higgins**. The name of the National Centre for Hereditary Coagulation Disorders was changed to the National Coagulation Centre. Work began on the site for the new national children's hospital. A number of events were held to mark the centenary of the 1916 Rising.	**Paul Lennon** as consultant otolaryngologist. **Grainne McDermott** as consultant anaesthetist. **Ann McKenna** as consultant plastic surgeon. **Stephen O'Connor** as consultant cardiologist. **Ciara Ryan** as consultant histopathologist. **Paul Staunton** as consultant in emergency medicine.	

Appendix

Chairmen of the Board, St James's Hospital, 1971–2018

July 1971–August 1972	Deputy P.J. Burke
August 1972–August 1973	Prof. D.I.D. Howie
August 1973–August 1974	Cllr. H.P. Dockrell
August 1974–August 1975	Prof. D.I.D. Howie
August 1975–August 1976	Cllr. H.P. Dockrell
August 1976–August 1977	Prof. D.I.D. Howie
August 1977–August 1978	Cllr. H.P. Dockrell
August 1978–August 1979	Prof. D.I.D. Howie
August 1979–August 1980	Dr J. Behan
August 1980–August 1981	Prof. D.I.D. Howie
August 1981–August 1982	Dr J. Behan
August 1982–August 1983	Prof. D.I.D. Howie
August 1983–August 1984	Dr J. Behan
August 1984–April 2002	Prof. D.I.D. Howie
May 2002–April 2011	Prof. T.N. Mitchell
April 2011–December 2014	Prof. D. Shanley
September 2015–Present	Mr P. Donnelly

Notes

Chapter One

1   J.T. Gilbert, *Calendar of ancient records of Dublin* (Dublin, 1896), vi, p. 179.

2   B. Fitzgerald, *The Anglo-Irish* (St Albans, 1952), p. 305.

3   D. Dickson, *New foundations: Ireland, 1660–1800* (Dublin, 2000), p. 115.

4   M. Hennessy, 'The priory and hospital of New Gate: the evolution and decline of a medieval monastic estate' in W. Smyth and K. Whelan (eds), *Common ground: essays on the historical geography of Ireland* (Cork, 1988), pp 41–54.

5   C. McNeill, 'Hospitals of St John without the New Gate, Dublin' in H. Clarke (ed.), *Medieval Dublin* (Dublin, 1990), pp 77–82. M.V. Ronan, *The Reformation in Dublin* (London, 1926), pp 187–92.

6   Gilbert, *Calendar of ancient records of Dublin*, iii, p. 225. G. Nicholls, *A history of the Irish poor law* (London, 1856), p. 28.

7   Gilbert, *Calendar of ancient records of Dublin*, v, p. 61.

8   39 Eliz. 1, c.3. An Act for the relief of the poor (1601).

9   Nicholls, *A history of the Irish poor law* (London, 1856), p. 13.

10   F. Powell, 'Dean Swift and the Dublin Foundling Hospital', *Studies*, 70: 278–9 (1981), 162–70.

11   J. Swift, 'A proposal for giving badges to the beggars in all the parishes of Dublin' in Temple Scott (ed.), *The prose works of Jonathan Swift*, 12 vols (London, 1905), vii, pp 325–35.

12   J. O'Carroll, 'Contemporary attitudes towards the homeless poor, 1725–1775' in D. Dickson (ed.), *The gorgeous mask: Dublin 1700–1850* (Dublin, 1987), p. 65.

13   Gilbert, *Calendar of ancient records of Dublin*, v, p. 586.

14   Ibid., pp 207–8.

15   'Proposals concerning a workhouse, 1681' in *Calendar of the manuscripts of the marquess of Ormond* (London), vi, p. 69.

16   T.K. Moylan, 'Vagabonds and sturdy beggars', *Dublin Historical Record*, 1:3 (1938), 41.

17   D. Keenan, *Eighteenth-century Ireland, 1703–1800: society and history* (Bloomington, 2014), p. 274.

18   'Heads of proceedings (1725–1726)', Marsh's Library, Dublin, MS.Z 3.1.1, 155.

19   Gilbert, *Calendar of ancient records of Dublin*, vi, p. 90.

20   Ibid., pp 90–1.

21   Ibid., pp 90 and 179.

22   Ibid., p. 179.

23   Ibid., p. 214. E. Malcolm, *Swift's hospital: the history of St Patrick's Hospital, Dublin, 1746–1989* (Dublin, 1989), pp 16–17.

24   Gilbert, *Calendar of ancient records of Dublin*, vi, p. 219.

25   Ibid., p. 282.

26   2 Anne, c.19. An Act for erecting a workhouse in the city of Dublin for employing and maintaining the poor thereof (1703).

27   Ibid.

28   Ibid.

29   Ibid.

30   G. Miege, *The present state of Great Britain and Ireland* (London, 1718), iii, pp 48–9.

31   J. Vernon, *Remarks on a paper, entituled, An abstract of the state of the work-house for maintaining of the poor of the city of Dublin* (Dublin, 1716), pp 1–12.

32   J. Warburton, J. Whitelaw and R. Walsh, *History of the City of Dublin*, 2 vols (London, 1818), i, p. 578.

33   W. Harris, *The history and antiquities of the city of Dublin* (Dublin, 1766), p. 370.

34   E. McParland, *Public architecture in Ireland, 1680 to 1760* (London, 2001), pp 75–9.

35   Vernon, *Remarks on a paper*, pp 1–12.

36   'Accounts of the workhouse, 1710', Marsh's Library, Dublin, MS.Z 3.1.1, 31.

37   C. Casey, *Dublin* (London, 2005), pp 642–4.

38   'Workhouse, Dublin: report of the lord mayor, and seven assistants of their proceedings for the year ending this fourth day of June, Dublin, 1705', Marsh's Library, Dublin, MS.Z 3.1.1, 31.

39   'Accounts of the workhouse, 1710', Marsh's Library, Dublin, MS.Z 3.1.1, 31.

40   'From the commencement of the Workhouse Act 1706', Marsh's Library, Dublin, MS.Z 3.1.1, 31.

41   W.D. Wodsworth, *A history of the ancient Foundling Hospital of Dublin from the year 1702* (Dublin, 1876), pp 3–4.

42   Ibid.

43   'A list of the poore in the City Workhouse from their several parishes with their age and qualitys, 1725–1726.' Marsh's Library, Dublin, MS.Z 3.1.1, 31.

44   J. Hawkesworth, *Letters written by the late Jonathan Swift, D.D., dean of St Patrick's, Dublin and several of his friends* (London, 1746), iii, pp 107–16.

45   Wodsworth, *A history of the ancient Foundling Hospital*, p. 4.

46   Workhouse Papers (1708), Marsh's Library, Dublin, MS.Z 3.1.1, 31.

47   Wodsworth, *A history of the ancient Foundling Hospital*, pp 3–4. *Dublin Evening Post*, 9 Dec. 1732.

48   Swift, 'A proposal for giving badges to the beggars' in Scott (ed.), *The prose works of Jonathan Swift*, vii, p. 326.

49   'Observations on the present state and condition of the workhouse, 6 Apr. 1726', Marsh's Library, Dublin, MS.Z 3.1.1, 31.

50   Ibid.

51   'A list of the poore in the City Workhouse', Marsh's Library, Dublin, MS.Z 3.1.1, 31.

52   Ibid.

53   O'Carroll, 'Contemporary attitudes towards the homeless poor, 1725–1775' in Dickson (ed.), *The gorgeous mask*, p. 77.

54   1 Geo. II, c.17. An Act for the better regulating of the Workhouse of the City of Dublin, and to regulate and provide for the poor thereof (1727).

55   Ibid.

56   Ibid.

57   Ibid.

58   T. Sheridan, *The works of the Rev. Jonathan Swift*, 24 vols (London, 1803), xviii, pp 258–64.

59   J. Swift, *Verses on the death of Doctor Swift* (Bathurst, 1739), pp 3–22.

60   E. Malcolm, *Swift's hospital: the history of St Patrick's Hospital, Dublin, 1746–1989* (Dublin, 1989), pp 32–103.

61   Swift, 'A proposal for giving badges to the beggars' in Scott (ed.), *The prose works of Jonathan Swift*, vii, p. 326.

62   L. Damrosh, *Jonathan Swift: his life and his world* (New Haven, 2013), p. 417.

63   *Dublin Evening Post*, 9 Dec. 1732.

64   J. Robins, *The lost children: a study of charity children in Ireland, 1700–1900* (Dublin, 1980), pp 6–8.

65   J. Kelly, 'Infanticide in eighteenth-century Ireland', *Irish Economic and Social History*, 19 (1992) 2–25.

66   K.H. O'Connell, *Irish peasant society* (Oxford, 1968), pp 31–86.

67   Robins, *The lost children* (Dublin, 1980), pp 12–13.

68   1 Geo. II, c.17. An Act for the better regulating of the Workhouse of the City of Dublin, and to regulate and provide for the poor thereof (1727).

69   J. Swift, *A modest proposal for preventing the children of poor people from being a burthen to their parents or the country, and for making them beneficial to the publick* (Dublin, 1729), p. 5.

70   Powell, 'Dean Swift and the Dublin Foundling Hospital', *Studies*, 70:278/9 (1981), 162–70.

71   Swift, *A modest proposal*, p. 7.

72   Ibid., p. 11.

73   Ibid., p. 14.

74   Robins, *The lost children*, p. 14.

75   3 Geo. II, c.17, Ir Stat. An Act for the better enabling of the governors of the Workhouse of the City of Dublin to provide for and employ the poor therein, and for the more effectual punishment of vagabonds: and also for the better securing of and providing for lunatics and foundling children (1729).

76   J. Swift, *A proposal for giving badges to the beggars in all the parishes of Dublin* (London, 1737), p. 4.

77   Wodsworth, *A history of the ancient Foundling Hospital*, pp 4–5.

78   W. Wright, *The Brontës in Ireland* (London, 1894), pp 15–31.

79   E. Chitham, *The Brontës' Irish background* (London, 1986), pp 123–33.

80   E. Chitham, *Western winds* (Dublin, 2015), pp 180–2.

Chapter Two

1   W.D. Wodsworth, *A history of the ancient Foundling Hospital of Dublin from the year 1702* (Dublin, 1876), p. 4.

2   D. Kertzer, *Sacrificed for honor: Italian infant abandonment and the politics of reproductive control* (Boston, 1993), p. 81.

3   J. Boswell, *The kindness of strangers: the abandonment of children in Western Europe* (New York, 1988), p. 421.

4   Wodsworth, *A history of the ancient Foundling Hospital*, p. 56.

5   *Instructions to the officers and servants of the Workhouse of the City of Dublin*, Haliday Collection of Pamphlets, National Library of Ireland, pp 3–14.

6   Ibid.

7   R. Moore, *Leeches to lasers: sketches of a medical family* (Killala, 2002), pp 39–58.

8   J. Swift, *A short view of the state of Ireland* (Dublin, 1727), p. 15.

9   Lord Tullamore, *A report from the lords committees appointed to enquire into the state of the workhouse of this city* (Dublin, 1737).

10   B. Twomey, *Dublin in 1707: a year in the life of the city* (Dublin, 2009), p. 10.

11   Wodsworth, *A history of the ancient Foundling Hospital*, pp 4–5.

12   Ibid., pp 1–2.

13   Ibid., p. 27.

14   J. Bell, *Travels from St Petersburg in Russia to diverse parts of Asia* (London, 1764), pp 118–19.

15   Wodsworth, *A history of the ancient Foundling Hospital*, p. 32.

16   Ibid., p. 4.

17   9 Geo. II, c. 25, An Act for rebuilding the cathedral church of St Finbarry, in the city of Cork, and for erecting a workhouse in the city of Cork … (1735).

18   J. Warburton et al., *History of the city of Dublin*, 2 vols (London, 1818), i, p. 582.

19   Wodsworth, *A history of the ancient Foundling Hospital*, pp 26–7.

20   Ibid.

21   Ibid., p. 27.

22   The Tholsel was a merchants' hall where the city assembly met, and it also functioned as a courthouse in the eighteenth century.

23   *Pue's Occurrences*, 31 (16 Apr. 1754) and 33 (23 Apr. 1754).

24   Wodsworth, *A history of the ancient Foundling Hospital*, p. 29.

25   Ibid.

26   J. Robins, *The lost children: a study of charity children in Ireland, 1700–1900* (Dublin, 1980), p. 19.

27   Ibid.

28   J. Swift, *A proposal for giving badges to the beggars in all the parishes of Dublin* (London, 1737), p. 9.

29   Ibid., p. 8.

30   Ibid., pp 13–14.

31   Ibid., p. 11.

32   I. Ehrenpreis, *Swift: the man, his works and the age* (London, 1983), pp 813–16.

33   D. Dickson, *Arctic Ireland: the extraordinary story of the Great Frost and forgotten famine of 1740–1741* (Belfast, 1998), p. 1.

34   Ibid., pp 37–8.

35   Ibid., p. 57.

36   Warburton et al., *History of the city of Dublin*, 2 vols (London, 1818), i, pp 583–5.

37   A. Crookshank and D. Webb, *Paintings and sculptures in Trinity College Dublin* (Dublin, 1990), p. 23.

38   23 Geo. II, c. 11. An Act to provide for begging children, and for the better regulation of charity schools, and for taking up vagrant and offensive beggars in the city of Dublin and liberties thereof, and the liberties thereto adjoining (1749).

39   Robins, *The lost children*, p. 20.

40   C. DeLaselle, 'Les enfants abandonnés à Paris au XVIII. siècle', *Annales, Économies, Sociétés, Civilisations*, 30 (1975), 187–218.

41   *Instructions to the officers and servants of the Workhouse of the City of Dublin*, Haliday Collection of Pamphlets, National Library of Ireland, pp 3–14.

42   Wodsworth, *A history of the ancient Foundling Hospital*, p. 33.

43   'A report from the committee appointed to enquire into the state and management of the fund of the workhouse of the city of Dublin, and into the conduct of the officers and servants of the said house, for ten years last past' (Dublin, 1758), pp 4–7.

44   *Instructions to the officers and servants of the Workhouse of the City of Dublin*, pp 3–14.

45   'A report from the committee appointed to enquire into the state and management of the fund of the workhouse of the city of Dublin, pp 4–7.

46   M. Hayden, 'Charity children in eighteenth-century Dublin', *Dublin Historical Record*, 3 (1943), 92–107.

47   'A report from the committee appointed to enquire into the state and management of the fund of the workhouse of the city of Dublin', pp 4–7.

48   Wodsworth, *A history of the ancient Foundling Hospital*, p. 29.

49   J. Whitelaw, *An essay on the populations of Dublin being the result of an actual survey in 1798* (Dublin, 1805), pp 50–1.

50   C. Maxwell, *Dublin under the Georges* (London, 1956), pp 138–80.

51   *Dublin Journal*, 30 Sept. 1758.

52   Robins, *The lost children*, p. 26.

53   *Saunders's Newsletter*, 2 Feb. 1774.

54   *Freeman's Journal*, 3–5 May 1770.

55   11–12 Geo III, c. 11. An Act for better regulating the foundling hospital and workhouse in the city of Dublin and increasing the fund for the support thereof (1772).

56   Robins, *The lost children*, pp 23–4.

57   Wodsworth, *A history of the ancient Foundling Hospital*, p. 34.

58   Robins, *The lost children*, pp 24–5.

59   *Dublin Journal*, 25 Mar. 1760.

60   W. Henry, *The cries of the orphans: a sermon preached in the parish church of St Michael, on Sunday April 27th* (Dublin, 1760), pp 3–24.

61   *Freeman's Journal*, 7–10 June 1766.

62   Ibid., 6–9 May 1769.

63   Wodsworth, *A history of the ancient Foundling Hospital of Dublin from the year 1702* (Dublin, 1876), p. 34.

64   M.P. O'Malley, *Lios-an-Uisce* (Dublin, 1982), p. 51.

65   *Instructions to the officers and servants of the Workhouse of the City of Dublin*, pp 3–14.

66   *Freeman's Journal*, 19–22 Oct. 1765.

67   Anon., *An introduction to the reading of the Holy Bible, composed for the use of the Foundling Hospital in Dublin and the charity schools of Ireland* (Dublin, 1765), pp 116–125.

68   *Dublin Journal*, 6 Oct. 1764.

69   *Freeman's Journal*, 25–9 Apr. 1769.

70   C. Orr, 'Aunts, wives, courtiers: the ladies of Bowood' in N. Aston and C. Orr (eds), *An enlightened statesman in Whig Britain: Lord Shelbourne in context* (Woodenbridge, 2011), pp 67–8.

71   Robins, *The lost children*, p. 25.

72   O'Malley, *Lios-an-Uisce*, pp 51–2.

73   Orr, 'Aunts, wives, courtiers' in Aston and Orr (eds), *An enlightened statesman*, pp 67–8.

74   *Freeman's Journal*, 20–3 July 1765.

75   B.B. Butler, 'Lady Arbella Denny', *Dublin Historical Record*, 9:1 (1947) 1–20.

76   *Dublin Chronicle*, 29 Jan. 1788.

Chapter Three

1   W.D. Wodsworth, *A history of the ancient Foundling Hospital of Dublin from the year 1702* (Dublin, 1876), p. 111.

2   R. Woodward, *An argument in support of the right of the poor in the kingdom of Ireland to a national provision in the appendix to which an attempt is made to settle a measure of the contribution due from each man to the poor, on the footing of justice* (Dublin, 1768), pp 1–55.

3   S. Millin, 'Slums: a sociological retrospect of the city of Dublin', *Journal of the Statistical and Social Inquiry Society of Ireland*, 13:94 (1913–14), 130–57.

4   11 and 12 Geo. III, c. 11. An Act for better regulating the foundling hospital and workhouse in the city of Dublin (1772).

5   Ibid.

6   J. Robins, *The lost children: a study of charity children in Ireland, 1700–1900* (Dublin, 1980), p. 29.

7   11 and 12 Geo. III, c. 11. An Act for better regulating the foundling hospital and workhouse in the city of Dublin (1772).

8   Governors of the Foundling Hospital and Workhouse, 'Rules, orders and by-laws made by the governors of the Foundling Hospital and Workhouse in the City of Dublin for the better regulation and preserving decency and order among the owners, drivers and keepers of hackney-coaches, landaus, chariots, post-chaises, Berlins etc.' (Dublin, 1774), National Library of Ireland 1772 (326).

9   11 and 12 Geo. III, c. 11. An Act for better regulating the foundling hospital and workhouse in the city of Dublin (1772).

10   15 and 16 Geo. III, c. 25. To amend an act passed in the 11th and 12th years of his Majesty's reign entitled, An Act for better regulating the foundling hospital and workhouse in the city of Dublin (1775).

11   Millin, 'Slums', 139.

12   Robins, *The lost children*, p. 29.

13   J. Howard, 'An account of the principle lazarettos in Europe, together with further observations on some foreign prisons and hospitals and additional remarks on the present state of those in Great Britain and Ireland' (London, 1789), pp 82–3.

14   W. Carleton, *The autobiography of William Carleton* (London, 1968), pp 95–6.

15   Wodsworth, *A history of the ancient Foundling Hospital*, pp 48–9.

16   Ibid., p. 22.

17   'Foundling Hospital in the city of Dublin' in *Reports from the commissioners of the Board of Education in Ireland: eighth report* (London, 1813), pp 168–215.

18   J. Warburton et al., *History of the city of Dublin*, 2 vols (London, 1818), i, p. 584.

19   Robins, *The lost children*, p. 31.

20   'Report of the committee appointed to enquire into the state and management of the Foundling Hospital', *Commons Journal* (1792), 1–30.

21   Ibid.

22   *Freeman's Journal*, 31 May 1796.

23   J.A. Froude, *The English in Ireland in the eighteenth century*, 3 vols (London, 1872–4), iii, p. 243.

24   'Report from the committee of the house of commons appointed to inquire into the management and state of the Foundling Hospital, May 1797, appended to reply of the governors etc. (1816), National Library of Ireland, pp 50–81.

25   C. Cameron, *History of the Royal College of Surgeons in Ireland* (Dublin, 1886), p. 104.

26   *Report of the committee of the house of commons appointed to inquire into the management and state of the Foundling Hospital, May 1797*, pp 50–81.

27   Ibid.

28   Ibid.

29   Ibid.

30   Froude, *The English in Ireland in the eighteenth century*, iii, p. 30.

31   Wodsworth, *A history of the ancient Foundling Hospital*, p. 45.

32   38 Geo. III, c. 35. An Act for the better management of the workhouse and foundling hospital in Dublin (1798).

33   C. Maxwell, *Dublin under the Georges* (London, 1956), p. 186.

34   J. Barrington, *Personal sketches of his own times*, 2 vols (London, 1827), i, pp 189–90.

35   Cameron, *History of the Royal College of Surgeons*, p. 319.

36   Wodsworth, *A history of the ancient Foundling Hospital*, p. 45.

37   Cameron, *History of the Royal College of Surgeons*, pp 360–1.

38   Wodsworth, *A history of the ancient Foundling Hospital of Dublin*, p. 26.

39   Ibid., p. 47.

40 Ibid., p. 89.

41 Cameron, *History of the Royal College of Surgeons*, p. 333.

42 *Literary Panorama and National Register*, 1 July 1815.

43 Warburton et al., *History of the city of Dublin*, ii, p. 744.

44 J. Creighton, 'Report (on inoculation) laid before the governors of the Foundling Hospital', *Medical and Physical Journal*, 34:142 (1810), 522–3.

45 Cameron, *History of the Royal College of Surgeons*, pp 360–1.

46 'Report of the Cow-Pock Institution Dublin', *Medical and Physical Journal*, 34:142 (1810), 518–21.

47 Warburton et al., *History of the city of Dublin*, i, pp 585–7.

48 C. Casey, *Dublin* (London, 2005), p. 642.

49 Warburton et al., *History of the city of Dublin*, i, pp 585–7.

50 J.J. McGregor, *New picture of Dublin* (Dublin, 1821), p. 250.

51 D. O'Grada, *Georgian Dublin: the forces that shaped the city* (Dublin, 2015), p. 18.

52 P. Henchy, 'Francis Johnston, architect', *Dublin Historical Record*, 11:1 (1949), 1–16.

53 G.N. Wright, *An historical guide to the city of Dublin* (London, 1825), p. 230.

54 Warburton et al., *History of the city of Dublin*, i, p. 582.

55 Board of Governors, 'Rules for conducting the education of the female children in the Foundling Hospital' (Dublin, 1800), pp 3–23.

56 Wodsworth, *A history of the ancient Foundling Hospital*, p. 55.

57 E. Wakefield, *An account of Ireland, political and statistical*, 2 vols (London, 1812), ii, pp 427–31.

58 Robins, *The lost children*, pp 40–1.

59 S. Grimes, *Ireland in 1804* (Dublin, 1980), p. 30.

60 J. Carr, *The stranger in Ireland* (Philadelphia, 1806), p. 491.

61 A. Plumptre, *Narrative of a residence in Ireland during the summer of 1814 and that of 1815* (London, 1817), p. 42.

62 Carr, *The stranger in Ireland*, pp 315–16.

63 Wakefield, *An account of Ireland*, ii, p. 435.

64 Warburton et al., *History of the city of Dublin*, i, p. 583.

65 Ibid., pp 583–5.

66 Ibid., p. 588.

67 T. Cromwell, *Excursions through Ireland* (London, 1820), pp 131–3.

68 M. Ryan, 'Lectures on the physical education and diseases of infants and children', *London Medical and Surgical Journal*, 5:120 (1834), 490–5.

69 Warburton et al., *History of the city of Dublin*, i, p. 592.

70 *Poor Law Commissioners: eighth annual report* (London, 1842), p. 339.

71 Wodsworth, *A history of the ancient Foundling Hospital*, pp 23–4.

72 Ibid., pp 13–22.

73 T. Malthus, *An essay on the principle of population*, 4 vols (London, 1803), ii, p. 220.

74 Warburton et al., *History of the city of Dublin*, i, pp 595–6.

75 Wodsworth, *A history of the ancient Foundling Hospital*, p. 49.

76 D. Dickson, *The gorgeous mask: Dublin, 1700–1850* (Dublin, 1987), p. 7.

77 M. Maguire, 'A study of poor law relief in Dublin between 1770 and 1830 with specific reference to the Foundling Hospital and the House of Industry' (BA, St Patrick's College, Maynooth, 1980).

78 'Reply of the governors of the Foundling Hospital to a memorial of the lord mayor etc. together with other documents' (Dublin, 1816), National Library of Ireland, pp 36–7.

79 W.J. Fitzpatrick, *The life of Charles Lever* (London 1896), pp 57–8.

80 J. Griscom, *A year in Europe*, 2 vols (New York, 1824), ii, pp 317–18.

81 Papers relating to the Foundling Hospital of Dublin, HC 1824 (281) xxi, 1–8.

82 Griscom, *A year in Europe*, ii, pp 318–19.

83 Robins, *The lost children*, pp 52–3.

84 'Charitable institutions (Dublin): reports of George Nicholls on the Foundling Hospital and House of Industry', Dublin, HC 1842 (389) xxxviii, 1–16.

85 Ibid.

86 Wodsworth, *A history of the ancient Foundling Hospital*, p. iii.

Chapter Four

1   M. de Nie, *The eternal paddy: Irish identity and the British press* (Madison, 2004), p. 105.

2   G. Nicholls, 'Commissioners' third report' in G. Nicholls, *A history of the Irish poor law* (London, 1856), p. 132.

3   *Third report of the commissioners for inquiry into the condition of the poorer classes in Ireland* (Dublin, 1836), Appendix (c), Part 11, 'Report on the City of Dublin', p. 27.

4   R.B. McDowell, 'Ireland on the eve of famine' in R.D. Edwards and T.D. William (eds), *The Great Famine: studies in Irish history, 1845–52* (Dublin, 1994), p. 44.

5   J. O'Connor, *The workhouses of Ireland* (Dublin, 1995), p. 279.

6   G. Nicholls, *Poor laws – Ireland: three reports* (London, 1838), pp 8–9.

7   P. Gray, *The making of the Irish poor law, 1815–43* (Manchester, 2009), pp 131–72.

8   F. Corrigan, 'Dublin workhouses during the Great Famine', *Dublin Historical Record*, 29:2 (1976), 59–65.

9   A. Clifford, *Poor law in Ireland* (Belfast, 1983), p. 96.

10   J. Robins, *Custom House people* (Dublin, 1993), pp 52–5.

11   P.J. Meghen, 'Building the workhouses', *Administration*, 3:1 (1955), 42–6.

12   T. Cuffe, 'Past and present associations of St James's parish' in *St James's church centenary record* (1952), 55–60.

13   G. Wilkinson, 'Report of the progress of workhouses in Ireland' in *Sixth annual report of the Poor Law Commissioners* (London, 1840), p. 232.

14   *Sixth annual report of the English Poor Law Commissioners* (London, 1840), p. 739.

15   Ibid., p. 232.

16   O'Connor, *The workhouses of Ireland*, p. 101.

17   Minutes of the meeting of the board of guardians of the South Dublin Union, 18 Jan. 1844.

18   H. Burke, *The people and the poor law in nineteenth-century Ireland* (Littlehampton, 1987), p. 163.

19   Minutes of meeting of the board of guardians of the South Dublin Union, 20 July 1848.

20   Register of admission and discharge, South Dublin Union, National Archives BG 79/G 1A.

21   *Seventh annual report of the English Poor Law Commissioners* (London, 1841), pp 4–7.

22   Minutes of the meeting of the board of guardians of the South Dublin Union, 4 Aug. 1840.

23   Nicholls, *A history of the Irish poor law*, p. 262.

24   Minutes of the meeting of the board of guardians of the South Dublin Union, 26 June 1845.

25   Ibid., 25 Aug. 1845.

26   Nicholls, *A history of the Irish poor law*, p. 226.

27   *Bengal Catholic Herald*, 6 Nov. 1841.

28   M. Dufficy, 'The story of St James's church, James's Street, Dublin', *Dublin Historical Record*, 29:2 (1976), 66–9.

29   Nicholls, *A history of the Irish poor law*, p. 264.

30   Minutes of the meeting of the board of guardians of the South Dublin Union, 16 Oct. 1845.

31   *Sixth annual report of the English Poor Law Commissioners* (London, 1840), p. 239.

32   M. Powell, 'The workhouses of Ireland', *University Review*, 3 (1965), 11–13.

33   Poor Law (Ireland). Copies of the correspondence between the Poor Law Commissioners in Ireland and the boards of guardians of the North and South Dublin Unions, relative to the duties and payment of the medical officers of those Unions, HC 1842 (274), 1–12.

34   Ibid.

35   Ibid.

36   C. Cameron, *History of the Royal College of Surgeons in Ireland* (Dublin, 1886), p. 616.

37   *Eleventh annual report of the English Poor Law Commissioners* (London, 1845), p. 351.

38   E.D. Mapother, 'The Dublin hospitals: their grants and governing bodies', *Journal of the Statistical and Social Inquiry Society of Ireland*, 5:37 (1870), 130–42.

39   Cameron, *History of the Royal College of Surgeons*, pp 631–2.

40   R. Mayne, 'Observations on pericarditis', *Dublin Journal of Medical Science*, 7 (1835), 255–78.

41   W. Stokes, *Diseases of the heart and aorta* (Dublin, 1854), pp 9–50.

42   Ibid., p. 601.

43 Minutes of the meeting of the board of guardians of the South Dublin Union, 30 May 1844.

44 R. Gaffney, 'Women as doctors and nurses' in O. Checkland and M. Lamb (eds), *Health care as social history* (Aberdeen, 1982), p. 139.

45 Ibid.

46 Minutes of the meeting of the board of guardians of the South Dublin Union, 14 Mar. 1844.

47 Ibid., 13 Dec. 1845.

48 C. O'Brien, 'A history of two Dublin hospitals', unpublished manuscript (Dublin, n.d.), pp 19–20.

49 Minutes of the meeting of the board of guardians of the South Dublin Union, 26 Aug. 1841.

50 Corrigan, 'Dublin workhouses', 59–65.

51 O'Connor, *The workhouses of Ireland*, p. 265.

52 Ibid., pp 182–3.

53 Minutes of the meeting of the board of guardians of the South Dublin Union, 11 Jan. 1844.

54 Ibid., 6 Nov. 1845.

55 Nicholls, *A history of the Irish poor law*, p. 265.

56 Minutes of the meeting of the board of guardians of the South Dublin Union, 29 Feb. 1844.

57 Ibid.

58 Ibid.

59 Burke, *The people and the poor law*, p. 92.

60 Minutes of the meeting of the board of guardians of the South Dublin Union, 29 Aug. 1844.

61 Ibid., 22 Aug. 1844.

62 Ibid., 29 May 1845.

63 Ibid., 18 Sept. 1845.

64 Ibid., 14 Sept. 1848.

65 Ibid., 10 June 1844.

66 Ibid., 27 May 1844.

67 Ibid., 15 May 1845.

68 Ibid., 29 May 1845.

Chapter Five

1 W. Wilde, 'Census of Ireland for the year 1851', Parliament Papers, part V, vol. 1 (Dublin, 1856), pp 246–7.

2 W. Smyth, 'Mapping the people: the growth and distribution of the population' in J. Crowley, W.J. Smyth and M. Murphy (eds), *Atlas of the Great Irish Famine* (Dublin, 2012), pp 13–22.

3 F. Corrigan, 'Dublin Workhouses during the Great Famine', *Dublin Historical Record*, 29:2 (1976), 59–65.

4 Minutes of the meeting of the board of guardians of the South Dublin Union, 6 Nov. 1845.

5 Ibid., 29 Nov. 1845.

6 *Twelfth annual report of the English Poor Law Commissioners* (London, 1846), p. 30.

7 Minutes of the meeting of the board of guardians of the South Dublin Union, 13 Nov. 1845.

8 Ibid., 5 Mar. 1846.

9 Ibid., 26 Mar. 1846.

10 Ibid., 9 Apr. 1846.

11 Ibid., 14 May 1846.

12 Ibid., 4 June 1846.

13 M. O'Mahony, *Famine in Cork city* (Dublin, 2005), pp 65–95.

14 Minutes of the meeting of the board of guardians of the South Dublin Union, 12 Nov. 1846.

15 Ibid., 31 Dec. 1846.

16 Ibid.

17 R. Mayne, 'Observations on the late epidemic of dysentery in Dublin', *Dublin Quarterly Journal of Medicine*, 7 (1849), 294–308.

18 R. Mayne, 'Observations on chronic dysentery', *Dublin Quarterly Journal of Medicine*, 10 (1850) 353–72.

19 Sir W.P. MacArthur, 'Medical history of the Famine' in R.D. Edwards and T.D. Williams (eds), *The Great Famine* (Dublin, 1994), pp 263–315.

20 T.W. Guinnane and C. Ó Gráda, 'The workhouses and Irish Famine mortality', WP00/10, Centre for Economic Research, University College Dublin (2000), pp 1–25.

21 Minutes of the meeting of the board of guardians of the South Dublin Union, 15 July 1847.

22 Ibid., 11 Nov. 1847.

23 Ibid., 25 Nov. 1847.

24 R.B. McDowell, 'Ireland on the eve of the Famine' in R.D. Edwards and T.D. Williams (eds), *The Great Famine* (Dublin, 1994), pp 46–7.

25 Minutes of the meeting of the board of guardians of the South Dublin Union, 16 Mar. 1847.

26 Ibid., 7 Jan. 1847.

27   C. Tunney and P. Nugent, 'Liverpool and the Great Irish Famine' in J. Crowley, W.J. Smyth and M. Murphy (eds), *Atlas of the Great Irish Famine* (Dublin, 2012), pp 504–10.

28   R.J. Raymond, 'Dublin: the Great Famine, 1845–1860', *Dublin Historical Record*, 33:3 (1980), 98–105. C. O'Gráda, *Black '47 and beyond: the Great Irish Famine in history, economy and memory* (Princeton, 1999), p. 173.

29   A. Nicholson, *Annals of the Famine in Ireland* (Dublin, 1998), pp 43–4.

30   L. Atthill, *Recollections of an Irish doctor* (London, 1911), pp 133–4.

31   T. Willis, *The social and sanitary condition of the working classes in Dublin* (Dublin, 1845), p. 31.

32   Ibid., pp 42–5.

33   Minutes of the meeting of the board of guardians of the South Dublin Union, 14 Jan. 1847.

34   J. Robins, *The miasma; epidemic and panic in nineteenth-century Ireland* (Dublin, 1995), p. 132.

35   Minutes of the meeting of the board of guardians of the South Dublin Union, 12 Aug. 1847.

36   B.B. Butler, 'Thomas Pleasants and the Stove Tenter House 1815–1944', *Dublin Historical Record*, 7:1 (1944), 16–21.

37   Robins, *The miasma*, p. 132.

38   Wilde, 'Census of Ireland for the year 1851', 246–7.

39   Robins, *The miasma*, p. 134.

40   J. O'Rourke, *The Great Irish Famine* (Dublin, 1989), pp 219–24.

41   R. Cowen, *Relish: the extraordinary life of Alexis Soyer, Victorian celebrity chef* (London, 2006), pp 108–34.

42   O'Rourke, *The Great Irish Famine*, pp 219–24.

43   J.D.H. Widdess, *A history of the Royal College of Physicians of Ireland* (Edinburgh, 1963), p. 176.

44   Minutes of the meeting of the board of guardians of the South Dublin Union, 22 Mar. 1847.

45   Cowen, *Relish*, pp 108–34.

46   C. Woodham-Smith, *The Great Hunger* (London, 1962), pp 178–9.

47   Minutes of the meeting of the board of guardians of the South Dublin Union, 2 Dec. 1847.

48   Ibid., 12 Aug. 1847.

49   *First report of the Irish Poor Law Commissioners* (1848), pp 389–90.

50   Minutes of the meeting of the board of guardians of the South Dublin Union, 11 Sept. 1847.

51   Ibid., 23 Aug. 1847.

52   Ibid., 16 Dec. 1847.

53   Ibid., 6 Jan. 1848.

54   Ibid., 27 Jan. 1848.

55   Ibid., 13 Jan. 1848.

56   Ibid., 15 Jan. 1848.

57   Ibid., 20 May 1848.

58   Ibid., 4 Mar. 1848.

59   H. Burke, *The people and the poor law in nineteenth-century Ireland* (Dublin, 1987), p. 142.

60   Ibid., p. 147.

61   Minutes of the meeting of the board of guardians of the South Dublin Union, 1 Jan. 1846.

62   Ibid., 25 Oct. 1847.

63   Ibid., 1 Apr. 1847.

64   Ibid., 9 Feb. 1848.

65   Ibid., 4 May 1848.

66   Ibid., 30 Nov. 1848.

67   Ibid.

68   Ibid., 17 June 1847.

69   Ibid., 2 Sept. 1848.

70   Ibid., 8 May 1851.

71   Ibid., 22 Apr. 1852.

72   Ibid., 29 Apr. 1852.

73   Ibid., 28 Oct. 1847.

74   Ibid., 21 Sept. 1848.

75   Ibid.

76   Robins, *The miasma*, p. 137.

77   Minutes of the meeting of the board of guardians of the South Dublin Union, 28 Dec. 1848.

78   Ibid., 8 Feb. 1849.

79   Ibid., 4 Jan. 1849.

80   Ibid., 8 Feb. 1849.

81   Ibid., 18 Jan. 1849.

82   Ibid., 15 Feb. 1849.

83   Ibid., 17 May 1849.

84   Ibid., 14 June 1849.

85   'Preface' in C.P. Meehan (ed.), *The poets and poetry of Munster* (Dublin, 1883).

86   J.C. Mangan, 'The Famine'. *Irishman*, 9 June 1849, p. 363.

87 J. Keegan, 'To the Cholera', *Cork Magazine*, 2:13 (1850).

88 *Irish Times*, 8 Nov. 2016.

89 J. Keegan, *Legends and poems*, ed. J. O'Hanlon, with memoir by D.J. O'Donoghue (Dublin, 1907).

90 Minutes of the meeting of the board of guardians of the South Dublin Union, 21 July 1849.

91 C. Cameron, *History of the Royal College of Surgeons in Ireland* (Dublin, 1886), p. 542.

92 Minutes of the meeting of the board of guardians of the South Dublin Union, 13 Sept. 1849. Ibid., 13 Nov. 1849.

Chapter Six

1 Minutes of the meeting of the board of guardians of the South Dublin Union, 11 Mar. 1852.

2 H. Burke, *The people and the poor law in nineteenth-century Ireland* (Littlehampton, 1987), p. 179.

3 J. Prunty, *Dublin slums* (Dublin, 1998), p. ix.

4 Minutes of the meeting of the board of guardians of the South Dublin Union, 13 Feb. 1851.

5 Ibid., 20 Feb. 1851.

6 L. Atthill, *Recollections of an Irish doctor* (London, 1911), pp 157–9.

7 Minutes of the meeting of the board of guardians of the South Dublin Union, 20 Feb. 1851.

8 Ibid., 24 Feb. 1848.

9 G. Nicholls, *A history of the Irish poor law* (London, 1856), pp 369–70.

10 *Third annual report of the commissioners for relief of the poor in Ireland* (1850), pp 133–4.

11 Minutes of the meeting of the board of guardians of the South Dublin Union, 17 July 1851.

12 Ibid., 3 June 1852.

13 Ibid., 4 May 1854.

14 Ibid., 28 May 1863.

15 M. Kohli, *The golden bridge: young immigrants to Canada, 1833–1939* (Toronto, 2003), p. 289.

16 Ibid., p. 290.

17 Minutes of the meeting of the board of guardians of the South Dublin Union, 28 Sept. 1882.

18 Ibid., 19 Oct. 1882.

19 D. McLoughlin, 'Workhouses and Irish female paupers, 1840–1870' in M. Luddy and C. Murphy (eds), *Women surviving* (Dublin, 1990), pp 117–47.

20 Minutes of the meeting of the board of guardians of the South Dublin Union, 12 Feb. 1852.

21 Ibid., 11 Mar. 1852.

22 Ibid., 15 Mar. 1852.

23 Ibid., 11 Mar. 1852.

24 Ibid., 3 June 1852.

25 Ibid., 17 Feb. 1853.

26 Ibid., 24 Feb. 1853.

27 Ibid., 3 Nov. 1853.

28 Ibid., 9 July 1863.

29 Ibid., 15 Dec. 1853.

30 Ibid., 20 Apr. 1855.

31 Ibid., 2 July 1857.

32 Ibid., 15 Sept. 1853.

33 Ibid., 23 Nov. 1854.

34 Ibid., 24 Nov. 1853.

35 Ibid., 2 Feb. 1854.

36 Ibid., 16 Apr. 1854.

37 Ibid., 19 Jan. 1854.

38 Ibid., 26 Jan. 1854..

39 Ibid., 16 Apr. 1854.

40 Ibid., 15 Aug. 1861.

41 *The Nation*, 5 Apr. 1851.

42 'Poor Employment (Ireland)', Hansard HC Deb., 118 (1851), 374–92.

43 Burke, *The people and the poor law*, p. 205.

44 *Eighth annual report of the commissioners for administering the laws for relief of the poor in Ireland* (Dublin, 1855), p. 636.

45 Ibid.

46 Minutes of the meeting of the board of guardians of the South Dublin Union, 14 May 1857.

47 Ibid., 1 Oct. 1857.

48 A. Clark, 'Wild workhouse girls and the liberal imperial state in mid-nineteenth-century Ireland', *Journal of Social History*, 39:2 (2005), 389–409.

49 Minutes of the meeting of the board of guardians of the South Dublin Union, 24 July 1862.

50 Ibid., 20 Nov. 1862.

51 *Cavan Observer*, 12 Feb. 1859.

52 Minutes of the meeting of the board of guardians of the South Dublin Union, 19 Feb. 1863.

53 J. Robins, *The lost children: a study of charity children in Ireland, 1700–1900* (Dublin, 1980), p. 267.

54 N. O'Cleirigh, *Hardship and high living: Irish women's lives, 1808–1923* (Dublin, 2003), p. 82.

55 Burke, *The people and the poor law*, p. 211.

56 Ibid., pp 212–13.

57 Minutes of the meeting of the board of guardians of the South Dublin Union, 9 Aug. 1860.

58 D. Coakley, *The importance of being Irish* (Dublin, 1994), pp 112–14.

59 P. Smyth, *140 years a growing: the Carmelite chaplaincy at St James's Hospital* (Dublin, 2001), pp 1–36.

60 D. Cosgrave, *Centenary souvenir, 1827–1927: Carmelite Fathers, Whitefriars Street, Dublin* (Dublin, 1927), p. 35.

61 Minutes of the meeting of the board of guardians of the South Dublin Union, 11 Dec. 1856.

62 H. Burke, *The people and the poor law*, p. 185.

63 Minutes of the meeting of the board of guardians of the South Dublin Union, 26 Jan. 1860.

64 D. Coakley, *The Irish School of Medicine: outstanding practitioners of the 19th century* (Dublin, 1988), pp 101–2.

65 Burke, *The people and the poor law*, p. 249.

66 Minutes of the meeting of the board of guardians of the South Dublin Union, 9 Feb. 1865.

67 Ibid., 13 June 1861.

68 Ibid., 14 Nov. 1861.

69 Obituary, *Dublin Journal of Medical Science*, 37 (1864), 499–504.

70 C. Cameron, *History of the Royal College of Surgeons in Ireland* (Dublin, 1886), pp 631–2.

71 Ibid., p. 607.

72 Minutes of the meeting of the board of guardians of the South Dublin Union, 14 Sept. 1865.

73 Ibid., 4 Oct. 1866.

74 Ibid., 8 Nov. 1866.

75 Ibid., 31 Oct. 1878.

76 Ibid., 19 May 1870.

77 Ibid.

78 *Annual report of the Irish Poor Law Commissioners* (1868), pp 55–6.

79 Minutes of the meeting of the board of guardians of the South Dublin Union, 29 Nov. 1877.

80 Ibid., 4 Feb. 1875.

81 Ibid., 2 Aug. 1866.

82 Ibid., 25 Oct. 1866.

83 J. Robins, *The miasma: epidemic and panic in nineteenth-century Ireland* (Dublin, 1995), p. 206.

84 Minutes of the meeting of the board of guardians of the South Dublin Union, 2 Nov. 1871.

85 Ibid., 10 Oct. 1872.

86 Ibid., 18 July 1880.

87 Ibid., 22 Jan. 1880.

88 Ibid., 16 Dec. 1880.

89 Ibid., 23 Oct. 1878.

90 Ibid., 8 May 1879.

91 Ibid., 8 Feb. 1866. Ibid., 27 Apr. 1871.

92 Ibid., 8 Nov. 1882.

93 Ibid., 7 Oct. 1869.

94 Ibid., 16 Mar. 1871.

95 Ibid., 20 Nov. 1890.

96 Ibid., 10 June 1869.

97 Ibid., 2 July 1868.

98 Cosgrave, *Centenary souvenir, 1827–1927*, p. 37.

99 M. Luddy, *Women in Ireland, 1800–1918: a documentary history* (Cork, 1999), pp 123–5.

100 B. Kennerk, *Temple Street Children's Hospital* (Dublin, 2014), pp 1–11.

101 Robins, *The lost children* (1980), p. 282.

102 Ibid., p. 302.

103 *Annual report of the Local Government Board for Ireland* (1901), pp vii–x.

104 Ibid.

105 Ibid.

106 F. Falkiner, *Transactions of the National Association for the Promotion of Social Science* (Dublin, 1881), p. 571.

107 L. Carroll, 'Our Pole Star is Truth', *TCD Journal of Post Graduate Research*, 6JR (2007).

108 M.E. Daly, *Dublin: the deposed capital* (Cork, 1984), pp 99–100.

109 Ibid., p. 90.

Chapter Seven

1 J. Plunkett, *Strumpet city* (London, 1978), p. 179.

2 A. Carroll, *Leaves from the annals of the Sisters of Mercy*, 3 vols (New York, 1881), i, p. 46.

3 Minutes of the meeting of the board of guardians of the South Dublin Union, 1 July 1880.

4   Ibid., 2 Sept. 1880.

5   Ibid., 11 Nov. 1880.

6   P. Scanlon, *The Irish nurse: a study of nursing in Ireland: history and education, 1718–1981* (Manorhamilton, 1991), p. 79.

7   Carroll, *Leaves from the Annals of the Sisters of Mercy*, i, pp 46–8.

8   C. O'Brien, 'A history of two Dublin hospitals', unpublished manuscript (Dublin, n.d.), p. 20.

9   Minutes of the meeting of the board of guardians of the South Dublin Union, 9 Feb. 1882.

10   Ibid., 17 Mar. 1898.

11   S. Lunney, *With mercy towards all* (Dublin, 1987), p. 175.

12   Minutes of the meeting of the board of guardians of the South Dublin Union, 4 Mar. 1897.

13   Lunney, *With mercy towards all* (Dublin, 1987), p. 175.

14   R. Gaffney, 'Women as doctors and nurses' in O. Checkland and M. Lamb (eds), *Health care as social history* (Aberdeen, 1982), pp 134–48.

15   Census of Ireland, 1911.

16   Minutes of the meeting of the board of guardians of the South Dublin Union, 2 July 1902.

17   Ibid., 15 July 1903.

18   Ibid., 28 July 1917. Minutes of the meeting of the board of guardians of the Dublin Union, 9 Nov. 1918.

19   Minutes of the meeting of the board of guardians of the South Dublin Union, 4 Nov. 1897.

20   Ibid.

21   *Irish Times*, 25 Mar. 1871.

22   L. Carroll, *In the fever king's preserves: Sir Charles Cameron and the Dublin slums* (Dublin, 2011), p. 77.

23   'Report on the nursing and administration of Irish workhouses and infirmaries, 1895–6: Dublin South', *British Medical Journal*, 2 (1896), 795–7.

24   Ibid.

25   Ibid.

26   Anon., *Ladies of the Liberties* (Dublin, 2002), pp 65–85.

27   R. Meath (ed.), *The diaries of Mary, countess of Meath* (London, 1990), pp 46–52.

28   Minutes of the meeting of the board of guardians of the South Dublin Union, 15 Apr. 1899.

29   *New York Times*, 4 Sept. 1902.

30   C. Scuffil, *The South Circular Road, Dublin, on the eve of the First World War* (Dublin, 1913), p. 11.

31   *Irish Times*, 21 Apr. 1900.

32   M. McCarthy, *Five years in Ireland* (Dublin, 1903), pp 482–564.

33   L.M. Geary, 'The medical profession, care and the poor law in nineteenth-century Ireland' in V. Crossman and P. Gray (eds), *Poverty and welfare in Ireland, 1838–1948* (Dublin, 2011), pp 189–222. J. O'Connor, *The workhouses of Ireland* (Dublin, 1995), pp 194–5.

34   Ibid., pp 195–7.

35   D. Durnin, 'Medicine in the city' in F. Devine (ed.), *A capital in conflict: Dublin city and the 1913 Lockout* (Dublin, 2013), pp 83–93.

36   J. Prunty, *Dublin slums* (Dublin, 1998), p. 163.

37   F. Dunne, 'Sanatoria and tuberculosis dispensaries' in Countess of Aberdeen (ed.), *Ireland's crusade against tuberculosis*, 2 vols (Dublin, 1907), ii, pp 57–66.

38   Ibid., pp 65–6.

39   Minutes of the meeting of the board of guardians of the South Dublin Union, 30 June 1915.

40   Ibid., 21 Apr. 1915.

41   Ibid., 10 Nov. 1915.

42   Ibid., 6 Mar. 1918.

43   D. Dickson, *Dublin: the making of a capital city* (Dublin, 2014), p. 418.

44   Minutes of the meeting of the board of guardians of the South Dublin Union, 4 Jan. 1908.

45   M.E. Daly, *Dublin: the deposed capital* (Cork, 1984), p. 92.

46   *Irish Times*, 4 Oct. 1910.

47   Ibid.

48   Minutes of the meeting of the board of guardians of the South Dublin Union, 15 Sept. 1908.

49   D. Cosgrave, *Centenary souvenir, 1827–1927: Carmelite Fathers, Whitefriars Street, Dublin* (Dublin, 1927), p. 35.

50   Daly, *Dublin*, p. 84.

51   Workhouse admission and discharge register, 1918. South Dublin Union, book 148.

52   Plunkett, *Strumpet city*, p. 179.

53   Ibid., p. 191.

54   F. Cullen, *Cleansing rural Dublin: public health and housing initiatives in the South Dublin Poor Law Union, 1880–1920* (Dublin, 2001), pp 6–7.

55   Minutes of the meeting of the board of guardians of the South Dublin Union, 15 July 1908.

56   Ibid., 16 June 1915.

57   Ibid., 13 Dec. 1916.

58   Ibid., 3 July 1918.

59   Minutes of the meeting of the board of guardians of the Dublin Union, 14 Aug. 1918.

60   Ibid., 16 Oct. 1918.

61   Ibid., 10 Sept. 1919.

62   Ibid., 18 Feb. 1920.

63   F. Kennedy, 'Frank Duff's search for the neglected and rejected', *Studies*, 91:364 (2002), 381–9.

64   F. Duff, *Miracles on tap* (New York, 1961), p. 2.

65   L. O'Broin, *Frank Duff: a biography* (Dublin, 1982), p. 4.

66   F. Kennedy, *Duff: a life story* (London, 2011), pp 61–8.

67   C. Hallack, *The Legion of Mary* (New York, 1950), pp 12–13. L. Suenens, *Edel Quinn* (Dublin, 1954), pp 30–2.

68   Kennedy, 'Frank Duff's search', 381–9.

69   N. Johnson, *Britain and the 1918–1919 influenza epidemic* (London, 2006), p. 82. I. Milne, 'The 1918–1919 influenza pandemic – a Kildare perspective', *Journal of the County Kildare Archaelogical Society*, 20 (2013).

70   M. Worobey, Han Guan-Zhu and Andrew Rambaut, 'A synchronized global sweep of the internal genes of modern avian influenza virus', *Nature*, 508 (2014), 254–6.

71   C. Foley, 'This revived old plague: coping with flu' in C. Cox and M. Luddy (eds), *Cultures of care in Irish medical history, 1750–1970* (London, 2010), pp 141–67.

72   I. Milne, 'Through the eyes of a child: "Spanish" influenza remembered by survivors' in A. Mac Lellan and A. Mauger (eds), *Growing pains* (Dublin, 2013), pp 159–74.

73   I. Milne, 'Influenza: the Irish local government boards last great crisis' in D. Lucey and V. Crossman (eds), *Healthcare in Ireland and Britain from 1850* (London, 2014), pp 217–36.

74   Ibid.

75   C. Foley, *The last Irish plague: the great flu epidemic in Ireland, 1918–1919* (Dublin, 2011), p. 141.

76   Ibid., p. 1.

77   Minutes of the meeting of the board of guardians of the South Dublin Union, 6 Nov. 1918.

78   Ibid., 16 Nov. 1918.

79   P.B. Gatenby, *Dublin's Meath Hospital* (Dublin, 1996), p. 95.

80   D.W. Macnamara, 'Memories of 1918 and "The Flu", *Journal of the Irish Medical Association*, 35 (1954), 208–13.

81   Cosgrave, *Centenary souvenir*, p. 37.

82   G.B. Kolata, *Flu: the story of the Great Influenza of 1918 and the search for the virus that caused it* (New York, 1999), p. 199.

Chapter Eight

1   Sir F. Vane, letters to his wife, April and May 1916, Cumbria Record Office.

2   D. Cosgrave, *Centenary souvenir, 1827–1927: Carmelite Fathers, Whitefriars Street, Dublin* (Dublin, 1927), p. 37.

3   A. Crowder, personal communication.

4   Minutes of the meeting of the board of Guardians of the South Dublin Union, 9 June 1915.

5   Ibid., 12 Aug. 1908.

6   B. Neary, *Lugs: the life and times of Jim Branigan* (Dublin, 1985), p. 3.

7   Ibid., p. 2.

8   M. Caulfield, *The Easter Rebellion* (Dublin, 1995), p. 50.

9   P.J. Hally, 'The Easter Rising in Dublin: the military aspects', *Irish Sword*, 1:7 (1966), 314–26.

10   F. McGarry, *The Rising, Ireland: Easter 1916* (Oxford, 2010), p. 188.

11   S. McCoole, *Easter widows* (Dublin, 2014), p. 115.

12   C. Townshend, *Easter 1916: the Irish rebellion* (London, 2005), p. 94.

13   M. Laffan, *Judging W.T. Cosgrave: the foundation of the Irish state* (Dublin, 2014), pp 27–38.

14   Witness statement of Miss Annie Mannion, BMH, WS297.

15   Anon., 'Events of Easter Week: fighting in the South Dublin Union', *Catholic Bulletin*, 8:3 (1918), 153–6.

16 Witness statement of P.S. Doyle, BMH, WS155.

17 A Volunteer, 'The South Dublin Union area', *Capuchin Annual*, 33 (1966), 201–13.

18 Witness statement of W.T. Cosgrave, BMH, WS268.

19 W. Henry, *Supreme sacrifice: the story of Eamonn Ceannt, 1881–1916* (Cork, 2005), p. 71.

20 Witness statement of James Coughlan, BMH, WS304.

21 Witness statement of P.S. Doyle, BMH, WS155.

22 N. Richardson, *According to their lights* (Dublin, 2015), p. 27.

23 S. Geoghegan, *The campaigns and history of the Royal Irish Regiment*, 2 vols (Edinburgh, 1927), ii, p. 102.

24 Anon., 'Events of Easter Week: the fighting in the South Dublin Union', *Catholic Bulletin*, 8:4 (1918), 205–8.

25 A. Kinsella, 'Alan Livingstone Ramsay, 1890–1916: from Ballsbridge to the South Dublin Union', *Dublin Historical Record*, 48:1 (1995), 6–14.

26 L. Kenny, 'Picture emerges of Naas fatality of the Easter Rising ... April 1916', *County Kildare Electronic History Journal*, www.kildare.ie/ehistory.

27 Anon., 'Events of Easter Week', *Catholic Bulletin*, 8:3 (1918), 153–6.

28 Sceilg, 'The South Dublin Union' in Piaras Beaslai (ed.), *Dublin's fighting story, 1916–1921* (Tralee, 1947), pp 29–38.

29 Anon., 'Events of Easter Week', *Catholic Bulletin*, 8:4 (1918), 205–8.

30 Witness statement of George Irvine, BMH, WS265.

31 Anon., 'Events of Easter Week', *Catholic Bulletin*, 8:4 (1918), 205–8.

32 Witness statement of James Burke, BMH, WS1758.

33 *Kildare Observer*, 27 May 1916.

34 M. Browne, 'On Garden Hill: a family remembers', *Federated Dublin Voluntary Hospitals annual conference and St James's Hospital annual conference brochure* (1982), 52–3.

35 Anon., 'Events of Easter Week', *Catholic Bulletin*, 8:4 (1918), pp 205–8.

36 Ibid., pp 201–13.

37 Anon., 'Events of Easter Week: the fighting in the South Dublin Union', *Catholic Bulletin*, 8:5 (1918), 257–60.

38 Witness statement of Patrick Smyth, BMH, WS305.

39 Anon., 'Events of Easter Week', *Catholic Bulletin*, 8:5 (1918), 257–60.

40 *Kildare Observer*, 27 May 1916.

41 Witness statement of Dan McCarthy, BMH, WS722.

42 A Volunteer, 'The South Dublin Union Area', 201–13.

43 Caulfield, *The Easter Rebellion*, p. 93.

44 Witness statement of Annie Mannion, BMH, WS297.

45 G.A. Hayes-McCoy, 'A military history of the 1916 Rising' in K.B. Nowlan (ed.), *The making of 1916* (Dublin, 1969), pp 255–338.

46 S. Collins, *The Cosgrave legacy* (Dublin, 1996), p. 10.

47 M. Fitzpatrick, *The parish of St James, James's Street, Dublin: celebrating 150 years, 1844–1994* (Dublin, 1994), p. 33.

48 Hayes-McCoy, 'A military history' in Nowlan (ed.), *The making of 1916*, pp 255–338.

49 Anon., 'Events of Easter Week', *Catholic Bulletin*, 8:5 (1918), 257–60.

50 Witness statement of Michael Lynch, BMH, WS511.

51 Witness statement of Liam O'Flaithbheartaigh, BMH, WS248.

52 Vane, letters to his wife, April and May 1916.

53 D. Ryan, *The Rising: the complete story of Easter Week* (Dublin, 1949), p. 179.

54 Vane, letters to his wife, April and May 1916.

55 Ibid.

56 Anon., 'Events of Easter Week: the fighting in the South Dublin Union', *Catholic Bulletin*, 8:6 (1918), pp 309–12.

57 M. Gibbon, *Inglorious soldier* (London, 1968), pp 58–9.

58 Vane, letters to his wife, April and May 1916.

59 Caulfield, *Easter Rebellion*, p. 223.

60 C. Housley, *The Sherwood Foresters in the Easter Rising: Dublin 1916* (Nottingham, 2015), pp 60–7.

61 Caulfield, *The Easter Rebellion*, p. 224.

62 W.C. Oates, 'The 2/8th Battalion, the Sherwood Foresters' in *The Great War, 1914–1918* (East Sussex, 1919; repr. 2009), p. 47.

63 J. Doolan, National Library of Ireland, MS 10915.

64 J.V. Joyce, 'Easter Week 1916: the defence of the South Dublin Union', *An t-Oglach* (June 1926), 3–5.

65 Anon., 'Events of Easter Week', *Catholic Bulletin*, 8:6 (1918), 309–12.

66 Witness statement of James Foran, BMH, WS243.

67 Caulfield, *The Easter Rebellion*, p. 229.

68 Vane, letters to his wife, April and May 1916.

69 M. Foy and B. Barton, *The Easter Rising* (Gloucestershire, 1999), p. 103.

70 Fitzpatrick, *The parish of St James*, pp 1–44.

71 Vane, letters to his wife, April and May 1916.

72 Ibid.

73 Witness statement of Annie Mannion, BMH, WS297.

74 Minutes of the meeting of the board of guardians of the South Dublin Union, 10 May 1916.

75 Ibid.

76 Ibid., 17 May 1916.

77 Ibid., 31 May 1916.

78 Cosgrave, *Centenary souvenir, 1827–1927*, p. 37.

79 B. Barton, *From behind closed doors: secret court martial records of the 1916 Easter Rising* (Belfast, 2002), pp 181–97.

80 Laffan, *Judging W.T. Cosgrave*, p 56–7.

Chapter Nine

1 Dáil Éireann, V123, 14 Dec. 1950.

2 Minutes of the meeting of the board of guardians of the South Dublin Union, 13 Mar. 1918. Ibid., June 1918.

3 J. O'Connor, *The workhouses of Ireland* (Dublin, 1995), p. 197.

4 Minutes of the meeting of the board of guardians of the Dublin Union, 5 Jan. 1921.

5 M. Browne, 'On Garden Hill: a family remembers', *Federated Dublin Voluntary Hospitals annual conference and St James's Hospital annual conference brochure* (1982), pp 52–3.

6 Minutes of the meeting of the board of guardians of the Dublin Union, 2 Feb. 1921.

7 Ibid., 9 Feb. 1921.

8 Ibid., 18 May 1921.

9 Ibid., 2 Nov. 1921.

10 Ibid., 6 Apr. 1921.

11 Ibid., 23 May 1922.

12 A. Parkinson, *Belfast's unholy war* (Dublin, 2004), pp 64–6.

13 Minutes of the meeting of the board of guardians of the Dublin Union, 14 June 1922.

14 Ibid., 3 July 1922.

15 Ibid.

16 Ibid., 12 July 1922.

17 Ibid., 2 Aug. 1922.

18 R.D. Edwards, *Patrick Pearse: the triumph of failure* (Dublin, 1990), p. 332.

19 Minutes of the meeting of the board of guardians of the Dublin Union, 29 Nov. 1922.

20 Ibid.

21 Ibid., 6 Dec. 1922.

22 Ibid., 13 Dec. 1922.

23 Ibid.

24 Ibid., 4 July 1923.

25 Ibid., 31 Oct. 1923.

26 P. Yeates, *A city in civil war: Dublin, 1921–4* (Dublin, 2015), pp 248–57.

27 Minutes of the meeting of the board of guardians of the Dublin Union, 21 Nov. 1923.

28 Ibid.

29 Ibid.

30 *Report of the commissioners for the Dublin Union*, 19 Nov. 1924, p. 156.

31 Ibid., 23 Nov. 1923, p. 435.

32 Ibid., 21 July 1924, p. 94.

33 J. Prunty, *Dublin slums* (Dublin, 1998), p. 198.

34 *Hospitals Commission: second general report, 1935 and 1936* (Dublin, 1937), p. 59.

35 B. Hensey, *The health services of Ireland* (Dublin, 1959), pp 10–11.

36 As late as 1950, it would be described in Dáil Éireann by a deputy as 'this anachronistic symbol of alien government'. Dáil Éireann, V123, 14 Dec. 1950.

37   D. Cosgrove, *Centenary souvenir, 1827–1927: Carmelite Fathers, Whitefriars Street, Dublin* (Dublin, 1927), p. 35.

38   *Irish Free State hospital year book and medical directory* (Dublin, 1937), p. 95.

39   *Irish Times*, 14 Nov. 1929.

40   Ibid.

41   National Archives, Department of Local Government and Public Health: Dublin Union, SA8/159.

42   Ibid.

43   Ibid.

44   Ibid.

45   E.L. Gavin, personal communication (2004).

46   Obituary, William Cremin, *Mungret Annual*, 18:2 (1948), p. 116.

47   Kirkpatrick Archives, Royal College of Physicians of Ireland.

48   Ibid.

49   Ibid.

50   D.K. O'Donovan, 'T.C.J. O'Connell: an appreciation of a surgeon', *Irish Journal of Medical Science*, 155:9 (1986), 311–16.

51   National Archives, Department of Local Government and Public Health: St Kevin's Hospital, A8/330.

52   *Hospitals Commission: second general report, 1935 and 1936* (Dublin, 1937), p. 59.

53   *Report of the commissioners for the Dublin Union*, 4 Jan. 1930, p. 1.

54   Ibid., 14 May 1930, p. 364.

55   Minutes of Proceedings of the Dublin Board of Assistance, 4 Dec. 1935.

56   Obituary, William P. Murphy, *British Medical Journal*, 2:3956 (1936), 900.

57   M.G. Magan, 'Mass radiography service in Dublin' in J.C. Carr (ed.), *A century of medical radiation in Ireland – an anthology* (Dublin, 1995), pp 216–26.

58   E. MacThomais, 'The South Dublin Union', *Dublin Historical Record*, 26:2 (Dublin, 1973), 54–61.

59   M. Fitzpatrick, *The parish of St James, James's Street, Dublin: celebrating 150 years, 1844–1994* (Dublin, 1994), pp 14–15.

60   T. Kinsella, *A Dublin documentary* (Dublin, 2006), pp 17–19.

Chapter Ten

1   'Proposals for reform of St Kevin's Institution', National Archives A8/159.

2   C.A. Barry, 'Irish regional life tables', *Journal of the Statistical and Social Inquiry Society of Ireland*, 16 (1941/42), 1.

3   *Irish Press*, 3 Oct. 1936.

4   D.S. Lucey and G.C. Gosling, 'Paying for health: comparative perspectives on patient payment and contributions for hospital provision in Ireland' in D.S. Lucey and V. Crossman (eds), *Health care in Ireland and Britain from 1850* (London, 2014), pp 81–100.

5   *Hospitals Commission: first general report, 1933–4* (Dublin, 1936), p. 92.

6   E. Nolan, *Caring for the nation: a history of the Mater Misericordiae University Hospital* (Dublin, 2013), pp 105–6.

7   M. Daly, 'An atmosphere of sturdy independence: the state and the Dublin hospitals in the 1930s' in E. Malcolm and G. Jones (eds), *Medicine, disease and the state in Ireland, 1650–1940* (Cork, 1999), pp 234–52.

8   Minutes of the meeting of the Dublin Board of Assistance, 4 Mar. 1936.

9   R. Barrington, *Health, medicine and politics in Ireland, 1900–1970* (Dublin, 1987), p. 117.

10   Minutes of the meeting of the Dublin Board of Assistance, 5 Feb. 1936.

11   'Discussion on the relationships of the teaching hospitals to the medical schools, the medical profession and the public', *Irish Journal of Medical Science*, 113 (1935), 193–216.

12   *Hospitals Commission: first general report, 1933–4* (Dublin, 1936), pp 11–17.

13   Ibid.

14   H. Moore, 'Future hospital policy in Dublin', *Irish Journal of Medical Science*, 126 (1936), 241–66.

15   Ibid.

16   Ibid.

17   *Hospitals Commission: second general report, 1935–6* (Dublin, 1937), p. 60.

18   'St Kevin's Hospital (Dublin Union)' in *Irish Free State hospital year book and medical directory* (Dublin, 1937), p. 95.

19 *Hospitals Commission: second general report, 1935–6* (Dublin, 1937), p. 291.

20 Ibid., p. 39.

21 D. McCarthy, 'Hospitals and the people's needs', *Ireland Today*, 11:10 (1937), 37–43.

22 *Hospitals Commission: third general report, 1937* (Dublin, 1938), p. 15.

23 Barrington, *Health, medicine and politics*, p. 122.

24 Daly, 'An atmosphere of sturdy independence' in Malcolm and Jones (eds), *Medicine, disease and the state*, p. 246.

25 *Hospitals Commission: fifth general report, 1939–41* (Dublin, 1943), p. 284.

26 *Hospitals Commission: seventh general report, 1945–7* (Dublin, 1948), pp 22–3.

27 Minutes of the meeting of the Dublin Board of Assistance, 24 Jan. 1940.

28 Ibid., 5 Feb. 1941.

29 St Kevin's Hospital, Dublin, National Archives, A8/331.

30 Memorandum of the commissioners appointed to administer the affairs of the Dublin Board of Assistance, National Archives, A8/331.

31 Ibid.

32 Dáil Éireann Debate, 'Dublin Union nursing staff', vol. 85, no. 5, 19 Nov. 1941.

33 *Hospitals Commission: seventh general report, 1945–7* (Dublin, 1948), p. 150.

34 Ibid., p. 304.

35 Ibid.

36 'General review and report on progress of the commissioners for the Dublin Board of Assistance', National Archives, A8/33.

37 'Proposals for reform of St Kevin's Institution', National Archives, A8/159.

38 Ibid.

39 St Kevin's Hospital, Dublin, National Archives, SA8/330.

40 *Evening Mail*, 18 Aug. 1945.

41 St Kevin's Institution, National Archives, SA8/331

42 St Kevin's Hospital, Dublin, 1945–54, National Archives, SA8/34.

43 C. O'Brien, 'A history of two Dublin hospitals', unpublished manuscript (Dublin, n.d.), p. 20.

44 C.S. Breathnach, personal communication.

45 Ibid.

46 B. O'Donnell, *Irish surgeons and surgery in the twentieth century* (Dublin, 2008), p. 322.

47 V. Coffey, 'Observations: female skin and mental wards', private collection.

48 'St Kevin's Hospital (Dublin Union)' in *Irish Free State hospital year book and medical directory* (Dublin, 1937), p. 95.

49 V. Coffey, personal communication.

50 Obituary, Dr Victoria Coffey, *Irish Times*, 9 August 1999.

51 Barrington, *Health, medicine and politics in Ireland, 1900–1970* (Dublin, 1987), p. 142.

52 J. Deeny, *To cure and to care* (Dublin, 1989), p. 142.

53 'Proposals in respect of chronic departments', St Kevin's Hospital, National Archives, SA 8/37.

54 D.K. O'Donovan, personal communication.

55 F.O.C. Meenan, *St Vincent's Hospital (1834–1994): an historical and social portrait* (Dublin, 1995), p. 118.

56 O'Donnell, *Irish surgeons and surgery*, pp 565–6.

57 St Kevin's Hospital, Dublin, National Archives, SA8/37. C.S. Breathnach, personal communication.

58 St Kevin's Hospital, Dublin, National Archives, SA8/37.

59 O'Donnell, *Irish surgeons and surgery*, p. 499.

60 E. Burke-Kennedy, 'Blind and deaf doctor who was hero for all', *Irish Times Health Supplement*, 24 Jan. 2012.

61 J. Hanlon, 'James Hanlon', *NCBI News* 13:3 (2010), pp 11–14.

62 J.K. Feeney, *The Coombe Lying-In Hospital* (Dublin, 1970), pp 153–4.

63 C.S. Breathnach, personal communication.

64 Ibid.

65 Ibid.

66 R.C. Geary, 'The mortality from tuberculosis in Saorstát Éireann: a statistical study', *Journal of the Statistical and Social Inquiry Society of Ireland*, 14:7 (1929/30), 67–103.

67 K. Kearns, *Dublin tenement life* (Dublin, 2006), pp 12–14.

68 Minutes of the meeting of the Dublin Board of Assistance, 25 Nov. 1936.

69 C.S. Breathnach and J.B. Moynihan, 'The academy's foray into the politics of phthisis (tuberculosis), 1940–1946', *Irish Journal of Medical Science*, 173:1 (2004), 48–52.

70 H. Hitchcock, *TB or not TB* (Galway, 1995), p. 105.

71 N. Browne, *Against the tide* (Dublin, 1986), p. 85.

72 C.S. Breathnach, personal communication.

73 C.S. Breathnach, 'The man who most influenced me', *British Medical Journal*, 311 (1995), 852

74 Ibid.

75 Kirkpatrick Archives, Royal College of Physicians of Ireland.

76 W.H. Fennell, 'Cardiovascular services development in the South of Ireland', *Heartwise* (Winter 2006), 28–9.

77 O'Donnell, *Irish surgeons and surgery*, pp 370–1.

78 Obituary, *Irish Times*, 21 May 2005.

79 O'Donnell, *Irish surgeons and surgery*, p. 376

80 H.J. Browne, 'The Richmond Surgical Hospital' in E. O'Brien, L. Browne and K. O'Malley (eds), *A closing memoir: the Richmond, Whitworth and Hardwicke Hospitals* (Dublin, 1988), pp 98–9.

81 A. Quinn, *Patrick Kavanagh: a biography* (Dublin, 2001), p. 343.

82 K. Shaw, personal communication.

83 Ibid.

84 U. Agnew, *The mystical imagination of Patrick Kavanagh* (Dublin, 2000), p. 36.

85 A. Quinn (ed.), *Patrick Kavanagh: selected poems* (London, 2000), p. 119.

Chapter Eleven

1 N. Browne, personal communication.

2 R. Barrington, *Health, medicine and politics in Ireland, 1900–1970* (Dublin, 1987), p. 201.

3 St Kevin's Hospital, National Archives of Ireland, A8/272.

4 C.E. Lysaght, 'Report on the Development of St Kevin's as a Hospital Centre', National Archives of Ireland (1949), H10/14/68.

5 Ibid.

6 St Kevin's Hospital, National Archives of Ireland, A8/330.

7 St Kevin's Institution, National Archives of Ireland, H10/14/68.

8 Local Government (Dublin) (Temporary) Act, 1948.

9 St Kevin's Institution, National Archives of Ireland, H10/14/68.

10 N. Browne, personal communication.

11 Dáil Éireann, vol. 123, 14 Dec. 1950.

12 St Kevin's Rehabilitation Programme, National Archives of Ireland, H10/14/68.

13 Ibid., HC10/14/12.

14 N. Browne, personal communication.

15 Barrington, *Health, medicine and politics in Ireland, 1900–1970*, p. 207.

16 J. McPolin, 'Commentary on report of consultative council set up by order of the minister for health, dated 4/11/1947 in connection with the proposed establishment at St Kevin's Hospital, Dublin, of a postgraduate medical school for medical officers of local authorities', *Journal of the Medical Association of Éire*, 26:155 (1950), 76–7.

17 Ibid.

18 St Kevin's Hospital, National Archives of Ireland, A8/330.

19 J. Deeny, *To cure and to care* (Dublin, 1989), p. 110.

20 St Kevin's Hospital, National Archives of Ireland, A8/272.

21 M.J. O'Donnell, 'The post-graduate school', *Journal of the Medical Association of Éire*, 26:156 (1950), 94.

22 Ibid.

23 Letter to the editor, *Irish Times*, 6 Oct. 1994.

24 Ibid.

25 Summary of recommendations of chief medical adviser as to future status and staffing of St Kevin's Institution, National Archives A8/159.

26 St Kevin's Hospital Rehabilitation Programme, National Archives of Ireland, H10/14/68.

27 Ibid., H10/14/16.

28 *Irish Press*, 14 Mar. 1956.

29 Ibid., 14 Sept. 1954.

30 C. O'Brien, 'A history of two Dublin hospitals', unpublished manuscript (Dublin, n.d.).

31 J.J. Nolan, review of development of St Kevin's Hospital 1953/54 and 1958/59 (1960), private collection.

32 St Kevin's Rehabilitation Programme, National Archives of Ireland, HC/10/14/12.

33 Obituary, *Irish Times*, 24 Mar. 1964.

34 St Kevin's Rehabilitation Programme, National Archives of Ireland, HC/10/14/16.

35 J. St L. O'Dea, 'The use of beds in St Kevin's Hospital', *Journal of the Irish Medical Association*, 56:333 (1965), 87–93.

36 Minutes of the meeting of the Dublin Board of Assistance, 9 Feb. 1938.

37 N. Browne, *Against the tide* (Dublin, 1986), pp 143–4.

38 Barrington, *Health, medicine and politics in Ireland, 1900–1970*, pp 201–21.

39 C. O'Brien, 'A history of two Dublin hospitals', unpublished manuscript (Dublin, n.d.).

40 N. Browne, *Against the tide* (Dublin, 1986), p. 144.

41 H.J. Browne, 'The Richmond Surgical Hospital' in E. O'Brien, L. Browne and K. O'Malley (eds), *A closing memoir: the Richmond, Whitworth and Hardwicke Hospitals* (Dublin 1988), pp 95–106.

42 O'Donnell, *Irish surgeons and surgery*, pp 312–13.

43 Obituary, *Irish Times*, 12 Sept. 1984.

44 St Kevin's Hospital, National Archives of Ireland, SA8/37.

45 K. Aboud and L. Hogan, 'Dr Thomas D. Hanratty', *Contacts: Eastern Health Board Staff Magazine*, 17:3 (1991), 2.

46 Ibid.

47 J. Fleetwood, personal communication.

48 M. Brady, 'Care of the aged female', *Journal of the Irish Medical Association*, 45 (1959), 126–35.

49 Health Authorities Act, 1960.

50 E.T. MacSearraigh, personal communication.

51 I. Browne, *Music and madness* (Dublin, 2008), pp 176–7.

52 *Irish Press*, 26 May 1966.

53 I. Browne, *Music and madness* (Dublin, 2008), pp 176–7.

54 *Irish Times*, 17 Feb. 1955.

55 P. Holland, 'The Department of Pathology' in O'Brien, Browne and O'Malley (eds), *A closing memoir*, pp 133–4.

56 St Kevin's Hospital, National Archives. SA/880.

57 Dáil Éireann, vol. 232, 14 Feb. 1968.

58 Ibid.

59 'Outline of the future hospital system', *Report of the Consultative Council on General Hospital Services* (Fitzgerald Report) (Dublin, 1968).

Chapter Twelve

1 J.S. McCormick, 'Message from the Eastern Health Board' in *10th anniversary celebration report: Federated Dublin Voluntary Hospitals and St James's Hospital* (Dublin, 1971), p. 12.

2 P. Gatenby, *The School of Physic, Trinity College, Dublin* (Dublin, 1994), p. 51.

3 I. Howie, 'The emergence of a hospital system to meet the challenges of 2000 and beyond' in D. Fitzpatrick (ed.), *The Feds* (Dublin, 2006), p. 25.

4 J.B. Lyons, 'Mercer's Hospital' in Fitzpatrick (ed.), *The Feds*, pp 107–13.

5 Gatenby, *The School of Physic of Trinity College Dublin*, p. 55.

6 J. Galvin, 'Anaesthesia' in D. Fitzpatrick (ed.), *The Feds* (Dublin, 2006), pp 151–9.

7 W.J.E. Jessop, 'The medical school' in *Federated Dublin Voluntary Hospitals and St James's Hospital conference report* (Dublin, 1972), p. 13.

8 Ibid.

9 P.B. Gatenby, 'History of the Federated Dublin Voluntary Hospitals' in *Federated Dublin Voluntary Hospitals and St James's Hospital*, pp 14–17.

10 Ibid.

11 'Outline of the future hospital system', *Report of the Consultative Council on General Hospital Services* (Fitzgerald Report) (Dublin, 1968).

12 D. Hourihane, 'Pathology' in Fitzpatrick (ed.), *The Feds*, p. 264.

13 Howie, 'The emergence of a hospital system to meet the challenges of 2000 and beyond', pp 25–42.

14 F. O'Ferrall, 'The formation of the Adelaide and Meath Hospital, Dublin, incorporating the National Children's Hospital' in Fitzpatrick (ed.), *The Feds*, pp 43–62.

15 Howie, 'The emergence of a hospital system' in Fitzpatrick (ed.), *The Feds*, pp 25–42.

16 C. Hohler, 'The badge of St James's' in I. Cox (ed.), *The scallop* (London, 1957), pp 51–70.

17   S. Murphy and T. Byrne, *St James's grave-yard, Dublin: history and associations* (Dublin, 1988), pp 12–30.

18   M. Dufficy, 'The story of St James's church, James's Street, Dublin', *Dublin Historical Record*, 29:2 (1976), 66–9.

19   B. Hensey, *The health services of Ireland* (Dublin, 1972), p. 35.

20   McCormick, 'Message from the Eastern Health Board' in *10th anniversary celebration report*, p. 12.

21   J.B. Lyons, *The quality of Mercer's: the story of Mercer's Hospital, 1734–1991* (Dublin, 1991). T.G. Moorhead, *A short history of Sir Patrick Dun's Hospital* (Dublin, 1942). T.P.C. Kirkpatrick, *The history of Doctor Steevens' Hospital* (Dublin, 1924). Fitzpatrick (ed.) *The Feds*. D. Coakley, *Baggot Street: a short history of the Royal City of Dublin Hospital* (Dublin, 1995). D. Coakley, *Dr Steevens' Hospital: a brief history* (Dublin, 1992).

22   P. Logan, *Medical Dublin* (Dublin, 1984), p. 62.

23   L. Landa, 'Jonathan Swift and charity', *Journal of English and Germanic Philology*, 44:4 (1945), 337–50.

24   T. Service, 'Handel's *Messiah* – the sound of our better selves', *The Guardian*, 17 Apr. 2014.

25   Logan, *Medical Dublin*, p. 63.

26   Lyons, *The quality of Mercer's*, p. 71.

27   C. Keane, 'Clinical microbiology' in Fitzpatrick (ed.), *The Feds*, pp 181–94.

28   Moorhead, *A short history of Sir Patrick Dun's Hospital*, p. 4.

29   Ibid., p. 66.

30   Ibid., p. 35.

31   D. Coakley, *Robert Graves: evangelist of clinical medicine* (Dublin, 1996), pp 87–102.

32   D. Coakley, *Irish masters of medicine* (Dublin, 1992), pp 143–48.

33   Ibid., pp 205–12.

34   T. Hennessy, 'General surgery' in Fitzpatrick (ed.), *The Feds*, pp 211–17.

35   J.B. Lyons, *An assembly of Irish surgeons* (Dublin, 1984), pp 34–9.

36   D.G. Weir, 'Sir Patrick Dun's Hospital' in Fitzpatrick (ed.), *The Feds*, p. 137.

37   D.G. Weir, personal communication.

38   D.G. Weir, 'Sir Patrick Dun's Hospital' in Fitzpatrick (ed.), *The Feds*, pp 133–44.

39   D. Coakley, *Irish masters of medicine* (Dublin, 1992), pp 73–80.

40   Coakley, *Baggot Street*, pp 8–9.

41   Ibid., p. 23.

42   G. Gearty, 'The Royal City of Dublin Hospital, Baggot Street' in Fitzpatrick (ed.), *The Feds*, p. 131.

43   I. Graham, 'Cardiology' in Fitzpatrick (ed.), *The Feds*, pp 166–70.

44   Obituary, *Irish Times*, 29 Mar. 2014.

45   Kirkpatrick, *The history of Doctor Steevens' Hospital*, p. 8.

46   M. Saffron, *Samuel Clossy, MD – the existing works* (New York, 1967), pp xxvii–lxxxvi.

47   Coakley, *Dr Steevens' Hospital*, p. 27.

48   Coakley, *Irish masters of medicine*, pp 263–70.

49   J.B. Prendiville et al., 'Plastic surgery and oral and maxillo-facial surgery' in D. Fitzpatrick (ed.), *The Feds*, pp 276–82.

50   D. Fitzpatrick, 'Dr Steevens' Hospital' in Fitzpatrick (ed.), *The Feds*, pp 80–1.

51   J. Galvin, 'Anaesthesia' in Fitzpatrick (ed.), *The Feds*, pp 151–9.

52   Department of Health, 'Report of the study group on children's hospital services' (Dublin, 1970), p. 1.

53   Ibid., pp 20.

54   Ibid., pp 1–93.

55   Minutes of the board of St James's Hospital (1980), B.46/80.5.

56   Ibid., 1981, B.15/81.

Chapter Thirteen

1   Minutes of the board of St James's Hospital, 14 Dec. 1971.

2   M. Butler, 'Urology' in D. Fitzpatrick (ed.), *The Feds* (Dublin, 2006), pp 289–98.

3   D. Malone, personal communication.

4   V.L. Beckett, *Living medicine: memoir snapshots* (Philadelphia, 2004), pp 108–26.

5   Minutes of the board of St James's Hospital, 29 May 1977.

6   *Irish Times*, 9 Feb. 1973.

7   I. Howie, 'The emergence of a hospital system to meet the challenges of 2000 and beyond' in Fitzpatrick (ed.), *The Feds*, pp 32–3.

8   K. Keating, 'Physiotherapy' in Fitzpatrick (ed.), *The Feds*, pp 272–5.

9   D. Oakley, *Hands-on for 100 years: a history of physiotherapy in Ireland* (Dublin, 2005), pp 4–14.

10   Obituary, *UCC Medical Alumni and Faculty*, 14 (2016), 18.

11   Howie, 'The emergence of a hospital system' in Fitzpatrick (ed.), *The Feds*, pp 25–42.

12   Obituary, *Irish Times*, 26 Oct. 2013.

13   Ibid.

14   'Prof. Neale, a dynamo of endless energy', *Irish Medical Times*, 17 Sept. 1976.

15   Ibid.

16   T. Hennessy, 'General surgery' in Fitzpatrick (ed.), *The Feds*, pp 211–17.

17   G. Shanik, 'Vascular surgery' in Fitzpatrick (ed.), *The Feds*, pp 299–301.

18   R. Kirkham, personal communication.

19   C. Keane, 'Clinical microbiology' in Fitzpatrick (ed.), *The Feds*, pp 181–7.

20   Ibid.

21   Minutes of the board of St James's Hospital, 29 Jan. 1982.

22   C. O'Morain, 'Gastroenterology' in Fitzpatrick (ed.), *The Feds*, pp 202–10.

23   www.tcd.ie/alumni/about/alumni/interviews/donald-weir.php.

24   A.V. Hoffbrand, 'Professor John Scott, foetal and neural tube defects', *British Journal of Haematology*, 164 (2014), 496–502.

25   I. Temperley, 'Haematology' in Fitzpatrick (ed.), *The Feds*, pp 224–33.

26   Howie, 'The emergence of a hospital system' in Fitzpatrick (ed.), *The Feds*, pp 25–42.

27   Temperley, 'Haematology' in Fitzpatrick (ed.), *The Feds*, pp 224–33. Report of the tribunal of inquiry into the infection with HIV and hepatitis C of persons with haemophilia and related matters (Dublin, 1999), p. 148. J.F.A. Murphy, 'The Lindsay Tribunal into HIV and hepatitis C infection in haemophiliacs', *Irish Medical Journal*, 95:9 (2002), 260–1.

28   Temperley, 'Haematology' in Fitzpatrick (ed.), *The Feds*, pp 224–33.

29   Department of the Taoiseach, 'Speech by the taoiseach, Mr Bertie Ahern, T.D., at the launch of "A vision of a cancer network 5 years on" in Collins Barracks on Monday, 7 April, 2008.

30   M. Webb, *Trinity's psychiatrists* (Dublin, 2011), pp 117–19.

31   B. Sheppard, 'Retirement of John Bonnar', *Trinity Medical News*, 20 (1999), 4.

32   J. Shannon, 'The birth of Irish fertility treatment', *Medical Independent*, 22 July 2010.

33   J.B. Lyons, *The quality of Mercer's: the story of Mercer's Hospital, 1734–1991* (Dublin, 1991), p. 175.

34   J.B. Lyons, 'Mercer's Hospital' in Fitzpatrick (ed.), *The Feds*, p. 118.

35   L. Clancy et al., 'Effect of air pollution on death rates in Dublin, Ireland: an intervention study', *The Lancet* 360 (2002), 1210–14.

36   Minutes of the board of St James's Hospital, 29 Sept. 1982.

37   Ibid., 16 Apr. 1987.

38   J.B. Prendiville, D.L. Lawlor and F. Brady, 'Plastic surgery and oral and maxillo-facial surgery' in Fitzpatrick (ed.), *The Feds*, pp 276–82.

39   I. Howie, 'Chairman's report', *St James's Hospital annual report* (Dublin, 1987), p. 4.

40   Howie, 'The emergence of a hospital system' in Fitzpatrick (ed.), *The Feds*, p. 41.

41   F.N. O'Keeffe et al., 'Acquired immunodeficiency syndrome with Kaposi sarcoma in Ireland', *Irish Journal of Medical Science*, 152:9 (1983), 353–7.

42   D. Freedman, *AIDS – the problem in Ireland* (Dublin, 1987), pp 68–70.

43   F. Mulcahy, personal communication (2006).

44   J. Gaffey, *Witnessing the pandemic: Irish print media and HIV/AIDS in Ireland and Sub-Saharan Africa* (Bethesda, 2007), pp 19–29.

45   J. O'Beirne, *St James's Hospital annual report* (1982), pp 17–18.

46   I. Howie, S. Grace and B.M. McCann, *Art in St James's Hospital* (Dublin, 2013), pp 4–83.

47   Ibid.

48   W. Watts, *William Watts, Provost Trinity College Dublin: a memoir* (Dublin, 2008), pp 161–2.

49   Lyons, *The quality of Mercer's*, p. 208.

50   Minutes of the board of St James's Hospital, 3 Feb. 1995.

Chapter Fourteen

1   T. Mitchell, 'Creating a world-class university hospital in Ireland', *St James's Hospital annual report* (2005).

2   Minutes of the board of St James's Hospital (1997), B.40/97.

3   J.B. Walsh, 'Clinical directorates are a major advance in hospital management', *Irish Medical News*, 12 July 1999.

4   Minutes of the board of St James Hospital (1983), B.51/83.

5   Ibid. (1980), B.117/80.

6   'Departmental reports', *St James's Hospital annual report* (1994), pp 18–19.

7   S. Carolan et al., 'Nursing services' in Fitzpatrick (ed.), *The Feds*, pp 240–52.

8   Minutes of the board of St James's Hospital, 5 Dec. 1996.

9   'St James's Hospital Foundation launched', *St James's Hospital Newsletter*, Sept. 1997.

10   *Orationes Comitiis*, University of Dublin, 1998.

11   E. Murphy, 'Maintaining the "gift of life" in a climate of a shrinking donor pool and increasing demand' (MSc, TCD, 2008).

12   J. O'Regan, *Scott Tallon Walker Architects: 100 buildings and projects, 1960–2005* (Kinsale, 2006), pp 206–9.

13   I. Temperley, 'Haematology' in Fitzpatrick (ed.), *The Feds*, pp 224–33.

14   P. Smyth, *140 years a growing: the Carmelite chaplaincy at St James's Hospital* (2001), p. 2.

15   *Irish Times*, 22 Jan. 2003.

16   T. Mitchell, 'Introduction from the chairman', *St James's Hospital annual report* (2002), p. 6.

17   Ibid., 2003, p. 6.

18   D. Coakley, *Medicine in Trinity College Dublin* (Dublin, 2014), pp 308–9.

19   Ibid., pp 308–9.

20   'The development of radiation oncology services in Ireland', Department of Health and Children (2003).

21   A. Farmar, *A haven in Rathgar: St Luke's and the Irish experience of cancer, 1952–2007* (Dublin, 2003), p. 153.

22   S. McCann, 'Clinical directorate reports', *St James's Hospital annual report* (2003), pp 33–4.

23   *Irish Times*, 11 May 2013.

24   National Cancer Forum, 'A strategy for cancer control in Ireland', Department of Health and Children (2006), pp 39–50.

25   *Irish Medical Times*, 21 Oct. 2016.

26   T. Mitchell, 'Introduction from the chairman', *St James's Hospital annual report* (2006), pp 6–8.

27   Minutes of the board of St James's Hospital, 1 April 2011.

28   D. Shanley, 'Introduction from the chairman', *St James's Hospital annual report* (2012), p. 13.

29   T. Mitchell, 'Introduction from the chairman', *St James's Hospital annual report* (2006), p. 8.

30   *Irish Medical Times*, 10 May 2016.

31   Ibid.

32   Department of Public Expenditure and Reform, 'Building on recovery: infrastructure and capital investment, 2016–2021' (Dublin, 2015), p. 31.

Bibliography

The records of the City Workhouse and of the Foundling Hospital were destroyed by an explosion in the Four Courts at the beginning of the Civil War in 1922. However, when William Dudley Wodsworth wrote *A brief history of the ancient Foundling Hospital* in 1876 he had access to these records, which included twenty volumes of the *Minutes of the governors* and various registries and 'mortality books'. According to Wodsworth, there were also tomes that recorded the regulations of the Foundling Hospital and its finances. As a consequence, one is dependent on Wodsworth's history and the reports of official inquiries for information relating to both of these institutions.

Primary sources

Bureau of Military Archives
Witness statements.

Cumbria Record Office, The Castle, Carlisle, England
Letters of Sir Francis Fletcher Vane.

Marsh's Library
Items relating to the workhouse (1705–26), MS.Z3.1.1 (144) to Z3.1.1 (155).

Mercy Congregational Archives, Dublin.
O'Brien, Sr Catherine of Siena, 'A history of two Dublin hospitals', unpublished manuscript (Dublin n.d.).

National Archives of Ireland
Minute Books of the South Dublin Union, BG79, A1–A127.
Register of Admission and Discharge, South Dublin Union, BG 79/G 1A.
Lysaght, C.E., 'Report on the development of St Kevin's as a hospital centre' (1949) H10/14/68.

St Kevin's Hospital, Resident Medical Superintendent, HC/10/14/12.

St Kevin's Rehabilitation Programme, HC10/14/12.

St Kevin's Rehabilitation Programme, HC10/14/16.

St Kevin's Rehabilitation Programme, H10/14/68.

St Kevin's Institution, H10/14/68.

Conference on St Kevin's Institution, H10/14/68.

St Kevin's Hospital, Dublin, 1945–54, A8/34.

St Kevin's Institution: Proposals for Reform of, A8/159.

St Kevin's Hospital, A8/272.

St Kevin's Hospital, Dublin, A8/330.

St Kevin's Hospital, A8/331.

St Kevin's Hospital: Proposals in Respect of Chronic Departments, SA8/37.

St Kevin's Hospital, Dublin, SA8/159.

National Library of Ireland

Instructions to the officers and servants of the Workhouse of the city of Dublin, Haliday Collection of Pamphlets, P751 (22).

Rules, orders and by-laws made by the governors of the Foundling Hospital and Workhouse in the city of Dublin for the better regulation and preserving decency and order among the owners, drivers and keepers of hackney-coaches, landaus, chariots, post-chaises, Berlins etc., (1774) 326.

Report from the committee of the house of commons appointed to inquire into the management and state of the Foundling Hospital, May 1797, appended to reply of the governors etc. (1816).

Private collection

Crowder, A., 'Frasers and McDowells', unpublished manuscript.

Royal College of Physicians of Ireland

Kirkpatrick Archives.

RTÉ Archive

Kavanagh, P., 'Hospital notebook', Radio Éireann, 1955.

St James's Hospital, Dublin

Minutes of the Board of St James's Hospital.

Secondary sources

Agnew, U., *The mystical imagination of Patrick Kavanagh* (Dublin, 1999).

Anonymous, *1916 Rebellion handbook* (Dublin, 1916; repr. 1998).

Anonymous, *Ladies of the Liberties* (Dublin, 2002).

Anonymous, *An introduction to the reading of the Holy Bible, composed for the use of the Foundling Hospital in Dublin and the charter schools of Ireland* (Dublin, 1765).

Aston, N. & Orr, C. (eds), *An enlightened statesman in Whig Britain: Lord Shelbourne in context* (Woodenbridge, 2011).

Atthill, L., *Recollections of an Irish doctor* (London, 1911).

Barrington, J., *Personal sketches of his own times* (London, 1827).

Barrington, R., *Health medicine and politics in Ireland, 1900–1970* (Dublin, 1987).

Barton, B., *From behind closed door: secret court martial records of the 1916 Easter Rising* (Belfast, 2002).

Bateson, R., *They died by Pearse's side* (Dublin, 2010).

Beaslai, P. (ed.), *Dublin's fighting story, 1916–1921* (Tralee, 1947).

Beckett, V.L., *Living medicine: memoir snapshots* (Philadelphia, 2004).

Bell, J., *Travels from St Petersburg in Russia to diverse parts of Asia* (2nd ed. London, 1764).

Boswell, J., *The kindness of strangers: the abandonment of children in Western Europe* (New York, 1988).

Brady, J. & Simms, A. (eds), *Dublin, 1745–1922: hospitals, spectacle and vice* (Dublin, 2006).

Brontë, E., *Wuthering Heights* (Oxford, 1981).

Brooking, C., *A map of the city and suburbs of Dublin* (London, 1728).

Browne, M., *A tale of two hospitals: St Finbarr's Hospital and Regional Hospital* (Cork, 1989).

Browne, N., *Against the tide* (Dublin, 1986).

Brugha, M., *History's daughter* (Dublin, 2005).

Burke, H., *The people and the poor law in nineteenth-century Ireland* (Littlehampton, 1987).

Burke, H., *The Royal Hospital Donnybrook: a heritage of caring* (Dublin, 1993).

Butler, T.C., *John's Lane: history of the Augustinian friars in Dublin* (Dublin, 1983).

Cameron, C., *History of the Royal College of Surgeons in Ireland* (Dublin, 1886).

Cameron, C., *How the poor live* (Dublin, 1904).

Carleton, W., *The autobiography of William Carleton* (London, 1968).

Carr, Sir John, *The stranger in Ireland: or, a tour in the southern and western parts of that country in the year 1805* (Philadelphia, 1806).

Carr, J.C. (ed.), *A century of medical radiation in Ireland – an anthology* (Dublin, 1995).

Carroll, A., *Leaves from the annals of the Sisters of Mercy* (New York, 1881).

Casey, C., *Dublin: the city within the Grand and Royal canals and the Circular Road with the Phoenix Park* (London, 2005).

Caulfield, J. *Portraits, memoirs and characters of remarkable persons* (London, 1819).

Caulfield, M., *The Easter Rebellion* (Dublin, 1995).

Checkland, O. & Lamb, M. (eds), *Health care as social history* (Aberdeen, 1982).

Chitham, E., *The Brontës' Irish background* (London, 1986).

Chitham, E., *Western winds: the Brontës' Irish heritage* (Dublin, 2015).

Clarke, H. (ed.), *Medieval Dublin* (Dublin, 1990).

Clifford, A., *Poor law in Ireland* (Belfast, 1983).

Coakley, D., *The Irish School of Medicine: outstanding practitioners of the 19th century* (Dublin, 1988).

Coakley, D., *Dr Steevens' Hospital: a brief history* (Dublin, 1992).

Coakley, D., *Irish masters of medicine* (Dublin, 1992).

Coakley, D., *Baggot Street: a short history of the Royal City of Dublin Hospital* (Dublin, 1995).

Coakley, D., *Robert Graves: evangelist of clinical medicine* (Dublin, 1996).

Coakley, D. & O'Doherty, M. (eds), *Borderlands: essays on literature and medicine* (Dublin, 2002).

Coakley, D., *Medicine in Trinity College Dublin* (Dublin, 2014).

Collins, J., *Life in old Dublin* (Cork, 1978).

Collins, S., *The Cosgrave legacy* (Dublin, 1996).

Collins, S., *Balrothery Poor Law Union, County Dublin, 1839–1851* (Dublin, 2005).

Coogan, T.P., *1916: the Easter Rising* (London, 2001).

Cosgrove, D., 'South Dublin Union' in *Centenary souvenir, 1827–1927: Carmelite Fathers, Whitefriars Street, Dublin* (Dublin, 1927).

Countess of Aberdeen (ed.), *Ireland's crusade against tuberculosis* (Dublin, 1907).

Cowen, R., *Relish: the extraordinary life of Alexis Soyer, Victorian celebrity chef* (London, 2006).

Cox, C. & Luddy, M. (eds), *Cultures of care in Irish medical history, 1750–1970* (London, 2010).

Cox, I. (ed.), *The Scallop* (London, 1957).

Cromwell, T. *Excursions through Ireland* (London, 1820).

Crookshank, A. & Webb, D., *Paintings and sculptures in Trinity College Dublin* (Dublin 1990).

Crossman, V. & Gray, P. (eds), *Poverty and welfare in Ireland, 1838–1948* (Dublin, 2011).

Crowley, J., Smyth, W.J. & Murphy, M. (eds), *Atlas of the Great Irish Famine* (Dublin, 2012).

Cuffe, T., 'Past and Present Associations of St James's parish' in *St James's church centenary record* (Dublin, 1952).

Cullen, F., *Cleansing rural Dublin: public health and housing initiatives in the South Dublin Poor Law Union, 1880–1920* (Dublin, 2001).

Daly, M.E., *Dublin: the deposed capital* (Cork, 1984).

Damrosh, L., *Jonathan Swift: his life and his world* (New Haven, 2013).

Deeny, J., *To cure and to care* (Dublin, 1989).

de Nie, M., *The eternal Paddy: Irish identity and the British press* (Madison, 2004).

Devine, F. (ed.), *A capital in conflict: Dublin city and the 1913 Lockout* (Dublin, 2013).

Dickson, D. (ed.), *The gorgeous mask: Dublin, 1700–1850* (Dublin, 1987).

Dickson, D., *Arctic Ireland: the extraordinary story of the great frost and forgotten famine of 1740–1741* (Belfast, 1998).

Dickson, D., *New foundations Ireland, 1660–1800* (Dublin, 2000).

Dickson, D., *Dublin: the making of a capital city* (Dublin, 2014).

Donnelly, J., *The Great Irish Potato Famine* (Stroud, 2002).

Duff, F., *Miracles on tap* (New York, 1961).

Edwards, O.D. & Pyle, F. (eds), *1916: the Easter Rising* (London, 1968).

Edwards, R.D., *Patrick Pearse: the triumph of failure* (Dublin, 1990).

Edwards, R.D. & Williams, T.D. (eds), *The Great Famine: studies in Irish history, 1845–52* (Dublin, 1994).

Ehrenpreis, I., *Swift: the man, his works, and the age* (London, 1983).

Farmar, T., *A haven in Rathgar: St Luke's and the Irish experience of cancer, 1952–2007* (Dublin, 2003).

Feeney, J.K., *The Coombe Lying-In Hospital* (Dublin, 1970).

Ferriter, D. (ed.), *Dublin's fighting story* (Dublin, 2009).

Finnane, M., *Insanity and the insane in post-Famine Ireland* (London, 1981).

Fitzgerald, B., *The Anglo-Irish* (St Albans, 1952).

Fitzpatrick, D. (ed.), *The Feds: an account of the Federated Dublin Voluntary Hospitals, 1961–2005* (Dublin, 2006).

Fitzpatrick, M., *The parish of St James, James's Street, Dublin: celebrating 150 years, 1844–1994* (Dublin, 1994).

Fitzpatrick, J., *The life of Charles Lever* (London, 1896).

Foley, C., *The last Irish plague: the great flu epidemic in Ireland, 1918–1919* (Dublin, 2011).

Foy, M. & Barton, B., *The Easter Rising* (Gloucestershire, 1999).

Freedman, D., *AIDS – the problem in Ireland* (Dublin, 1987).

Froude, J.A., *The English in Ireland in the eighteenth century* (London, 1874).

Gaffey, J., *Witnessing the pandemic: Irish print media and HIV/AIDS in Ireland and sub-Saharan Africa* (Bethesda, 2007).

Gatenby, P.B., *The School of Physic, Trinity College Dublin* (Dublin, 1994).

Gatenby, P.B., *Dublin's Meath Hospital* (Dublin, 1996).

Geoghegan, S., *The campaign and history of the Royal Irish Regiment* (Edinburgh, 1927).

Gibbon, M., *Inglorious soldier* (London, 1968).

Gilbert, J.T., *Calendar of ancient records of Dublin*, vols 3–7 (Dublin, 1892–1898).

Gray, P., *The making of the Irish poor law, 1815–43* (Manchester, 2009).

Grimes, S., *Ireland in 1804* (Dublin, 1980).

Griscom, J., *A year in Europe* (New York, 1824).

Hallack, C., *The Legion of Mary* (New York, 1950).

Hally, P.J., 'The Easter Rising in Dublin: the military aspects', *Irish Sword*, 1:7 (1966), 314–26.

Hardiman, N.P. & Kennedy, M., *Directory of Dublin 1738* (Dublin, 2000).

Harris, W., *The history and antiquities of the city of Dublin* (Dublin, 1766).

Hawkesworth, J., *Letters written by the late Jonathan Swift, D.D., dean of St Patrick's, Dublin and several of his friends* (London, 1746).

Hayden, M., 'Charity children in eighteenth-century Dublin', *Dublin Historical Record*, 3 (1943), 92–107.

Hegarty, S. & O'Toole, F., *The Irish Times book of the 1916 Rising* (Dublin, 2006).

Henry, W., *Supreme sacrifice: the Story of Éamonn Ceannt, 1881–1916* (Cork, 2005).

Henchy, P., 'Francis Johnston, architect', *Dublin Historical Record*, 1 (1949), 1–16.

Hensey, B., *The health services of Ireland* (Dublin, 1972).

Hitchcock, H., *TB or not TB?* (Galway, 1995).

Hopkinson, M., *Green against green: the Irish Civil War* (Dublin, 2004).

Hopkirk, M., *Nobody wanted Sam: the story of the unwelcomed child, 1530–1948* (London, 1949).

Housley, C., *The Sherwood Foresters in the Easter Rising: Dublin 1916* (Nottingham, 2015).

Howard, J., *The state of prisons* (London, 1780).

Howard, J., *An account of the principle lazarettos in Europe together with further observations on some foreign prisons and hospitals and additional remarks on the present state of those in Great Britain and Ireland* (London, 1789).

Howie, I., Grace, S. & Moore McCann, B., *Art in St James's Hospital* (Dublin, 2013).

Hughes, M., 'The Parnell sisters', *Dublin Historical Record*, 21:1 (Dublin, 1966), 14–27.

Inglis, H.D., *A journey throughout Ireland* (London, 1834).

Johnson, N., *Britain and the 1918–1919 influenza epidemic* (London, 2006).

Jones, G., & Malcolm, E. (eds), *Medicine, disease and the state in Ireland, 1650–1940* (Cork, 1999).

Jones, G., *Captain of all these men of death: the history of tuberculosis in nineteenth- and twentieth-century Ireland* (Amsterdam, 2001).

Kearns, K., *Dublin tenement life* (Dublin, 2006).

Keegan, J., *Legends and poems*, J. O'Hanlon (ed.), with memoir by D.J. O'Donoghue (Dublin, 1855).

Keenan, D., *Eighteenth-century Ireland, 1703–1800: society and history* (Bloomington, 2014).

Kennedy, F., *Duff: a life story* (London, 2011).

Kennerk, B., *Temple Street children's hospital* (Dublin, 2014).

Kertzer, D., *Sacrificed for honor: Italian infant abandonment and the politics of reproductive control* (Boston, 1993).

Kinsella, T., *A Dublin documentary* (Dublin, 2006).

Kirkpatrick, T.P.C., *The history of Doctor Steevens' Hospital* (Dublin, 1924).

Kissane, N., *The Irish Famine: a documentary history* (Dublin, 1995).

Kohli, M., *The golden bridge: young immigrants to Canada, 1833–1939* (Toronto, 2003).

Kolata, G.B., *Flu: the story of the great influenza of 1918 and the search for the virus that caused it* (New York, 1999).

Laffan, M., *Judging W.T. Cosgrave* (Dublin, 2014).

Laffan, W. (ed.), *The cries of Dublin, drawn from the life by Hugh Douglas Hamilton, 1760* (Dublin, 2003).

Logan, P., *Medical Dublin* (Dublin, 1984).

Lucey, D. & Crossman, V. (eds), *Healthcare in Ireland and Britain from 1850* (London, 2014).

Luddy, M. & Murphy, C. (eds), *Women surviving* (Dublin, 1989).

Luddy, M., *Women in Ireland, 1800–1918: a documentary history* (Cork, 1999).

Lunney, S., *With mercy towards all* (Dublin, 1987).

Lyons, J.B., *An assembly of Irish surgeons* (Dublin, 1984).

Lyons, J.B., *The quality of Mercer's: the story of Mercer's Hospital, 1734–1991* (Dublin, 1991).

Mac Lellan, A. & Mauger, A. (eds), *Growing pains* (Dublin, 2013).

MacThomais, E., 'The South Dublin Union', *Dublin Historical Record*, 26:2 (Dublin, 1973), 54–61.

McCarthy, D., 'Hospitals and the peoples' needs', *Ireland Today*, 11:10 (1937), 37–43.

McCarthy, M., *Five years in Ireland* (Dublin, 1903).

McCoole, S., *No ordinary women: Irish female activists in the Revolutionary Years, 1900–1923* (Dublin, 2004).

McCoole, S., *Easter widows* (Dublin, 2014).

McGarry, F., The *Rising: Ireland, Easter 1916* (Oxford, 2010).

McGregor, J.J., *New picture of Dublin* (Dublin, 1821).

McParland, E., *Public architecture in Ireland 1680 to 1760* (London, 2001).

Maguire, M., 'A study of poor law relief in Dublin between 1770 and 1830 with specific reference to the Foundling Hospital and the House of Industry' (BA, St Patrick's College, Maynooth, 1980).

Malcolm, E., *Swift's hospital: the history of St Patrick's Hospital, Dublin, 1746–1989* (Dublin, 1989).

Malcolm, E. & Jones, G. (eds), *Medicine, disease and the state in Ireland, 1650–1940* (Cork, 1998).

Malthus, T., *An essay on the principle of population* (London, 1803).

Manley, B., *Frank Duff: one of the best* (Dublin, 1980).

Marnham, N., 'Daniel Edward Heffernan's map of Dublin 1861', *Architecture Ireland*, 18 June 2016.

Maxwell, C., *Dublin under the Georges, 1714–1830* (London, 1956).

Meath, R. (ed.), *The diaries of Mary, countess of Meath* (London 1990).

Meehan, C.P. (ed.), *The poets and poetry of Munster* (Dublin, 1883).

Meenan, F.O.C., *St Vincent's Hospital (1834–1994): an historical and social portrait* (Dublin, 1995).

Miege, G., *The present state of Great Britain and Ireland* (London, 1718).

Molyneux, D. & Kelly, D., *When the clock struck in 1916: close-quarter combat in the Easter Rising* (Dublin, 2015).

Moore, R., *Leeches to lasers: sketches of a medical family* (Killala, 2002).

Moorhead, T.G., *A short history of Sir Patrick Dun's Hospital* (Dublin, 1942).

Moylan, T.K., 'Vagabonds and sturdy beggars', *Dublin Historical Record*, 1:3 (1938), 65–74.

Morash, C., *The hungry voice: the poetry of the Famine* (Dublin, 1989).

Murphy, E., 'Maintaining the "gift of life" in a climate of a shrinking donor pool and increasing demand' (MSc, TCD: 1985).

Murphy, S. & Byrne, T., *St James's graveyard, Dublin, history and associations* (Dublin, 1988).

Neary, B., *Lugs: the life and times of Jim Branigan* (Dublin, 1985).

Nicholls, G., *Poor laws – Ireland*, reports 1–3 (London, 1838).

Nicholls, G., *Charitable institutions (Dublin): reports on the Foundling Hospital and House of Industry, Dublin* (1842).

Nicholls, G., *A history of the Irish poor law* (London, 1856).

Nicholson, A., *Annals of the Famine in Ireland* (Dublin, 1998).

Nolan, E., *Caring for the nation: a history of the Mater Misericordiae University Hospital* (Dublin, 2013).

Nowlan, K.B. (ed.), *The making of 1916: studies in the history of the Rising* (Dublin, 1969).

Oakley, D., *'Hands on' for 100 years: a history of physiotherapy in Ireland* (Dublin, 2005).

Oates, W.C., *The Sherwood Foresters in the Great War, 1914–1918: 2/8th Battalion* (East Sussex, 2009).

O'Brien, E., Browne, L. & O'Malley, K. (eds), *A closing memoir: the Richmond, Whitworth and Hardwicke hospitals* (Dublin, 1988).

O'Brien, P., *Uncommon valour* (Dublin, 2010).

O'Broin, L., *Frank Duff: a biography* (Dublin, 1982).

O'Cleirigh, N., *Hardship & high living: Irish women's lives, 1808–1923* (Dublin, 2003).

O'Connell, K.H., *Irish peasant society* (Oxford, 1968).

O'Connor, J., *The workhouses of Ireland* (Dublin, 1995).

O'Donnell, B.P., *Irish surgeons and surgery in the twentieth century* (Dublin, 2008).

O'Farrell, M., *A walk through rebel Dublin 1916* (Cork, 1999).

O'Grada, C., *Ireland before and after the Famine* (Manchester, 1993).

O'Grada, C., *Black '47 and beyond: the Great Irish Famine in history, economy and memory* (Princeton, 1999).

O'Grada, D., *Georgian Dublin: the forces that shaped the city* (Dublin, 2015).

O'Mahony, C., *Cork's poor law palace: workhouse life, 1838–1890* (Cork, 2005).

O'Mahony, M., *Famine in Cork City* (Dublin, 2005).

O'Malley, M.P., *Lios-an Uisce*, (Dublin, 1982).

O'Regan, J., *Scott Tallon Walker Architects: 100 buildings and projects, 1960–2005* (Kinsale, 2006).

O'Rourke, J., *The Great Irish Famine* (Dublin, 1989).

O'Toole, F., *Judging Shaw* (Dublin, 2004).

Parkinson, A., *Belfast's unholy war* (Dublin, 2004).

Plumptre, A., *Narrative of a residence in Ireland during the summer of 1814 and that of 1815* (London, 1817).

Plunkett, J., *Strumpet city* (London, 1978).

Prunty, J., *Dublin slums* (Dublin, 1998).

Quinn, A. (ed.), *Patrick Kavanagh: selected poems* (London, 2000).

Quinn, A., *Patrick Kavanagh: a biography* (Dublin, 2001).

Quinn, T., *Flu: a social history of influenza* (London, 2008).

Reynolds, J., *Grangegorman: psychiatric care in Dublin since 1815* (Dublin, 1992).

Richardson, N., *According to their lights* (Dublin, 2015).

Robins, J., *The lost children: a study of charity children in Ireland, 1700–1900* (Dublin, 1980).

Robins, J., *Fools and mad: a history of the insane in Ireland* (Dublin, 1986).

Robins, J., *Custom house people* (Dublin 1993).

Robins, J., *The miasma; epidemic and panic in nineteenth-century Ireland* (Dublin, 1995).

Rocque, C., *An exact survey of the city and the suburbs of Dublin* (London, 1756).

Ronan, M.V., *The reformation in Dublin* (London, 1926).

Ryan, D., *The Rising: the complete story of Easter Week* (Dublin, 1949).

Saffron, M., *Samuel Clossy, M.D. – the existing works* (New York, 1967).

Scanlon, P., *The Irish nurse: a study of nursing in Ireland: history and education, 1718–1981* (Manorhamilton, 1991).

Scott, T. (ed.), *The prose works of Jonathan Swift*, vol. 7 (London, 1905).

Scuffil, C., *The South Circular Road: Dublin, on the eve of the First World War* (Dublin, 2013).

Shannon-Mangan, E., *James Clarence Mangan* (Dublin, 1996).

Sheridan, T., *The works of the Rev. Jonathan Swift*, vol. 18 (London, 1803).

SICCDA (South Inner City Community Development Association), *Ladies of the Liberties* (Dublin, 2002).

Smyth, P., *140 years a growing: the Carmelite chaplaincy at St James's Hospital* (Dublin, 2001).

Smyth, W. & Whelan, K. (eds), *Common ground: essays on the historical geography of Ireland* (Cork, 1988).

Stokes, W., *Diseases of the heart and aorta* (Dublin, 1854).

Suenens, L., *Edel Quinn* (Dublin, 1954).

Swift, J., *A modest proposal for preventing the children of poor people from being a burden to their parents or the country and for making them beneficial to the publick* (Dublin, 1729).

Swift, J., *A short view of the state of Ireland* (Dublin, 1727).

Swift, J., *A proposal for giving badges to the beggars in all the parishes in Dublin* (London, 1737).

Swift, J., *Verses on the death of Doctor Swift* (London, 1739).

Temperley, I., *Blood, toil and tears: my contribution to Irish haematology* (Dublin, 2013).

Townshend, C., *Easter 1916: the Irish rebellion* (London, 2005).

Trimmer, S., *An abridgement of the New Testament* (London, n.d.).

Twomey, B., *Dublin in 1707: a year in the life of the city* (Dublin, 2009).

Ua Ceallaigh, S., *Cathal Brugha* (Dublin, 1942).

Vane, F.F., *Agin the governments* (London, 1929).

Wakefield, E., *An account of Ireland, political and statistical* (London, 1812).

Warbuton, J., Whitelaw, J. & Walsh, R., *History of the city of Dublin*, 2 vols (London, 1818).

Watts, W., *Provost Trinity College Dublin: a memoir* (Dublin, 2008).

Webb, M., *Trinity's psychiatrists* (Dublin, 2011).

Whitelaw, J., *An essay on the populations of Dublin, being the result of an actual survey taken in 1798* (Dublin, 1805).

Widdess, J.D.H., *A history of the Royal College of Physicians of Ireland* (Edinburgh, 1963).

Wilde, W., *Austria: its literary, scientific and medical institutions* (Dublin, 1843).

Willis, T., *The social and sanitary condition of the working classes in Dublin* (Dublin, 1845).

Wilson, R, *The life and times of Queen Victoria* (London, 1887).

Wodsworth, W.D., *A history of the ancient Foundling Hospital of Dublin from the year 1702* (Dublin, 1876).

Woodham-Smith, C., *The Great Hunger* (London, 1962).

Woodward, R., *An argument in support of the right of the poor in the kingdom of Ireland: in the appendix to which an attempt is made to settle a measure of the contribution due from each man to the poor, on the footing of justice* (Dublin, 1768).

Wright, G.N., *An historical guide to the city of Dublin* (London, 1825).

Wright, W., *The Brontës in Ireland* (London, 1894).

Yeates, P., *A city in civil war: Dublin, 1921–4* (Dublin, 2015).

Index

Note: The **Chronology** section is not included in the Index;
page references in *italics* denote illustrations

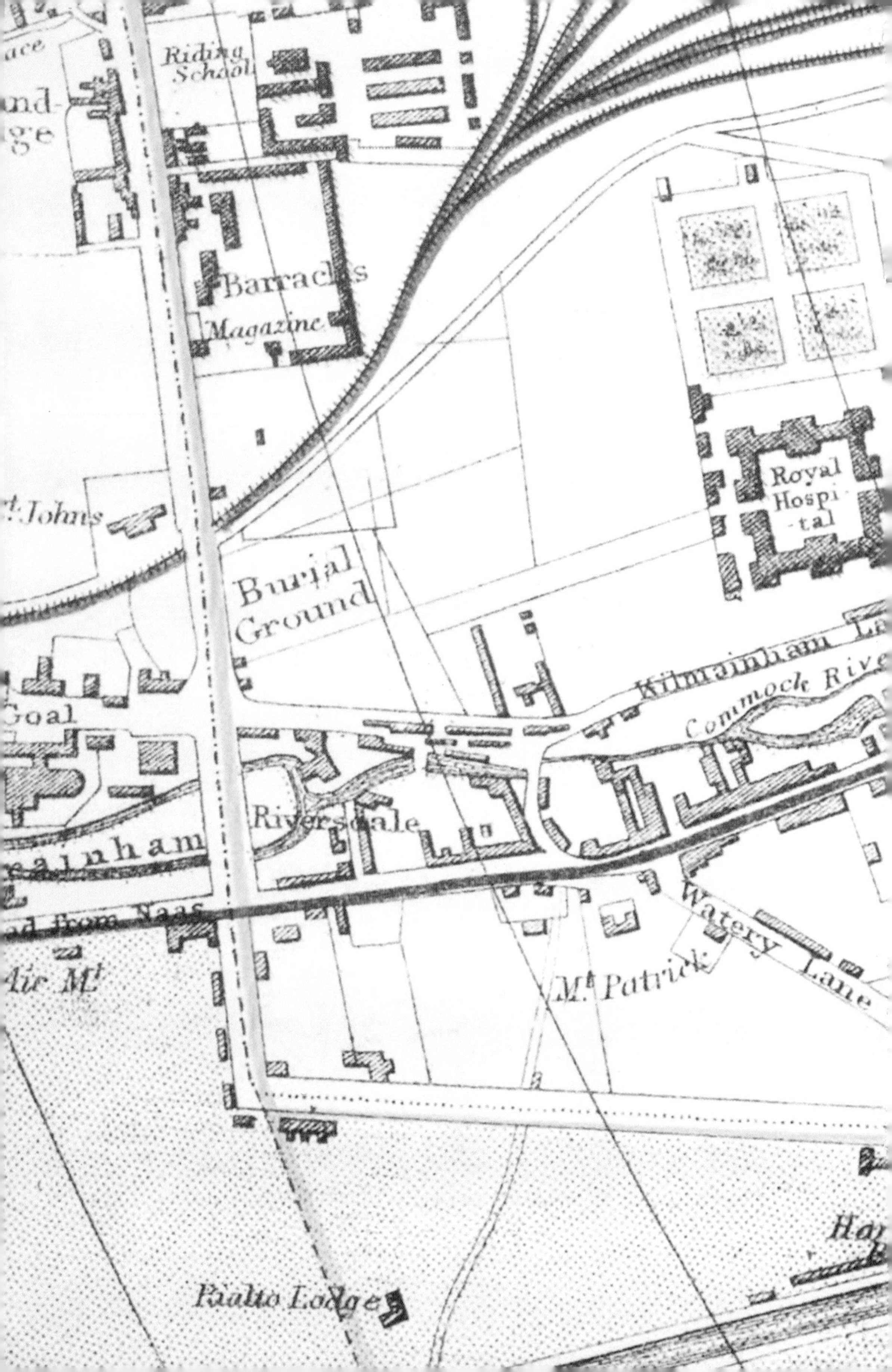

Riding School

Barracks

Magazine

St. Johns

Burial Ground

Goal

Riverscale

ainham

ad from Naas

Air M{t}

Rialto Lodge

Royal Hospital

Kilmainham La

Commock Rive

Watery Lane

M{t} Patrick

Ha